**Childhood Obesity
in America**

Laura Dawes

Childhood Obesity in America

Biography of an Epidemic

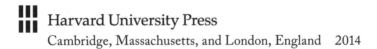 Harvard University Press

Cambridge, Massachusetts, and London, England   2014

Library of Congress Cataloging-in-Publication Data

Dawes, Laura, 1976–
Childhood obesity in America : biography of an epidemic / Laura Dawes.
    pages cm
Includes bibliographical references and index.
ISBN 978-0-674-28144-8
1. Obesity in children—United States. 2. Overweight children—United States. 3. Nutrition
policy—United States.   4. Health promotion—United States—Planning.   I. Title.
RJ399.C6D39 2014
618.92'398—dc23   2013039251

For Russell and Irene

Contents

**Childhood Obesity
in America**

Introduction

Charley weighs 174 pounds. He is still growing. Where he will stop no one knows. He smiles when asked this question, and says his ambition is to be a "big man."

> Celebrity fat boy, 174-pound, nine-year-old Charley Bilcher, 1896

Oh, Doctor, please have pity on me and answer this as soon as possible as I am getting so fat that I shall be ridiculous. Any boys that I shall meet will say, "Gee but you're fat!" And I cannot bear to hear that from a boy.

> "J," a fifteen-year-old girl, 142 pounds, writing to diet doctor Lulu Hunt Peters, 1924

I stuffed him like a goose.

> Mother of Francis Beach, aged six, weight 59 pounds, visiting an endocrine clinic, 1934

When they call you names, it hurts—Fatso, Tubby, even Tuba—it hurts. Of course, I don't cry, but I have to walk away. My main trouble is barbecued shrimp with lots of butter, and hot French bread dipped in butter.

> John Occhipinti, 151 pounds, eleven years old, attending Camp Tahoe "fat camp," 1967

I have been eating regularly at McDonald's restaurants since I was five years old. I ask my mother to take me to McDonald's. Between the ages of five and twelve I used to go to McDonald's approximately 3–4 times a week. I normally order the Happy Meal or sometimes a Big Mac. One of the reasons I went to McDonald's was because of the prizes.

> Ashley Pelman, fourteen years old, 170 pounds, suing McDonald's for promoting her obesity, 2002

Together, these five children, Charley, "J," Francis, John, and Ashley, span a century of childhood obesity in the United States. Each, however, grew up during a different stage in the history of how childhood obesity has been understood and treated, and what fatness in a child meant.

1

This book is about the changing environment of opinions, practices, and beliefs about childhood obesity in the twentieth century that surrounded and affected children like these—and many more like them.

For Charley, at the beginning of the century, childhood obesity was a rare condition and one that doctors didn't worry much about. Rather, a degree of plumpness in children was considered both attractive and beneficial. There was even some evidence that a degree of overweight in childhood protected children from infectious disease. Charley, his parents, and the *Chicago Daily Tribune* journalist who was interviewing them were proud that American-born Charley was fatter than another famous fat boy from Austria.

Fifteen-year-old "J" in 1924 found herself subject to a different set of understandings, and not just because she was a girl. In the 1920s, doctors in America began to see overweight in childhood as a worrying medical condition. Fat youngsters like "J" might be "good natured and amiable," thought one pediatrician, but were liable to suffer from "lessened powers of endurance and diminished activity" as a result of the strain the excess weight placed on heart and lungs. The main harms of the condition, were, however, considered to be social. "J" herself—a young teen—considered her fatness unattractive. She was a member of the first generation of children to turn to dieting as a way of losing weight.[1]

Little Francis Beach's doctors of the 1930s and 1940s believed his obesity to be caused by a *biological fault* in his endocrine glands and had sent him to a specialist endocrine clinic to be treated with injections of animal glands. One pediatrician he saw, however, had been trained in psychoanalysis, and she believed that Francis's condition was a sign of an angst-ridden family situation. Freudian explanations, widely popular in midcentury America, spoke to the role of *families* and *feelings* in causing a child's obesity.

Twenty years later, John Occhipinti was cruelly teased—"Tubby," "Tuba"—about his fatness. For him, obesity was both a social problem and a health one. Sociologists had begun to formally inquire into what it was like to be a fat child, and had confirmed what obese youngsters had known since the 1920s: they faced distressing stigmatization. Some doctors prescribed amphetamine diet pills to children like John as a way of altering the *energy balance* between caloric intake and outgo. Such metabolic or "energy balance" explanations broached the issue of personal responsibility—*behavior* as both the cause and treatment of childhood obesity—and made the condition ripe for commercial opportunities newly arrived on the child weight-loss scene: diet books specifically for children and summer "fat camps" like Camp Tahoe that John went to.

And lastly, at the end of the century, Ashley found herself in an environment in which childhood obesity ran and continues to run at epidemic proportions in the United States, particularly among African American and Hispanic children. For her, childhood obesity was (and is) attributed to *societal factors*—an environment of fast food, limited exercise, poverty and poor education, parental failure, regulatory failure, and rampant marketing targeted at children. Ashley was seeking to use the court system as a way of fighting against her obesity-causing environment.

For each of these children, the time when they were born made a difference in how their parents, their peers, their doctors, and they themselves understood their condition and what they did about it. In this book, "childhood" refers to the span from infancy through to age eighteen, and so encompasses babyhood through to adolescence. Our current fear that childhood obesity is at epidemic levels in the United States (and many other countries, too) can obscure the fact that childhood obesity has a history in America—and a long and varied one at that. This book is a biography of childhood obesity, chronicling its course in America from its first appearance as a medical concern, through to its maturation as full-fledged epidemic. It looks at the changing answers to critical questions about childhood obesity across the twentieth century and how they might be answered in the twenty-first. What causes obesity in childhood? How should the condition be diagnosed? Is childhood fat dangerous, and, if so, how and why? How can—and should—childhood obesity be treated?

The understanding of and approach to childhood obesity at any one period in the twentieth and twenty-first centuries is an amalgamation of prior thinking and beliefs. It is not that "better" or more correct ideas about childhood obesity replaced earlier, less correct ones, but rather that each new idea joined a mélange of existing ones. Older ideas sometimes became less important or were seen as applying only in a minority of cases, but they did not disappear. As childhood obesity became a bigger problem over the twentieth century, our ideas about it became more complex, more emotionally fraught. There are few conditions that involve so many people, so intensively—offering advice on it, researching it, framing policy to deal with it, treating it, making money from it, litigating about it, and, importantly, suffering with it.

Diagnosing childhood obesity involves drawing a line between children who are "normal sized" and those who are thought abnormal—"too large." Since diagnosis is integral to the way in which a condition is understood and approached, the first part of this book looks at how this boundary line has been drawn and how it has changed. The most fundamental criteria—and the oldest, historically speaking—for deciding if a child is too fat have been subjective, aesthetic factors: does the child *look* a healthy size and shape or not? Anyone who has raised an eyebrow—actually or figuratively—when seeing parents buy their 150-pound eight-year-old a dinner-plate-sized chocolate chip cookie will have been exercising a test of this nature. It is also the basis of "clinical impression," the most commonly used practice, both historically and today, in pediatric diagnosis of obesity. This diagnostic technique requires both looking and judging: the viewer has to interpret and assign significance to the child's body shape. Looking and judging, of course, requires some culturally calibrated standard to judge against. This aesthetic standard, however, changes over time and is different in different cultures.

Western culture has—until the very recent past in historical terms—held the belief that a healthy, happy, attractive, and delightful child is a chubby one. Chubby children were thought to have the "look" of health; and this "look" was attractive. But just as standards of attractiveness in women change over time (less so in men), so too the "look" of attractiveness and health in children has also changed, albeit less drastically. Since attractiveness is connected with rarity, and as childhood obesity has become more prevalent over the century, the dominant cultural ideal of the child body has become slimmer and more adult-like. But what "childhood obesity" looks like at the end of the century is also considerably fatter than "childhood obesity" at the start of the century. The standard for both the ideal and the obese child body has become more extreme. The fact that anyone—doctor or passerby—is steeped in these cultural standards for children's bodies and can therefore look at, judge, and diagnose a child as overweight is, of course, a feature of childhood obesity that adds to its emotional significance and misery. For most of the century, fatness exposed a child to judgment, and a harsh one at that.

Medical investigation, though, has also developed numerical—objective—criteria for answering the question "Is this child too fat?" This has been partly out of a professional value for precision, but also because diagnosis "by the numbers" is necessary for using the large-scale research methods that became the gold standard for medical research in the mid-twentieth century. *Measuring* a child's body had become a central tool in pediatric diagnosis by the 1930s. Parents and physicians became familiar with the scale, the tape measure, and the stadiometer (the instrument that measures height), and started using size—height and weight—as an indicator of the child's general health. This was a quiet revolution in the way children's health was assessed, a medical milestone testified by the countless doorframes across America notched at each passing birthday. Large-scale surveys since the 1870s produced tables of standard heights and weights against which a person could compare a child's growth, but with them brought a new aspect to parenting anxieties: parents would worry whether their child was "normal" or not, and they could test this question using height-weight tables.

Beyond family worries, height-weight standards also spoke to national pride, identity, and anxieties. School health surveys using the height-weight standards could give a good idea of how the future citizens of the nation were doing. Surveys of children's height and weight throughout the late nineteenth and twentieth centuries have consistently shown American children to be larger than those in other countries. Until the mid-1970s, that fact was a matter for national pride and satisfaction. Big children seemed a confirmation of patriotic ideals: the American way of life produced healthy, robust citizens. But since the 1970s, with the incidence of childhood obesity on the rise and American children still notably heftier than many of their international peers, the height-weight standard has become a more ambiguous expression of how American culture affects the bodies and health of children.

Obesity is, however, a condition of excess adiposity—of having too much body fat. As midcentury obesity researchers argued, height and weight measurements can give only an approximate indication of how fat a person is. In the second half of the twentieth century, the measures used to objectively identify childhood obesity shifted from assessments of body *shape*—its height, its weight—to measuring its *composition*. *Content*, not *contour*, became the goal of metrics for childhood obesity in the latter half of the twentieth century.

Technologies for investigating the composition of the human body have allowed researchers to derive diagnostic measures for childhood obesity that depend on body fat content rather than sheer bodily size. These technologies have been the fruit of some surprising research—research never intended for childhood obesity, but rather to keep navy divers alive or to test nuclear fallout patterns. However, there is a dilemma with basing the diagnosis of childhood obesity on body fat content: to get a direct, accurate measure of a person's body fat content, the person needs to be dead. If measuring a living child is the priority, then an approximation of body fat is as close as one can get. Despite this, researchers have pressed on, developing more and more techniques for approximating body fat content. Plethora, here, stands in for precision.

The most widely known and used technique for estimating body fat content these days is the body mass index (BMI), a convenient and easy calculation using height and weight measures. The index represents a broadly agreed upon compromise—a practical tool for the types of large-scale investigations that obesity researchers want to do and the best of the less-than-perfect options available for assessing body fat content. Moreover, the fact that BMI uses measurements (height and weight) with a long historical pedigree (allowing researchers to look back at changes in children's body fat content over a whole century of height-weight measuring) has played a big part in the BMI becoming accepted as the standard for quantifying childhood obesity.

———

As medical attention to childhood obesity has increased over the twentieth century, and as rates of childhood obesity have also increased, so too have perceptions of the causes and consequences of the condition changed. The second part of this book considers the changing understanding of and treatments for childhood obesity. Physicians began to pay attention to childhood obesity in the 1920s because they had come to understand the condition as harmful, and therefore part of medicine's purview. However, what these harms were thought to be has changed. Before about the midcentury, the dangers of obesity in children were thought to be different from and less serious than the dangers of obesity in adulthood. Insurance companies' actuarial data showed that obese adults suffered higher mortality rates than less weighty adults. Physicians believed that this might be because the large, metabolically inactive fat depot placed a lot of strain on a person's heart, lungs, and other organs, which would degrade over time under the constant pressure.

But researchers of the early twentieth century did not find strong evidence that overweight children suffered the same serious physical effects as adults. (This opinion would later be revised.) Rather, as one leading obesity researcher of the early twentieth century suggested, the harm of childhood obesity lay in the strain the excess bulk placed on posture and joints, and the fact that "fat children are the victims of continuous teasing, which in some is apt to initiate a feeling of inferiority resulting in serious behavior problems." That childhood obesity could inflict considerable pain of the emotional kind on its sufferers was, in fact, a new belief in the twentieth century. It was sufficiently radical an idea that doctors felt the need to tell parents that the jolly fat child was a figment of popular imagination. "I was an obese child myself, and I know that there is genuine mental suffering in being an obese child," said Lulu Hunt Peters, a famous diet doctor and newspaper columnist. "The fat child is not a happy child." In 1925, this was revelatory and had big implications for how Americans saw themselves and the issue of obesity in childhood.[2]

Whether childhood obesity wreaked *physical* harms as well as social ones was a more contentious matter for the early twentieth century. One theory that was widely popular in the 1920s through to the early 1940s was that fatness in childhood was a symptom of endocrine trouble. Glands were in vogue at this time—much as today we have a vogue for genetics. Childhood fatness was one condition that the exciting young field of endocrinology seized for its own. Malfunctioning glands might cause very serious problems for the child's physical and sexual development. Under this understanding, childhood obesity *was* connected with physical harms, although it was a symptom and not a cause of those harms. The gland idea declined in acceptance in the 1940s as metabolic tests showed that most fat children's glands were working fine, but the explanation "oh, it's a gland thing" lived on in popular understanding of childhood chubbiness well into the 1960s.

In the first half of the twentieth century, by far the most widely held belief about why childhood obesity was less worrisome than adult obesity was that the childhood condition was transitory: "most people who are fat in childhood and early youth become thin later." Puberty would sort things out. By the midcentury, however, this assurance in the temporary nature of childhood obesity was beginning to unravel. Partly this was due to a change in thinking about chronic illness. In adults, large-scale epidemiological studies like the Framingham Study and the Build and Blood Pressure Study presented the new concept of the "risk factor"—a marker, either a behavior (like smoking) or a physical measurement (like high blood pressure), that was associated with greater statistical likelihood of getting sick. These studies found evidence that overweight in adulthood (especially in combination with high blood pressure) was a risk factor for a number of health problems, such as heart attacks, stroke, and diabetes. Critically, the studies suggested that a long-range perspective was needed in assessing what risks might factor into these sorts of "lifestyle"-related diseases. And that meant looking more thoroughly at childhood precursors.[3]

A number of studies conducted in the 1950s aimed to provide data on childhood obesity's persistence into adulthood, most notably a 1958 British study and a 1960 study in the United States. The American study—an analysis of twenty years of data collected by the Public Health Service—gave childhood obesity one of its most widely quoted and most ominous statistics: fully 80 to 85 percent of overweight children would grow up to become overweight adults. The results dealt a major blow to the it'll-get-better-by-itself understanding of childhood fatness. In particular, it meant childhood obesity was not just harmful because of joint pains or teasing but also because it was a risk factor for adult obesity, and adult obesity was, in turn, a risk factor for heart disease, diabetes, and cancer. Summarized one pediatrician in 1973,

> The main difference that exists between the problems of fat children and those of fat adults is that, in general, the former do not suffer direct medical consequences of their obesity. What is of major concern to the paediatrician is [rather,] that nine out of ten fat children emerge as fat adults.[4]

Within the last decade, that opinion—that childhood obesity is risky mainly because of its persistence into adulthood rather than because it is dangerous in its own right—has also been revised. Recent evidence from epidemiological studies has shown that the comorbidities of adult obesity can also be found in young fat people (metabolic syndrome, diabetes, inflammation, cardiovascular disease, sleep apnea, asthma, fatty liver disease). The mechanism that causes these problems appears to be connected with the function of fat in the human body. The century-old idea that fat was simply a metabolically inactive energy store has recently been replaced by the idea that fat plays a very *active* role, emitting and responding to hormonal signals and regulating the body's internal economy. Excess fat is now considered to wreak its harms not just through mechanical strain but also by disrupting the chemical operation of a person's body. And beyond symptoms in common with obesity in adulthood, obese children may also suffer physical problems that are specific to obesity in childhood, notably leg and hip problems associated with the fact that their bones are still growing. Most research into the stigma of obesity has looked at adults and has reported discrimination against fat people in employment situations, by insurance companies, and by health-care practitioners. But there is also a growing body of research that documents discrimination against fat children by their peers, their teachers, and even their parents.[5]

So from fatness in children being seen as a temporary social hindrance, it has changed to being considered an obdurate condition, with both immediate and lasting physical and emotional harms. These factors are, however, not independent strands, but are intertwined. As the condition became more common, with more cases and more extreme examples of obese children for physicians and researchers to examine, so medical interest looked more closely at the condition, and so too did its harms seem more apparent. The coming together of these strands has produced a condition with heightened emotional significance: it is now believed that obese children may be marked for a lifetime of suffering.

"Suffering?" the fat acceptance movement asks. "Suffering??" This activist and advocacy movement argues that fat people only "suffer" because of society's negative and condemning attitudes toward fatness. They don't suffer *from* their fatness, but *because* of it. The peak body of the movement, the National Association to Advance Fat Acceptance (NAAFA), founded in 1969, calls for greater acceptance of a wide range of body sizes and shapes and for active protection of fat people from discrimination through legislation and awareness-raising. NAAFA's now-disbanded radical offshoot, Fat Underground, would disrupt Weight Watchers meetings, proclaiming "Fat Power" and down with dieting.[6]

Medicine is a particular target for the fat acceptance movement's ire because of its assertion that obesity is a risk factor for poor health and should be treated. The fat acceptance movement argues that the medicalization of obesity is just one symptom of a groundless "moral panic" about fat—a situation that is promoted by the self-serving interests of the diet, fashion, pharmaceutical, and cosmetic industries, and by obesity researchers who stand to gain kudos and funding. Further, the ensuing antifat bias in society (and in medicine) constitutes an abuse of fat people's human rights. Instead, the fat acceptance movement counsels a "health at every size" (HAES) philosophy. This approach is associated with nutritionist Linda Bacon, who explained her views in her 2008 book *Health at Every Size*. Bacon is against the preoccupation with weight and with weight loss as the goal. Instead, she says, if you eat healthily and exercise regularly and are happy, your weight should not matter. You can be healthy at any and every size.[7]

In regard to childhood obesity, NAAFA cautions against any public health effort which may have the effect of further stigmatizing fat children and recommends the HAES philosophy. NAAFA itself does not deny that there have been considerable increases in fatness among children (and adults), although some parts of the fat acceptance movement say that this is incorrect and that there is, in fact, no childhood obesity "epidemic." Mainstream medicine has some areas of agreement and some areas of disagreement with the fat acceptance movement's approach to childhood obesity. It agrees that efforts should not stigmatize fat children and that healthy eating and exercise should be part of a regular lifestyle rather than an occasional fad, but disagrees that it is possible to be healthy at every size. There are some sizes, says medicine, where it is simply not possible to be healthy.[8]

The fat acceptance movement, angry and frustrated, points to some of the dilemmas particular to obesity and to childhood obesity. While medicine has determined that the condition warrants medical intervention, as this history of its understanding and treatment shows, it has struggled to pin down the exact physiological mechanism by which it causes its harms and has to date failed to provide an effective solution that people can easily achieve.

————

Considering the changing plight of fat children as individuals is one perspective on the history of childhood obesity; this book moves between that and another perspective, concerned with children as a group or population. To return to the five fat children who opened this chapter, in 1967, an eleven-year-old American boy like John Occhipinti was, on average, about

4 inches taller and 16.5 pounds heavier than a boy of the same age in Charley Bilcher's era of 1880. This sort of increase in average heights and weights, called *secular change* (meaning change across successive time periods) was the case for both boys and girls of all ethnic groups living in the United States within this time, although the degree to which different groups gained in height and weight differs. Some evidence suggests that upper-class boys, like John (who had his larger-size clothes tailor-made for him) reached the maximum genetic potential for size in about 1930. The average size of children from less socioeconomically advantaged families continued to get bigger until at least 1960 or even 1970. Wealthier, white children were taller and, especially, heavier than poorer black and Hispanic children over the early to mid-twentieth century.[9]

Child health experts have interpreted secular change in children's heights and weights up to about the 1960s as a positive development. Most researchers agree that this increase was because of environmental changes, with better nutrition and improved sanitation being the most prominent causes. The gain in size was thought to reflect improved general health, with bigger being better. Increases up to about 1960 or 1970 were all to the good.

But after 1970, there was a growing sense among child health researchers that "the pendulum ha[d] however swung towards overnutrition." Secular increases in children's heights seemed to have slowed after the midcentury, or possibly stopped altogether (there is debate on this point). But children's weights continued to increase. That weight has continued to increase suggests that, while both height and weight are affected by improved nutrition, weight is the quality most sensitive to environmental changes. One study comparing Louisiana children in 1973 with children in 1994 found that five- to fourteen-year-olds had gained an average of 7.5 pounds in weight and 0.6 inches in height, but fifteen- to seventeen-year-olds had gained on average 12.3 pounds and *declined* in average height by 0.1 inches. Nationwide data from the 1960s through to the mid-1990s also showed that children were getting heavier more than they were getting taller and that the patterning by socioeconomic level was breaking down. The increases were also patterned by ethnic group, with African American and Hispanic children increasing in weight the most. While Charley and John, white kids from comparatively well-off families, were the typical fat children of the first half of the twentieth century, Ashley, an African American child from inner-city New York, is the exemplar of childhood obesity later in the century.[10]

The underlying process of secular change suggested that the entire distribution of children's heights and weights in the United States was shifting upwards. But along with this whole-population shift, the incidence of childhood obesity—the topmost section of the weight distribution where Charley, Francis, "J," John, and Ashley were to be found—seemed to be increasing in size as well. (In other words, the *shape* of the weight distribution was also changing.) Clinicians of the 1950s onward had a sense that childhood obesity was becoming "unduly common" and that it "must be recognized as an important public health problem."[11]

Within the commercial sector—always alert to expanding potential markets—children's clothing retailers like Sears Roebuck felt there was sufficient demand to introduce a girls' "Chubby" fit (now more appealingly called "Pretty Plus" fit), which was optional on some of their clothing range from 1940 and standard from 1960. The equivalent fit for boys, "Husky" fit, was available from 1960. Although there are no nationwide estimates for this period (nor any agreement on how to diagnose childhood obesity), studies from the 1930s to the late 1960s suggested that between 10 to 15 percent of the child population of the United States was obese, with this rate holding steady or slightly increasing, up until about 1970.[12]

Massive government health surveys conducted from the 1960s onwards—the National Health (and Nutrition) Examination Surveys (NHES and NHANES)—provided the first nationally representative data on the incidence and changes in prevalence of childhood obesity. Statisticians have analyzed these data and found that the prevalence of childhood obesity has increased since the data was first collected. (The exact size of the increase calculated depends on what baseline is chosen to compare with later data.) The most recent estimate is that in excess of three times more children aged between two and nineteen years were obese in the 2000s than were in the 1960s.[13]

The increase in prevalence has been especially large in Native American, African American and Hispanic children, of whom over 40 percent are considered overweight and around 20 percent obese. Asian children are the least likely to be obese. Surprisingly, unlike in adults, obesity in childhood is not always associated with low family income. How childhood obesity varies with socioeconomic level differs by ethnic group. For example, poor white children are more likely to be obese than wealthier white children; but in African American children the relationship is reversed, with wealthier

African American children (and especially girls) more likely to be fat than children from poorer families. In childhood, obesity is not simply a matter of class.[14]

Rather, this complex patterning by ethnicity and by socioeconomic standing suggests that different groups respond differently to the changing environment. Researchers are beginning to investigate the nature of these differences, and have found that there are both biological and cultural factors at play. From a biological standpoint, different ethnic groups have different body shapes and store fat differently. (This also has implications for how obesity is diagnosed in different ethnic groups.) From a social standpoint, different ethnic groups—even within the same larger cultural environment—have different attitudes toward, say, food or body shape. Both biology and culture are therefore intertwined in shaping the increase and pattern of childhood obesity in the United States.[15]

In 1985, researchers from the Harvard School of Public Health gave the worrisomely high rate of childhood obesity a particular description: "these data indicate that obesity is epidemic in the pediatric population." The term "epidemic" has typified how childhood obesity has come to be spoken about, both in popular culture and in medical circles, since the late 1980s. This word "epidemic" is an interesting one, with two meanings. One colloquial meaning is "prevalent," but "epidemic" also has a specialized meaning of "widespread, fast-spreading *infectious* disease." In describing childhood obesity as an "epidemic," the researchers were not only claiming that childhood obesity was common but also that public health mechanisms should be brought to bear on the condition, as if it were an infectious disease. The third, and final, part of the book deals with this contemporary epidemic of childhood obesity, its causes, and our responses.[16]

Although there is no virus or bacteria or parasite that seems to be the cause of the epidemic of childhood obesity, the condition nevertheless does have some features in common with infectious disease. Childhood obesity seems to be passed along family and social networks and within communities: fat children tend to have fat friends; whole neighborhoods of children are obese. And the epidemic levels of the condition seem to be the result of *catching* obesity from the modern environment: "the vectors of subsidized agriculture and multinational companies providing cheap, highly refined fats, oils, and carbohydrates, labor-saving mechanized devices, affordable motorized transport, and the seductions of sedentary pastimes, such as television." Much of the discussion of the childhood obesity epidemic is a lament of modernity—a sense of bittersweet regret and historical irony that progress has created an "obesogenic" environment. The epidemic of childhood obesity is commonly described as, in medical historian Charles Rosenberg's phrase, a "pathology of progress."[17]

Childhood obesity is, however, not a problem limited to the United States, or even to developed countries alone. Since 1997, when the World Health Organization (WHO) held a conference on obesity, that body has called attention to the increasing rate of childhood obesity in many countries around the world—both developed and developing. WHO uses the language of a global epidemic: a pandemic. Egypt, Argentina, Malawi, Nigeria, Uzbekistan, Peru, Qatar, and Jamaica all exceed the United States in the prevalence of childhood overweight and obesity. Urbanization, dietary change (the "nutritional transition" to Westernized diets), and changing physical activity to more sedentary work and leisure activities are thought to be driving the spread into developing countries.[18]

These changes, while implicated with childhood obesity, have traditionally been viewed as positive signs of development, and something that people have aspired to. The standard thinking up until now has been that poverty-linked infectious diseases—the "age of pestilence and famine"—should drop away as a country develops, and more people should live into old age and suffer instead the degenerative diseases that accompany long life. But the increasing rate of childhood obesity in developing countries shows that this is not the case. Instead, developing countries are facing a "double burden" of disease, with infectious disease not replaced but joined by the "age of degenerative and man-made [that is, lifestyle] diseases."[19]

This recent framing of childhood obesity as being connected with "good things" (cheap food, mechanized transport, high consumption) makes it seem that an epidemic of childhood obesity was inevitable, the natural corollary of development—childhood obesity as "collateral damage" of modernity. But here a historical perspective about childhood obesity makes a considerable contribution. As this biography shows, there was a substantial period of time during which the United States (and other developed countries) was "modern" *and* had low rates of childhood obesity. Childhood obesity has not been at epidemic levels until quite recently; the United States has been modern and developed for much longer than that. The complicated patterning of childhood obesity whereby low socioeconomic status doesn't always correlate with increased obesity is a telling sign. It is the particular *choices, decisions,* and *policies* shaping American society of the second half of the twentieth century that have fostered increases in childhood obesity, rather than modernity or development per se.[20]

In March 2009, First Lady Michelle Obama and students from Bancroft Elementary School broke ground on a vegetable garden at the White House. It was the second time in American politics that a vegetable patch had served in affairs of state: Eleanor Roosevelt had a "Victory Garden" during World War II as part of the home-front efforts to win the war. For the Obamas, growing vegetables at the White House was the homey side of Barack Obama's major domestic policy ambition of reforming health care. When the first harvest of the vegetable garden was gathered (to media accompaniment), the first lady spelled out the connection:

> The President and Congress are going to begin to address health care reform, and these issues of nutrition and wellness and preventative care is [sic] going to be the focus of a lot of conversation coming up in the weeks and months to come. And these are issues that I care deeply about, especially when they affect America's children.
>
> Obesity, diabetes, heart disease, high-blood pressure are all diet-related health issues that cost this country more than $120 billion each year. That's a lot of money. While the dollar figure is shocking in and of itself, the effect on our children's health is even more profound. Nearly a third of the children in this country are either overweight or obese, and a third will suffer from diabetes at some point in their lifetime. In Hispanic and African American communities, those numbers climb even higher so that nearly half of the children in those communities will suffer the same fate. Those numbers are unacceptable.
>
> . . .
>
> This gorgeous and bountiful garden that you saw over there has given us the chance to not just have some fun, which we've had a lot of it [sic], but to shed some light on the important—on the important food and nutrition issues that we're going to need to address as a nation.[21]

The first lady noted that "not eating right" and "not moving their bodies" were the factors that contributed to the problem of childhood obesity. The garden, along with the model of activity and family togetherness that the Obama family presented, were the implied cures. The Obamas were presenting the changes *their* family had made as a model for what families across America could do. The students of Bancroft Elementary School, the immediate audience for the first lady's remarks, were representative of the larger audience she was addressing. (Bancroft Elementary has a high proportion of Hispanic and black students. Bancroft therefore represents the ethnic groups that have, disproportionately, the highest incidence of childhood obesity in the United States.) The White House vegetable garden was the beginning of a series of policy initiatives championed by the first lady to address childhood obesity in America.

That the president and the first lady are offering advice on the issue of childhood obesity is a clear sign of how encompassing the condition has become over the course of the twentieth century. (The issue is not, however, politically clear-cut. Although the far right of the political spectrum in the United States has attacked the first lady's antiobesity initiatives as an example of "a nanny state run amok," many prominent Republicans have supported federal efforts on this issue, while some Democrats voted against measures that would make school lunches healthier.) The understanding of the condition has expanded from initially being one of an internal bodily dysfunction or a question of personal responsibility, growing to becoming a family failing, and then expanding further to become a societal problem. In particular, the history of childhood obesity in America touches on important values and facets of American life—the nature of childhood, parents' responsibilities, economic and political duties, family values, pediatric medicine, economics and consumption, and the nature of progress and of scientific achievement.[22]

Like polio, its predecessor as the major scourge of child health at the midcentury, childhood obesity is connected with lasting harms into adulthood and gives its sufferers visually obvious—and (to many people) unattractive—signs of their affliction. Both conditions owe something of their heightened emotional valence to the fact that they attack the idea of childhood as a healthy, vital, active time. However, where they differ is in terms of how the condition and society's response to it reflect cultural values and self-perceptions. The polio story has become so famous because it seemed to confirm tropes of American ingenuity, the power of science, and the success of people working together with great leaders to achieve a common goal. The polio vaccine was gift from the United States to the rest of the world and a Cold War victory. As historian Allan Brandt has written of the episode, it was interpreted as a "triumph of . . . the American system," showing "the promise of the American life." Things "worked out right" in the end and the standard narrative of progress was confirmed.[23]

By contrast, childhood obesity questions those certainties: the condition is implicated with the American way of life and commercial freedoms, science has failed to provide an easy fix for the condition, and efforts to address the condition are marked by dissent, disagreement, and antagonism as vested interests clash with reformist aims. The American way of life is not bringing a welcome gift to the world this time. "Progress" is moving in the wrong direction when children might—controversially—not live as long as their parents. If polio was the childhood health threat of an optimistic America in the 1950s, childhood obesity is the childhood health condition for a more skeptical, less assured time.[24]

The way in which we as individuals and as a society respond to children's illness shows how medicine understands and explains illness, but also how society as a whole values children and childhood health. The comparison of childhood obesity and polio as major stages in the history of child health illustrates a worrying trend in how we respond to child sickness. This book traces an increase in children having to manage their own bodily health as one aspect of such a response. Over the century, obese children have come to be required to treat their own condition, through reading diet books, following an exercise and eating regime, and making good dietary choices, even educating their own parents about healthy behavior. This increase in child responsibility is partly a pragmatic adjustment, reflecting the changing nature of American childhood toward children becoming more independent and the practicalities of being able to reach children in schools more easily compared to educating adults. But it also reflects an erosion of childhood as a protected stage—American childhood is a much more exposed time than it historically has been—and an increasing unwillingness to hold adults to account for children's health.[25]

As just one part of the public health approach to containing the polio epidemic in the 1940s, children were encouraged to change their behavior and wash their hands regularly. In contrast, by far the majority of approaches to contain the childhood obesity epidemic demand children's individual action and personal responsibility. *Children* need to learn about nutrition. *Children* need to exercise more. *Children* need to know about the lure of advertising. Those are useful skills, but how effective can they be when our contemporary understanding of the causes of the childhood obesity epidemic implicates America's social, political, and economic *environment?* This environment is made and controlled by adults—governments, parents, corporations. *Children* suffer the effects of adults' choices, so making children the ones to take mitigating action seems hypocritical, at best. Historical experience in public health also suggests it is likely to be ineffective. Teaching children about healthy eating choices and encouraging physical activity is a worthy mission. But adults also need to take responsibility for the environment in which children live so that children do not have to be tender experts on all things related to eating and exercise.

This book is not just about the contemporary epidemic of childhood obesity. Indeed that forms only the last part of this biography of a medical condition. Nor does it claim to account for all the factors, historical and modern, that may "explain" the epidemic. But by appreciating a century's worth of childhood obesity—its diagnosis, its causes, its harms, its treatments, its meanings—we can find the gaps between understanding and response, the inconsistencies between theory and practice. In bridging those gaps, and resolving the inconsistencies, we can find ways to act more effectively against the condition.

PART 1

Measurement and Diagnosis

CHAPTER 1

How Big Is Normal?

Quantifying Children's Body Size

While we do not know much about obesity in babyhood and childhood, we do know that it not a matter to be bragged about.

W. A. Evans, physician, 1932

How did childhood obesity come to be a condition requiring medical attention? Fat children existed before the twentieth century. But great fatness in a child was rare enough to be considered a titillating deviation from the much slimmer norm. Indeed, some very large children became famous for their unusual size. In 1896, nine-year-old Charley Bilcher was a local celebrity in his hometown of Catasauqua, Pennsylvania, having overtaken Anton Mochty of Austria and brought home to the United States the title of "fattest boy in the world." Or there was "fat-boy prodigy," young Irwin O. Schell (aged eleven) of Reading, Pennsylvania, whose huge hands measured eleven inches over the knuckles. Or Blanche Gray of Detroit, who exhibited herself in traveling shows as "the fat girl." When Blanche died at age seventeen, her young husband sold her "mammoth cadaver" to a curious surgeon for twenty-five dollars. Extremely fat "prodigies" of the nineteenth century like Charley, Irwin, and Blanche were regarded as astonishing, even newsworthy—but not especially medically worrying in spite of Blanche's death at an early age. Speaking to the newspapers, Charley's parents were rather proud of their massive son's size: "Step forward, Charley, and have your picture taken," said his father. As was popularly believed at the time, they felt that Charley's fatness reflected favorably on his health and how well they provided for him. Moreover, they didn't think Charley's rotundity signified he was sick. In fact, they thought quite the opposite: Charley's bigness was considered a sign of abundant—nay, overflowing—good health. More moderate (and more common) degrees of fatness in childhood than Charley's impressive heft were seen as healthy and attractive and were popularly believed to confer greater resistance to infectious disease, which was then such a prominent childhood experience. *Under*weight children—those spindly, rachitic, unattractive specimens—they were the ones doctors and parents of the late nineteenth century worried about.[1]

Although newspapers of the 1880s and 1890s reported famous fat children as local sensations, just thirty years later such children would be taken to the doctor rather than feted. In that thirty-year span, fatness in a child had become medically worrying—no longer a cause for triumph for the fat child, nor something "to be bragged about" by his parents either. Why the change? Why did "prodigies" become patients? This chapter is concerned with the process by which youthful corpulence was medicalized as childhood obesity and with the influences and currents that saw fatness in childhood enter the list of pediatric ills. Two of these influences, and the subject of this chapter, were, firstly, the introduction of the idea that height and weight had medical significance and, secondly, the development of standards or norms for child body size and weight against which children could be compared. Measuring a child's height and weight and interpreting those measures as both socially and medically significant were critical steps in creating childhood obesity as a clinical condition.

––––––––––

Pity the pediatrician. The physician who specializes in treating sick children—a medical discipline that emerged in about the 1870s—has a considerable problem. A prominent early American "pediatrist" (an older term) described the dilemma thus:

> We usually begin by asking our adult patient how he feels or where he has pain if any be present, but our little patients may be too young to speak or if they do speak the pains and discomforts may be referred to in a misleading manner . . . All the information we are in the habit of getting from the patient's description of his discomfort may thus utterly fail us. The distress may be as great or even greater, but the infant crying in the night, however definite, however obscure, however complex, or however varied the nature of his misery may be, has nought but a cry.[2]

In other words, pediatricians are not able to rely on their child patients reporting symptoms correctly or accurately. Consequently, from its inception this specialty has used other means of diagnosis. Birth weight—routinely recorded for births in lying-in hospitals since about 1860—was, and is, used as a diagnostic sign of how well the infant was at birth and as a prognostic sign for its early growth. A child's "failure to thrive" has long been recognized by physicians, midwives, and parents as a "danger signal" that all was not well. To track the infant's and older child's general health, nineteenth-century pediatric textbooks like William Dewees's *Treatise on the Physical and Medical Treatment of Children* (1825) and Job Lewis Smith's *Treatise of the Diseases of Infancy and Childhood* (1841) (both popular guides that ran to multiple editions) counseled using *appetite* as the gauge. "Good appetite" was a "favorable prognostic sign." "Appetite" was a subjective quantity that relied on a parent's assessment of what "normal" eating was.[3]

But as relatively cheap, small scales became available late in the nineteenth century for home use, pediatric text books from about 1890 onward began to cast *weight* in the role that appetite had formerly fulfilled as an indicator of a child's general health. "A most important point in the estimation of the development and actual condition of children consists in weighing them," wrote pediatrist James Finlayson in 1889. Weight had benefits over appetite as a measure. It was objective; it could be recorded and tracked over time (handy, given changes in medical practice to seeing more patients, less frequently); it gave information on how a child was growing as well as the child's health at any one moment; and it could be assessed in patients too young to describe their own symptoms, and so at least partly answered the pediatrician's essential dilemma. Early pediatric textbooks like Finlayson's encouraged physicians to use the tape measure and the scale as part of their standard practice in examining child patients. By the 1920s, taking height and weight was a sufficiently standard part of the pediatric diagnostic work-up to make the scale and the stadiometer (the instrument used for measuring height with a vertical ruler and a sliding crossbar lowered to the crown of the child's head) stereotypical features of the doctor's office—recognized badges of office like the stethoscope and white coat. That height and weight became central to pediatric diagnostics was one of the quietest innovations in twentieth century medicine.[4]

Slews of height-weight studies of children have been carried out—the first, in 1871, is the intellectual progenitor of the now ongoing National Center for Health Statistics and the Center for Disease Control's rolling child health surveys. Reams of height-weight tables and graphs, each claiming

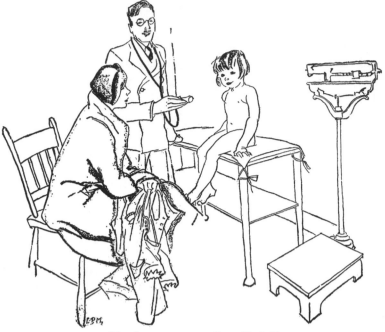

The doctor examines the well child

Figure 1.1 What to expect at a typical pediatric consultation, post-1920. The location (a pediatrician's office) is indicated by the examination table and the balance scale.

Source: Children's Bureau. *The Child from One to Six,* Children's Bureau Publication. Washington, DC: United States Department of Labor, Government Printing Office, 1937, 12. Courtesy of Ebling Library for the Health Sciences, University of Wisconsin–Madison.

status as a standard, have been produced from these huge number-gathering exercises. Why such a repeated effort to measure children? For one, the effort speaks to ongoing anxieties about children's health, although exactly what parents, researchers, physicians, teachers, and public servants commissioning surveys or using height-weight tables were anxious about has changed over time from the prevalence of underweight to overweight in children. For another, the repeated effort was an attempt to get the best data possible to address perceived problems with prior surveys or to use new methods and techniques in data gathering and analysis. And researchers also understood that the population of the United States was changing over time. Children were, in general, getting bigger, so new studies were needed to keep the results applicable to "modern" children. And lastly, the continual updating of studies reflects hard-fought battles over the philosophical question that is fundamental to developing any standard: *who* ought to be measured? That is, who ought to be the *reference population?* Beyond questions of childhood obesity and its diagnosis, the different answers to this apparently simple question trace researchers' changing thinking about how medicine relates to society, what its role ought to be, and where childhood health fits in with these aspirations.[5]

In the United States, the foundations for investigating children's height and weight were established in the years between 1870 and 1895 by three notable height-weight surveys. These studies provided the first indications of the range of American children's sizes and established *auxological* (body measurement) investigation as a research discipline in the country. Such studies produced quantitative descriptions of children's heights and weights—and started a trend toward establishing the dimensions of the normal child body and pathologizing deviations from this norm.

Henry Pickering Bowditch's study of Boston schoolchildren in 1871 was the first large-scale study of children's weight and height carried out in the United States and shows what the anxieties about child health were in the late nineteenth century. Bowditch was a physician, a member of Boston's Brahmin elite, and Harvard University's first professor of physiology. His comfortable career spanned private practice, university teaching and administration, and what was then referred to as "state medicine" or what we would now call public health. Bowditch's research interests were therefore substantial, covering both the scholarly question of human growth and development and the practical problems of community health.[6]

Bowditch's first motivation for measuring Boston children was nationalistic. He had read about similar investigations carried out earlier in the century in Belgium by statistician and sociologist Alphonse Quetelet, who had inventively applied statistical analysis techniques to various social phenomena, and in England by Charles Roberts, a fellow physician. Bowditch wanted to know how American children compared with their European peers—whether the American way of life with its opportunities, its egalitarianism, and its spacious freedom was written on children's bodies. And, being chair of the Massachusetts State Board of Health, Bowditch wanted to know how the health of Boston's immigrant children (mostly from Ireland, England, and Germany) compared with that of children from established American families. Quetelet's and Roberts's studies, in line with prevailing belief, showed that people's bodies, even if they were from the same racial stock, were shaped by the country of their upbringing. Native-born American children tended to be larger than Europeans. What then, asked Bowditch, would be the "effect of transplantation into new climatic conditions" on a child's growth? Would an immigrant child "attain to a stature resembling that of the natives of the States to which they emigrate" and become American in blood and bone and body, as well as citizenship? Or would the children of immigrants always, worrisomely, remain a group apart, an undersized nation within a nation? Reflecting his upper-crust anxieties about the influx of immigrants, Bowditch believed studying the heights and weights of Boston children could offer answers to this worry about assimilation.[7]

Beyond national inquiry—or, rather, national one-upmanship—there was also an intellectual aspect to Bowditch's interest in children's sizes. Quetelet's and Roberts's studies had produced contradictory evidence about how children grew. Quetelet's data seemed to show that Belgian boys were, on average, always bigger than girls of the same age. But Roberts's English data quite clearly showed that for a few years during puberty—the brief "period of female superiority"—girls were larger. Could *both* Roberts and Quetelet be right—did children of different countries grow differently? Or was one of them wrong and girls and boys did in fact grow differently? wondered Bowditch. Did American children grow in the same pattern as Belgian children or as English children?[8]

Bowditch also envisaged his results having a practical application. In the 1870s, physicians, educationalists, and feminists were waging a heated argument in Massachusetts social club halls over a theory concerning children's physical and mental growth. The contentious theory was that a child had only a fixed amount of energy available for both physical and mental growth, with the implication that "at those periods when the forces of the organism are engaged in producing rapid growth and development of the physique, the requirements in the way of mental effort should be reduced." Heavy emphasis on the "Three Rs" should therefore be scheduled during a child's slower growth times. Feminists were against this theory because of the implications it might have for girls' education. Harvard medical school professor Edward Clarke had given a talk entitled "Sex in Education or, A Fair Chance for Girls" to the New England Women's Club, in which he argued that girls "being educated and worked just like boys" risked the "healthy development of the ovaries and other accessory organs." The health of the nation, he argued, required that girls not be educated as wearyingly as boys. If physical and mental growth were antithetical to one another (and Bowditch said he would leave *that* to others to decide), data on how girls and boys grew could be useful for setting each sex's educational pace.[9]

National fortitude, clinical diagnosis, educational theory, and public health—all these issues could be helped, argued Bowditch, by surveying children's heights and weights. Testing the waters, Bowditch first conducted a small experiment measuring his own family members. From measurements on "thirteen individuals of the female, and twelve of the male sex" (his was a large family), Bowditch felt that the Roberts study in England was more likely to be right than Quetelet's Belgian study: between about the ages of twelve and a half to fourteen and a half, girls did indeed, on average, seem to be taller and heavier than boys. And, gratifyingly, American children did seem to be impressively large in comparison to their European cousins. Addressing the Boston Society of Medical Sciences, Bowditch proposed conducting "more extended observations" to find out more about the effect of "stock" or "ethnical group" and "climatic conditions" on children's growth.[10]

Bowditch got permission to do his extended study from the Massachusetts School Board in 1875. He, however, didn't lift a tape measure. He had class teachers from Boston schools measure their students' weight and height without shoes, but with the children remaining clothed out of consideration for logistics and contemporary mores about the appropriateness of children undressing. Bowditch supplied the schools with specially printed forms on which to record the information. Teachers were also asked to note whether each child showed any "deformity," and (under the same heading) to note "the fact of color . . . in order that negro and mulatto children might be distinguished from white children of American parents." This would allow Bowditch to separate the data along racial lines, with the data from poorer, smaller, African American children separated from wealthier, larger, white children. Although Bowditch did not say as much, if he compared only white Americans with Europeans he was more likely to find that "American" children were bigger than if he included black children in the "American" measurements. Teachers also had to record the nationality and occupation of each of the child's parents. If the child or teacher didn't know this information, Bowditch obtained it from the police. For a well-connected researcher like he was, state resources were made available. Privacy was not a concern in the experimental ethics of 1870. Nearly 11,000 girls and 13,700 boys were measured.[11]

Once the data cards were returned to him, Bowditch sent the figures to accountants across Boston for analysis. Dividing the labor of calculations in this way was necessary to handle such a large data set, since the "computing" power of the 1870s was limited to the slide rule. The accountants calculated averages (means) for the different measurements for each age, nationality, and sex and the ratio of weight to height for each child—an index, in Bowditch's opinion, of the "stoutness" of the child.

When he came to analyze the results, Bowditch's primary assumption was that bigger was better. He referred to tallness and heaviness as being "superior" to shortness and lightness. (Boys were therefore mostly "superior" to girls; Americans—at least white ones—were "superior" to immigrants.) Bowditch did not, however, mention the possibility of there being children who were *too* big: overweight or excessive nutrition was not a concern for him. The underweight child was what he saw as the potential problem.[12]

With his large sample, Bowditch found, as both his and Roberts's English study had earlier, that on average girls started to grow rapidly about four years before boys did and then stopped growing earlier as well, so that boys eventually surpassed them in height and weight. "The fact that these periods [of rapid growth] occur at different ages in the two sexes," said Bowditch, "may therefore be regarded as an argument against the co-education of boys and girls, except during the earlier years of life in which rates of growth are practically the same." However, he cautioned, "how much importance is attached to this argument" (and therefore to the resolution of the *Sex in Education* controversy) would need to be answered with data on mental development.[13]

From Bowditch's account of his analysis, it is not clear what he did with the data on African American children. One thing is apparent, however: he did *not* analyze that data as a group. There are no tables or graphs for the heights and weights of African American children in Bowditch's work. Given the categories he did in fact use for his analysis—"German," "Irish," "Russian," "English," and "American" parentage—and the fact that teachers were asked to record whether a child was African American in the same section as "deformities," it may be that Bowditch simply discarded the data from African American children. Alternatively, he also mentions that

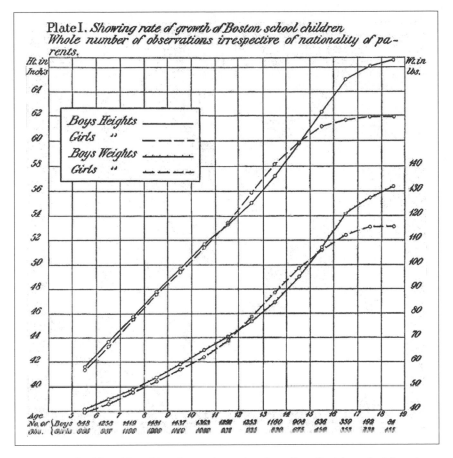

Figure 1.2 Girls' and boys' heights and weights from Bowditch's study. Note the "period of female superiority" from about age twelve to fifteen.

Source: Bowditch, H. *The Growth of Children.* Boston: Albert J. Wright, State Printer, 1877, foldout chart.

"observations on children of parents of any other single nationality [other than Irish or American] were not found to be numerous" and were therefore sometimes "thrown together into a single group of unclassified nationalities" for analysis. This data, Bowditch said, did not "throw any additional light on the question[s] under consideration," and so he did not publish it. So it is therefore also possible that, because of the racial mix in Boston in the 1870s, there was too little data on African American children for Bowditch to analyze it as a separate category.[14]

On the issue of "stock," Bowditch found that children whose parents were born in America were taller and heavier than the children of immigrants, although the difference seemed to narrow after just one generation. This, Bowditch suggested, was because the United States enjoyed "a more abundant distribution of comforts" than other countries, and that these comforts were reflected in the larger bodies of even the first generation born in the United States. Moreover, the pronounced class correlations that Roberts had found in England—children of professional-class parents (architects, clergymen, students, musicians, teachers) being taller and heavier than the children of unskilled laborers (firemen, pavers, sailors, and watchmen, in Bowditch's classification)—were not so apparent in the American data. This was a source of nationalistic pride for the American physiologist—"the American community" was less divided by class than "English society," and this showed in children's bodies. Most interestingly, Bowditch found that the social and environmental influences in the United States,

> which give a growing boy in this community greater height and weight than are attained by an English boy of the same age, affect the weight more powerfully than the height, and that the Boston boy is therefore by no means to be described as tall and thin in comparison with his English cousin.[15]

In other words, Boston boys were stockier than their English counterparts—their "more abundant comforts" went more to their poundage than to adding inches to their height. (Girls, too, showed this tendency.) Although Bowditch could not have anticipated this, his discovery is notable in light of secular changes in children's heights and weights over the course of the twentieth century, with children getting both taller and heavier, but more heavy than tall. Weight appears to be more plastic in regard to nutritional change than height. We do not, therefore, currently have an epidemic of tallness in children.

———

Bowditch's tables and graphs commenced the ensuing century's worth of work on establishing how tall and how heavy American children were. His work was followed by child measurement studies carried out in 1890–1892 in Worcester, Massachusetts, by Franz Boas (who, later in his career, became famous as "the father of American anthropology"). Boas's work, mainly intended to uncover more information about how children grew, illustrated levels of sophistication in the analysis and interpretation of data on children's body size beyond Bowditch's. Boas had intended to collect data for a number of years, but opposition from local newspapers whose editors could see no point to the then-novel idea of measuring children—other than for salacious reasons—made the young researcher leave town after just two years. Boas, however, continued to work with the data he had collected, sometimes combining it with other researchers' findings, reanalyzing it and investigating different aspects of child growth for the next forty years. The Bowditch and Boas studies were joined in 1892 by a study conducted in St. Louis, Missouri, by physician William Porter. Porter was particularly interested in the ramifications of growth patterns for educational pacing and intended his results to add a Midwest element to the otherwise New England–derived data.[16]

Bowditch, Boas, and Porter's work would, however, have remained merely an interesting intellectual inquiry into children's growth had it not been for the fact that their results were published in the most influential pediatric guide of the century, with height and weight measurements given clinical significance.

Luther Emmett Holt, Professor of the Diseases of Children at the College of Physicians and Surgeons, was the preeminent American pediatrician of the early twentieth century. Advisor to New York's Department of Health and the Child Health Organization (later the American Child Health Organization), founding member and sometime president of the American Pediatric Society (est. 1881), longtime editor of *The Archives of Pediatrics* (America's first journal devoted to pediatrics), and head physician at New York's Babies Hospital, Holt enjoyed a substantial professional and public reputation and had contributed much to nurturing pediatrics in the United States. He was well regarded, but not warmly liked, by his colleagues, who found him stuffy and distant—he apparently never said good morning—but he got on well enough with his child patients. Holt's professional reputation was based not on his personal charms but on two books that made him one of the first celebrity doctors in the United States, and, at the same time, helped make comparing a child's height and weight measurements against a standard a crucial diagnostic act.[17]

Diseases of Infancy and Childhood was a textbook Holt wrote for fellow pediatricians. It was first published in 1898 and ran to an impressive number of editions (eight during Holt's lifetime) and reprintings. *Diseases* surpassed all other pediatric texts in sales two years after its release and maintained a selling lead over all rival textbooks throughout Holt's lifetime. In this book, Holt advocated measurement and record keeping in pediatric diagnosis: tables, charts, and statistics were the essence of his systematic teaching style. Holt himself measured all his patients, even those coming to see him for warts, and he suggested that this practice was critically important for all pediatricians.[18]

In *Diseases*, Holt advised measuring children weekly for the first six months, then fortnightly up to one year, and then monthly. But not only that: Holt also gave a table of measurements with which he recommended physicians *compare* their patients. The table, which showed averages for boys' and girls' weight, height, chest, and head circumference for birth up to sixteen years, used data from Holt's personal observations on infants and Bowditch's figures for older children, and noted the differences compared with Boas's and Porter's figures. (Over the course of subsequent editions, Holt revised the height-weight estimates upward, saying that it had been his experience in private practice that children were in fact even heavier than Bowditch had found and much heavier than Porter's findings. Normalcy was getting bigger.)[19]

The second of Holt's two famous books told the public about the importance of measurement and comparison with standards. Long before Dr. Benjamin Spock's *Baby and Child Care* raised so many baby boomers, Holt's 1894 parent advice manual, *The Care and Feeding of Children: A Catechism for the Use of Mothers and Children's Nurses*, was given the extravagant moniker of "infant bible of the nation." The *New York Times*' book review of 1946 listed it (and its later editions) as one of most influential books on American life and culture, putting it in what today seems far more glamorous and prestigious company with Harriet Beecher Stowe's *Uncle's Tom's Cabin*, Nathaniel Hawthorne's *The Scarlet Letter*, and Benjamin Franklin's *Almanac*. When one of the Board of Lady Managers at the hospital where he worked suggested the hospital could raise money by running a training school for nursery maids, Holt devised the teaching material for the training program. He was asked by friends to make the material more widely available: *Care and Feeding* was the result.[20]

Care and Feeding spread the new gospel of weighing and measuring to mothers and to children's nurses. In successive editions of the book, weighing and measuring became increasingly central and increasingly defined by reference to quantified norms—the figures Bowditch, Boas, and Porter had found in their studies. Although in the first edition mothers were told the ages by which a healthy baby should have doubled and then trebled its birth weight, by the third edition in 1903, Holt had greatly expanded the section on measuring and changed from a self-referential approach to recommending comparison with his table of average measurements. (The third edition gave measures only for birth to ten years for boys; the fourth edition and thereafter gave weights for both sexes, up to fourteen years.) Holt's guide was adamant about how important weight, in particular, was as a clinical signifier.

Of what importance is the weight of a child?

asked the guide. And answered it:

Nothing else tells so accurately how well it is thriving.[21]

Parenting guides like Holt's and its ilk of the early twentieth century were so earnest about this new practice of weighing and measuring that they counseled mothers-to-be who were shopping to equip the nursery that, along with the layettes, and bibs, and cribs, they should also buy a scale. They even gave helpful pictures and recommended brands. An exceptionally well-fitted-out nursery might also include a special measuring board to make taking baby's length easier than measuring against the wall or the edge of a table. Mothers were being educated that their child's size was regarded as medically important.[22]

The process that Bowditch, Boas, Porter, and Holt had created and promoted had imbued children's heights and weights with clinical meaning. Holt's work in particular had suggested that pediatricians and parents should use measures of body size in their assessment of a child's health. But between the measurement studies and the way Holt had suggested their results be used in clinical settings was an interpretive gap that pediatricians and parents were encouraged to jump over. Bowditch, Boas, and Porter presented their work as *describing* what was *normal*—quantifying in inches and pounds what size and heft supposedly healthy children's bodies were. (There was, in fact, little effort given to ensuring the children being measured were actually healthy other than simply ruling out those with an obvious physical deformity. The implication was that the large numbers involved in the survey would balance any other health variations.) His own work, Bowditch said, was a first "rough approximation" for "establishing a normal standard of development." When it came to using the data, however, Holt (and later others) interpreted it not as descriptive but as prescriptive. While the Bowditch/Boas/Porter data gave a picture of the group of children measured, it would subsequently be used and promoted to physicians, parents, and school health officers as a standard against which a single child could be compared. Many children to one child; descriptive to prescriptive; research to clinical investigation; auxologists to parents, physicians, and class teachers. In shifting applications, interpretations, settings, and users, height-weight measurements took on new meanings and significance. Not only was normalcy quantified, not only did height and weight carry clinical meaning, but a child's body could be tested and judged as to how well it matched the descriptive criteria.[23]

One phenomenon more than any other of the early twentieth century illustrates these developments in quantifying normalcy, vesting height and weight with clinical significance, and judging children's bodies against the Bowditch/Boas/Porter size standards. "Better Babies" contests were held across America from the early teens to the 1920s. These contests were one example of a wider social anxiety about child health in the early twentieth century. Sparked by concerning levels of infant mortality, government and philanthropic efforts sought to address the matter through a range of means such as improved sanitation, child nutrition, and parent education. Better Babies contests were backed by women's committees and clubs, such as the Congress of Mothers and the American Medical Association's Committee for Public Health Education among Women, and supported by the popular magazine the *Woman's Home Companion*. The contests aimed at encouraging and rewarding child health and educating mothers about how to achieve it. Community groups like milk committees, state fair organizers, church clubs, agricultural organizations, and individuals could write to the *Woman's Home Companion* for advice and help in running a contest—the magazine would even help with prize money and a handsome medal picturing two "perfectly formed babies" for the winner. "Save the Babies" was the catchcry.[24]

Organizers hoped that the combination of free child-raising information and competitive spirit would drive mothers to raise "better" babies. And not just "babies"—the competitions covered children up to school age. Organizers also hoped that, in contrast to children's beauty contests, which were well known to be catty affairs, the scientific ideals of the Better Babies contests would encourage mothers of winners to share their recipes for raising pedigree kids. Measuring the young contestants' height and weight was an important (and the only impartial) aspect of the judging process.

Better Babies was hugely popular. In just one year (1914), the *Woman's Home Companion* sponsored contests in twenty-three states. Several organizers noted the wide demographic range of participants, particularly in the large metropolises like New York and Washington, D.C. Along with the clubby bastions of white middle- and upper-class women, contests were also organized by organizations with a particular ethnic bent, such as the Hebrew Institute in Chicago, the Kickapoo Indian Produce Fair in Horton, Kansas, and by African American community and church groups. The concept of the "better baby" clearly had broad appeal.[25]

In some towns, Better Babies contests arose out of baby beauty contests, but Iowa's 1911 baby contest (which lays claim to being one of the earliest in America) was modeled on its state agricultural fair. In the same way a fat, glossy pig could win the blue ribbon, a physically perfect (meaning both attractive and healthy) baby scored high. Judges—in this case physicians, rather than farmers—would mark children on a special scorecard. Scores would then be totted up to find the healthy winner.[26]

> Iowa has long excelled in prize crops of hogs and corn. She is not to be outdone when it comes to the higher order of creation. She is starting to show the world how to raise a prize crop of better babies.[27]

Similarly, Denver held its Better Babies competitions at the stockyards. Run by the National Western Live Stock Association, at the 1913 contest, Buffalo Bill rode around the ring with the two winners (one boy, one girl) on his saddle. It was a day out for the whole family.

Contest organizers would advertise through local newspapers and their own newsletters. Over the sometimes several days of the contest, mothers would bring their children to the contest location—often a pavilion within the state fair—for judging. Moving through different stations, and wearing only a cloth diaper or underwear, contestants would be measured, weighed, and scored on other points of physical and mental development.

Better Babies contests, parents were advised, were not meant to be like baby beauty contests. They were "scientifically based," with prizes for the *healthiest* specimens of babyhood. In practice, however, cultural standards have long conjoined child attractiveness with child health: a healthy child is considered attractive; an attractive child is likely to be healthy. And, to help decide on winners among large numbers of contestants based only on brief examination, Better Babies physician judges did incorporate what we would consider today as simply aesthetic standards. To one mother's "pathetic grief," her child was marked down for the "defect" of sticking out ears. Marks could be struck off for other unattractive features that had no pathological significance and also for supposedly troubling features of mental development, such as crying. Not just healthy, Better Babies winners also had to be pretty and charming.[28]

And the other common features of Better Babies winners were that they were tall for their ages—and chubby. As early measurement studies had shown, medicine of the early twentieth century was worried about the underweight child who failed to thrive and must therefore be sick; the corollary was that the chubby child with his rosy cheeks and dimpled knees epitomized the picture of health. And that was what Better Babies selected for: scoring systems selected winners who were large and heavy. That was achieved by comparing contestants' height and weight measures with tables of standard heights and weights.[29]

The two most widely used baby contest scorecards were those supplied by the *Woman's Home Companion* and by the American Baby Health Contest Association. Both scorecards used Holt's table of measurements against which children's heights and weights were compared. Under the scoring scheme, "physical development" (which height and weight reflected) counted for as much as 80 percent of the total marks. However, after a number of contests, organizers found that many entrants were scoring very highly against the Holt measures, making it difficult to clearly pick winners. The figures, based on regular babies and schoolchildren, were proving to be too low for the plump, pedigree children being entered in Better Babies. The *Woman's Home Companion* therefore issued new scorecards with tables of measurements that were arbitrarily larger than the Holt values. The magazine editor explained why they had settled on the new, larger standard:

> We believed that the highest possible standard should be set for babies entering these contests, even if these standards were above the measurements of the average child. We therefore set as our standard a height which was an inch to an inch and a half greater . . . and a weight which was one

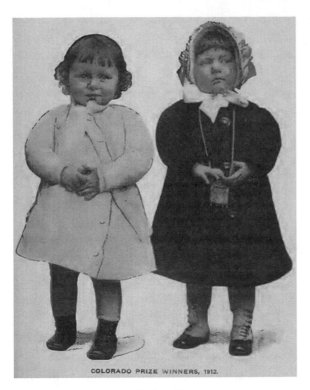

Figure 1.3 Plump and perfect. Better Babies Prize winners.
Source: North Carolina State Board of Health. "Colorado Prize Winners, 1912." *The Health Bulletin* 28, no. 6 (1913): 57.

to one and a half pounds greater than [the Holt] standard. The other measurements were correspondingly increased, except in the case of the circumference of the head, a large head often being an indication of rickets or other diseased condition.[30]

So the standards promoted by the Better Babies competitions, although based on the Bowditch-cum-Boas work, were an intellectual step away from those progenitors. The Holt tables were devised as a description of *normal* children and were intended to be used as a standard against which to judge whether a particular child was *normal*. Instead, the Better Babies tables would be an indication of what was *ideal*. Better Babies marked a subtle shift toward using height-weight tables as aspirational standards, based not on regular, normal children but on ideally healthy, pedigree children. The

Woman's Home Companion and the American Medical Association collected copies of the scorecards from the competitions and had a statistician, Frederick S. Crum of the Prudential Insurance Company, analyze them. The tables Crum produced were based on over ten thousand Better Babies contestants, ranging from six months to four years of age, making them the first height and weight standards developed in the United States that drew from a national—although not representative—sample. The Crum tables were adopted by the American Medical Association (AMA) and by the federal Children's Bureau and given out to parents as an indication of how big children *should* be.[31]

As medical practice, parenting advice, and the cultural phenomena of Better Babies contests in the opening decades of the twentieth century began to make American society sensitive to children's heights and weights, other areas of life also encouraged parents to take a good hard look at their children's bodily measurements. Going shopping also brought home to parents the growing significance of children's body size in American culture. Since the late nineteenth century, shop-bought or "ready-to-wear" clothing for children had been increasing in popularity and availability, first boys' clothing and then later girls'. Shopping for ready-to-wear clothes increasingly made parents aware of their child's size. Clothing assistants at Macy's were equipped with a tape measure to help the young customer into properly fitting clothes; Bergdorf Goodman gave customers a special card where a child's waist, height, chest, leg, and sleeve measurements were recorded.[32]

But it was the big catalogue sellers, like Sears Roebuck, whose business practices really drove home to parents the need to know how big their child was and also how their child's body compared with that of his or her peers. In early editions of the Sears *Big Book* catalogue, parents ordering clothes for their children were instructed to "be particular to always give the height, weight and age in young men's, boy's and children's orders, along with the rest of the information [chest, waist, and inner seam measures], as these are very important." The catalogue even came with a tape measure to make sizing up the child easy.[33]

From 1910, Sears introduced an innovation in clothes ordering: standard sizes. Sears saw standard sizes as an important way to increase buyers' confidence in purchasing clothes and, they hoped, to reduce the costly number of returns for poor fit. (Sears famously offered a money-back guarantee: "Satisfaction guaranteed or your money back.") With standard sizes, parents not only had to know their child's bodily dimensions but then also had to compare the measurements with a table of standards for what was considered—by Sears—to be "normal" size for the child's age. Sears's sizing designations were based on children's ages: a size 8 was meant to be the size for an average eight-year-old, so parents could get a clear sense of how their child compared with these newly devised norms. (This type of sizing system is sometimes called "age sizing.") Sears, being America's biggest catalogue seller, led the industry in developing sizing standards in the 1910s, and the practice became commonplace across all ready-to-wear children's clothing manufacturers by the 1930s. Each store devised its own sizing "standards" depending on its own particular tailoring practices.[34]

Although age sizes were meant to fit children of particular ages, the sizes were not based on, say, a formal survey of children's body measurements. Rather, clothing sizes were developed from in-house pattern makers' rules of thumb, trial-and-error, passed down "like recipes handed down through families." Only after a 1939 study by the Bureau of Home Economics was there a move toward developing sizing standards for children's clothes based on survey measurements. World War II prevented the widespread adoption of new sizing standards, however. It would be 1949 before the Mail Order Association of America—the trade organization for catalogue sellers such as Sears—adopted sizing standards based on the bureau's measurement survey. Parents suffering through the increasingly common experience of buying readymade children's clothes were having to assess whether their child was too skinny, too fat, or just right according to the particular store's sizing standards. Clothing sizing therefore contributed to making children's body size noticeable and important in American life (but didn't make clothes shopping any easier).[35]

―――――――――

The Bowditch/Boas/Porter/Holt and Crum tables started an ongoing process of surveying large groups of American children's heights and weights and presenting them as tabulated or graphed standards. These were sometimes smaller studies, sometimes considerably larger studies, like the massive federal survey of children for Children's Year in 1918 in which 7.5 million scorecards were used, 2 million were analyzed, and new standards drawn up based on nearly 200,000 children. Ethnic-group-specific studies were carried out from the 1920s to investigate physiological questions—did different ethnicities follow different patterns of growth?—and social questions—did impoverishment show up in the bodies of ethnic groups? These studies raised the still on-going question of whether there ought to be different standards for different ethnic groups.[36]

Parenting guides and pediatric textbooks routinely included tables and graphs, using one of the available studies—Holt, Crum, and the Children's Year data were all popular choices—as the recommended standard against which to compare a child's height and weight. The federal Children's Bureau published its own series of mailing pamphlets on child and infant health called *Infant Care* and *Your Child from One to Six,* which gave the Children's Year data as its standards. Parents were therefore federally advised to assess their child's height and weight. The normal child had been quantified and described in tabular form.[37]

By 1920, the idea that parents and physicians wouldn't know the significance of a child's height and weight measurements—a problem Boas contended with when trying to persuade people to support his study in 1892—was unthinkable. Physical dimensions were firmly established as the preeminent markers of a child's well-being—and of a parent's ability and skill in caring for them. Both pride and anxiety about children's health could be quantified by these measures. American society had been sensitized to a child's height and weight. A child's body measurements *meant something*—something both medical and social—and could, and should, be judged. This new propensity to measure and judge child bodies was a critical step in framing childhood obesity as a medical condition. The practices of measuring and recording children's bodily dimensions would shape the way childhood obesity came to be diagnosed, conceptualized, and experienced.

CHAPTER 2

Measuring Up

Height-Weight Standards and Diagnosis

Though we all know a really fat child when we see one, it is not easy to provide a good definition of obesity.

R. S. Illingworth, physician, 1958

By 1920, American society had been sensitized to a child's height and weight. Widely available technologies of scales and stadiometers made it easy to pin down a child's measurements. A visit to the doctor, a flick through a magazine, a trip to the department store; all of these activities brought home to parents that their child's body size mattered and meant something. But what, exactly, did it mean? If your child was big, should you be worried—or proud? And if worried, worried for what reason? Was a fat child a sick child, or just socially disadvantaged? The answers to those questions changed after 1890, but it was a gradual and patchy process, and one that is still not universally in agreement. Pediatricians of the nineteenth and early twentieth century had worried about children whose heights and weights fell below the norms being described by height-weight standards like Bowditch's or Holt's—*under*weight, not overweight was the troubling condition. But in the 1920s, influential pediatricians began to suggest that the other end of the spectrum—the overweight child—should also be a concern. Clinical equilibrium implied that children whose stats fell above the norm might also be something to worry about. "Too big" was a possibility. "The overweight boy," wrote one pediatrician in 1924, ought to be considered "as much of a problem as the underweight."[1]

Overweight in adults was already established as something that warranted medical attention. Over the course of the nineteenth century, obesity in adults had changed from being considered a desirable sign of prosperity and power to being increasingly regarded as, first, a problem of appearance; second, a sign of lax character; and, third, tagging along behind, a medical trouble. A sign of the changing times in regard to adult plumpness was the

41

diet guide *Letter on Corpulence, addressed to the public,* by a British under-taker, William Banting, in 1863. In his little book, Banting described how he had once suffered from the "distressing" and "lamentable disease" of obesity. He tried various remedies including Turkish baths, rowing, and taking the cleansing waters of Harrogate and Cheltenham spas to no avail, but, as he recounted in his *Letter,* he succeeded in losing weight by dieting. (The diet Banting followed, prescribed by his doctor, was what we would call today a "low-carb," "high protein" diet—the historical forebear of the famous Atkins diet.) Banting's guide also set out what it was about obesity that were considered the troubling aspects—social harms such as the "the sneers and remarks of the cruel and injudicious," physical inconveniences such as not being able to tie his shoes "without considerable pain and difficulty," and medical problems with his knees and ankles, sight, and hearing. By dieting, he had gone from 202 pounds to 167 pounds in nine months, and many of his troubles had cleared up with the lost weight. Banting's *Letter* was hugely popular, not only in his native England, but in America as well, showing that by the later years of the nineteenth century, obesity in adults was seen as a social and physical problem requiring a concerted effort on the part of both doctors and their fat patients to solve it.[2]

But in children, concern about fatness had lagged behind worries about fatness in adults. There was really no medical attention given to fat children up until the 1920s, and in fact, before this time if people thought about fatness in children it was seen as conferring social and physical benefits.

Exactly why this situation should change—why overweight in children became a topic of medical interest and concern—is difficult to pin down with any precision, but there are indications of certain factors and influences that may have contributed to the change. One factor that contributed to childhood corpulence becoming medicalized as childhood obesity was connected with increased anxiety about overweight in adults. Other reasons related to that most amorphous and diaphanous of historical changes: ideas about attractiveness and how embonpoint might reflect health in childhood. Still other factors were connected with changing thinking about the benefits of overweight in childhood.

In the nineteenth century and into the early twentieth, it was popularly believed that mild degrees of plumpness in childhood would help protect the child from infectious disease or, in the event the child did become sick, provide a safety margin against the loss of appetite during the illness. At the closing years of the nineteenth century, that possibility—that extra poundage conveyed protection from the major child-killers of diarrhea, diphtheria, scarlet fever, and tuberculosis—was a very powerful offer indeed. Scarlet fever alone had in the 1850s reached a death rate of up to 272 per 100,000 of the population; it killed 22 percent of toddlers who caught it. But as the nineteenth century finished and into the early decades of the twentieth, the threat of infectious disease in childhood receded, and childhood mortality rates dropped. Historians have argued about why this was the case. Improved nutrition, sanitation, and housing, and, to a lesser extent, improved medical care and vaccination may all have played a role in prompting the considerable decline in childhood deaths from infectious disease in the early twentieth century. The infectious diseases themselves may also have attenuated and become less virulent. As a case in point, infant mortality in New York City declined 40 percent between 1898 and 1911; mortality from measles, scarlet fever, and diphtheria dropped by 43 percent.[3]

As infectious disease became less of a threat to children, the perceived benefit of chubbiness declined in importance. A reduced threat from infectious disease meant less reason to value fatness in children. While this change did not make childhood obesity a medical *problem*, it made space for rethinking whether it was a good thing or not. In a scant twenty or so years, the belief that slight overweight in childhood had a protective effect and was a boon during illness had been replaced by its complete opposite: that overweight children were *more* susceptible to illness and, as one pediatrician said in the 1920s, were "less likely to recover from pneumonia or other acute illness" than slimmer children.[4]

Another factor that may have helped create childhood obesity as a medical problem was shifting taste in what was considered attractive in a child. For the early part of the twentieth century, roundedness and dimples were typical features of pretty children—children shown in art, advertising, and film. For example, the Gold Dust Twins (1897), the Uneeda biscuit boy in the yellow rain slicker (1899), the sweetly saccharin Pears Soap ads, the Jello Girl (from 1904), the Fisk tire tired toddler (1907), the Morton Salt Girl (1911)—all were chubby cherubs. Similarly, in film and on television, some of the biggest youthful box office names of the first half of the twentieth century—Shirley Temple, Jackie Cooper, Jackie Coogan, Baby Leroy—were dimpled darlings. The pretty child of the prewar era was a plump one.[5]

Plump children not only looked attractive in the reckoning of the time; they were also the picture of health. Clear, bright eyes; smooth, even-toned skin; plump, well-fed form: all these are what pediatrician Louis Starr (1849–1925) referred to as the "features of health," as well as being the features of childish attractiveness. The triumvirate of health, chubbiness, and attractiveness was made explicit in the drawings of the Campbell Kids, who advertised Campbell's Soup from 1904. Graphic artist Grace Wiederseim (later Drayton), who invented the Kids and drew them until 1916, intentionally made them fat to suggest to buyers that tinned soup was as nutritious as homemade: "Give Vigor and Strength" was the slogan.[6]

In comparison, advertising images of children and child stars of the latter half of the twentieth century have generally had slimmer, more angular and adult-like features—Jody Foster, Tatum O'Neal, Haley Joel Osmet, and so forth. The Morton Salt Girl with her umbrella and canister of trailing salt made her first appearance in 1914 as a tubby toddler. But she was redrawn several times after that and got taller, slimmer, and a little older each time. Her current incarnation, which dates from 1968, is as a slightly built seven- or eight-year-old. Attractiveness in a child has changed from chubby to slim over the course of the twentieth century.[7]

There are still fat child stars today—Honey Boo Boo (Alana Thompson), the reality television personality, and Rico Rodriguez from the television show *Modern Family* are two current instances. But this is nowhere near the uncritical love affair audiences had with the cute, chubby moppet of prewar entertainment. Also note that both Honey Boo Boo and Rico Rodriguez capture current anxieties about the childhood obesity epidemic—as worryingly connected with poverty, poor education, and gormless parenting in Honey Boo Boo's case, and with ethnic groups, in Rodriguez's case. By far the greatest bulk of famous chubby children in film, television, and advertising appeared well before 1940.

The change in what was considered pretty in a child from chubby to slim seems to have happened around the midcentury, significantly later than the 1920s, when fatness in a child started to be thought of as medically worrying. Popular culture lagged behind medical opinion in regarding childhood chubbiness in a positive way, but it is also possible that the aesthetic appeal of chubbiness in a child was already beginning to decline before the midcentury, helping make way for medical worries to take hold. In children, appearance and health circle one another.

Another factor that contributed to worry about overweight being extended to children was increasing concern about obesity in adults. Although life insurance companies had known since the late nineteenth century that considerably overweight adults were more risky insurance prospects than slimmer adults, this connection was made sharply apparent in 1913 by data from the Association of Life Insurance Companies and the Actuarial Society of America looking at the connection of weight to life expectancy. What the data showed was that adults who were considerably in excess of average weight had greater morbidity and mortality—were more likely to be sick and more likely to die—than average to slightly overweight people. Insurance companies recommended that adults be considered "obese" if their weight was in excess of 20 percent above the average for their height (and be levied higher insurance premiums or refused cover as a consequence). The 20 percent cutoff value demarcating the point where a person should be considered "obese" was an arbitrary one, based on choosing a level of mortality that was felt to be "too high" a risk for the insurers.[8]

Although the precise physical mechanism for what obesity did to the body was not clear, the impression was that obesity created strain on the body and its organs: strain on the heart trying to pump blood around that too-large body, strain on the lungs trying to oxygenate all that blood, strain on the legs and hips to support the weight, and so on. This ongoing strain presumably wore the body down, and so caused sickness and early death, which were shown in the insurance figures.[9]

The new insurance data on obesity in adults provided convincing evidence that obesity—at least in adulthood—was bad for one's health. Although the data only related to adulthood, it also created what could really only be described as a niggling feeling on the part of doctors that if obesity was bad for you in adulthood, perhaps—perhaps—it was not that good in childhood either. But there was a critical difference: there was no specific evidence that excess weight in children was associated with higher morbidity or mortality. Children did not buy insurance policies. Nor was there, at that time, any other sort of study looking at the long-term effects of obesity in children. And obesity in children was still relatively rare. "So far as we know," wrote one doctor in 1924, "the degenerative changes that go with obesity in the adult do not occur in childhood; but whether carrying around excessive weight early in life predisposes to a similar condition in adult life is another question." Possibly, wrote another pediatrician at this same time, "the tax put upon the heart and other vital organs by the extra burden of weight carried [produces] lessened powers of endurance and diminished activity," and maybe the "extra burden put upon the lungs and circulation . . . makes [fat children] less likely to recover from pneumonia or other acute illness." But what evidence there was on obesity in childhood suggested that, unlike in adults, the condition in children "has no such apparently physical defects." Rather, if obesity in children was a problem— and maybe it was, maybe it wasn't—its harms seemed to be in the social realm. "In games requiring more skill, such as baseball and tennis, [fat children] are decidedly awkward and backward as a group and hence we find them with the tendency to withdraw from competitive play and loaf," said a school doctor. Clumsiness and poor sporting performance made the fat child the butt of teasing, and this, for doctors of the 1920s and 1930s, was one of the most serious harms of obesity in childhood. Fat children might not suffer direct physical consequences of their fatness in the ways fat adult did, but they suffered nonetheless because their body size marked them out as different and as apparently less sporty than the slim child. The social suffering of fat children, combined with the possibility that, like fat adults, fat children might suffer physical harms, combined to make a case that doctors should take note of fat children and treat them.[10]

––––––––––

Height-weight standards set out the numerical parameters for a normal child body. Parents and pediatricians were invited to use the tables as a standard against which to judge children. In this way, height-weight standards had an important effect: they brought childhood obesity to greater awareness and prominence. Defining a norm or a standard meant that measurements below the norm were concerning—the undernourished children that pediatricians of the nineteenth and early twentieth centuries had worried about—but also that measurements *above* the norm might be troubling as well. A norm defined what was "just right," but it also defined "too small"—and "too big."

Consequently, from about 1920, pediatricians started using height-weight tables to define quantitatively what was meant by obesity in children. The tables seemed to offer the tantalizing prospect of a consistent, objective means of diagnosis that the whole medical profession might agree upon. And, if agreement on how to diagnose childhood obesity was settled, the profession could concentrate on causes and cures. The Boston pediatrician William Emerson was one of the earliest to suggest how height-weight tables for children might be used to define the condition. In adults, he said,

clinical evidence . . . corroborates the experience of life insurance companies that twenty per cent. above the average now in use may be considered the limit of normal weight, and any excess should be investigated. In certain children there is a natural tendency to excess of fatty tissue, just as in others, to bony structure or to muscular development; but when the excess passes beyond twenty per cent. we call the condition obese.[11]

That obesity in children should be defined as an excess of 20 percent above height-weight averages was therefore based on adult experience. In spite of the lack of data on children and overweight, Emerson's recommendation that obesity in children be thought of as weight in excess of 20 percent of average was taken up in its general terms. Pediatricians from the 1920s through to the 1970s used a percentage of average weight-for-height taken from height-weight standards to diagnose childhood obesity. The exact percentage that pediatricians used, however, ranged from 10 percent in excess of average up to Emerson's recommended 20 percent. Twenty percent was, however, the most commonly used cutoff and so was the de facto standard for defining childhood obesity quantitatively. Which tables were used in the diagnosis also varied. Common choices were the Bowditch, Holt, Children's Year, Crum (Better Babies) tables and the very popular 1923 Baldwin-Wood tables, which were based on a specially selected sample of middle- and upper-class white children from Iowa. (Baldwin described his tables as reflecting the "superior child"—physical standards to be aspired to).[12]

The use of tabulated standards and a 20 percent definition of childhood obesity did *not*, however, replace older methods of diagnosing obesity. Rather, older methods of diagnosis by eyeball—classifying children as obese because they were "clearly" or "obviously" or "frankly" so, or according to "clinical observations" or because of "the general appearance of the patient"— were often used either in tandem with the newer measurement-based methods or as the basis for an initial diagnosis later confirmed with the scale and the stadiometer. This aesthetically determined method of selecting obese children was considered perfectly valid because it rested on what was obvious to the beholder. As R. S. Illingworth explained, "we all know a really fat child when we see one." For example, in a 1942 study of obesity in children, the researchers chose their test subjects because they were children with "obvious obesity." That is, these children were initially diagnosed by eye as obese. Only in their analysis did the researchers use tabulated standards to verify that the children were beyond a certain cutoff marker. (In this case, all the children were over 55 percent in excess of average weight for height.)[13]

Both table-based and diagnosis-by-eye methods for determining whether a child was obese had advantages. Which method—or both—was most suitable to use depended on who was doing the diagnosing, where it was happening, and what purpose it was for. In the doctor's office, the physician could use tables and also his or her clinical judgment to factor in body build and muscular development—things that standard tables did not indicate. The 20 percent cutoff, wrote one pediatrician,

> holds for the majority, [but] one must keep in mind the occasional young "husky" of splendid build and muscular development, who may exceed that limit over the average, and yet not be obese.[14]

Indeed, a 2002 survey of medical and allied medical practitioners showed that, in a clinical setting—the one-on-one meeting of a patient with his or her physician—most practitioners relied *solely* on clinical judgment to decide if a child patient was too fat.[15]

However, in school health surveys or in mass epidemiological surveys where the experience of the measurer in making clinical judgments may not be substantial, or where an objective measure is desirable because of methodological standards, or simply where the press of time makes looking and assessing too onerous, table-based diagnoses had the benefit of precision. Tables could offer a cookie-cutter way of deciding whether a child was obese or not by precisely delineating the line between normality and overweight.

As using tables to judge children's bodies and make obesity diagnoses became more common, practical problems and issues began to be apparent. There was sufficient ire about tables that the 1930s and 1940s saw a considerable backlash against them—the Children's Bureau, for one, removed height-weight tables from their parental advice literature and warned parents against using them. One issue was a professional concern that parents and teachers were stepping too far into the doctor's sphere and that tables should be only one part of investigating a child's medical condition—an investigation that only a pediatrician was competent to do. Another problem was a practical one, stemming from a misunderstanding and lack of instruction on how the tables ought to be used for diagnostic purposes. Some school health programs interpreted the standards as meaning that, say, an eight-year-old who was forty-six inches tall *had* to weigh the weight given in the table—forty-eight pounds—to be normal. If the child weighed fifty pounds, he or she was diagnosed as obese. One Harvard auxologist lamented this common misunderstanding:

> There are zealous, if misguided, schoolmasters and mistresses still to be found sending home notices to gullible, phlegmatic or annoyed parents to the effect that their children are over- or underweight, if the children deviate by so much as a pound from the norms.[16]

Researchers developing new standard tables in the 1930s and 1940s tried different formats that would make the tables easier to use as diagnostic aids. One common solution was to specify a zone of normality rather than giving just a single average weight. Children falling below this zone were underweight; those above the zone were obese. (There were different ways of specifying the zone, such as using percentages, percentiles, or standard deviations about the mean.) The zone of normality idea was in fact the natural extension of defining obesity as weight in excess of 20 percent of average. Such a definition would imply that weights *up to* 20 percent of average were normal. Using the tables in this way to diagnose obesity therefore also reflected what could be considered normal variation in children's weights.[17]

When the American Medical Association and the National Education Association invited auxologist Howard Meredith to develop a new, definitive set of height-weight standards in 1947, he was instructed to also develop instructions for interpreting the tables such that they could be used "by the school nurse, the physical education instructor, or the one room rural school teacher" to identify under- and overweight children. Meredith's tables drew on the data from the same long-running study that the popular Baldwin-Wood tables from 1923 were based on, namely "superior" (that is, supposedly ideally healthy, ideally brought-up) white children living in Iowa.[18]

To help with interpretation, Meredith expressed the data as percentiles and gave names to the different percentile zones. Children falling in the 1st to 10th percentile band were "light"; children on the other end of the scale, from the 90th to 99th percentiles, were "heavy." Meredith also gave additional guidance as to how the tables could be used for diagnosing obesity. He advised users that children whose height measurement and weight measurement fell in the same percentile bracket were normal because they were in proportion, but, say, a boy whose height was in the "average" range but whose weight was in the "heavy" range "may be a healthy boy of stocky build or he may be "overweight" and in need of endocrine therapy, an especially prescribed diet, or a marked change in his daily regimen."[19]

Measures falling in different bands "may indicate normal stockiness or may reflect an undesirable state of health," and therefore the child should be referred to a physician for further examination. Meredith's tables could therefore give a preliminary diagnosis of obesity in one of two ways: either if the child's weight was above the 90th percentile or if his weight percentile was much larger than his height percentile. Meredith's instructions on how to diagnose obesity in children were a notable early attempt to quantify the idea that obesity wasn't simply heavy weight or bodily largeness, but a distortion of normal body proportions.[20]

Diagnosing obesity in childhood as an abnormal deviation from average weight given by a table of standards had certain advantages in terms of simplicity and objectivity. Basing diagnosis on measurement and numbers was also in line with the increasingly preferred style of medical research using large group studies rather than small case reports. But this way of diagnosing childhood obesity had one great problem: a child who weighed more than 20 percent over average could be rotund (and medically worrying) or could be tall or muscular (and a superb example of healthy youth). Tables alone couldn't tell these two physiques apart. There was always the issue of that "splendid young husky" who was heavy, but muscular rather than obese. Pediatric researchers investigating childhood obesity needed precise ways of delineating between the worryingly massive and the superbly large.

One early approach was to try to find a way of quantifying a person's build. Also variously called "physique," "constitution," "bodily habitus," "somatic form," and "morphogenotype," the sheer range of terms employed by researchers investigating potential measures covered an essential lack of precision and agreement about what in fact was being measured. But investigators agreed it had something to do with shape.

Separately, height or weight measurements gave a sense of only a single dimension of a person's body. But put together in an index or ratio, the two qualities could be combined to give information about the body's three-dimensional shape, "putting flesh on the bones" of one-dimensional measurements.

By the first decade of the twentieth century, three weight-height indices using different exponential powers of height or weight were being used by auxologists. Alphonse Quetelet, the inventive young Belgian statistician whose work in the mid-nineteenth century had helped inspire Henry Bowditch's study of children's heights and weights in the United States, had experimented with a simple index of weight divided by height (w/h) as an abstract indication of how weight changed with height as people grew. Bowditch had used this same index in his 1877 study. It was, he said, a measure of "stockiness."[21]

The second of the three widely used weight-height indices was weight divided by the square of height (w/h^2). The index was (and is) sometimes used with a scaling factor (a number that multiplies the index, i.e., $s \times w/h^2$) to make the results more convenient to work with than small decimals. Quetelet had also dabbled with this index and had observed,

> Following numerous experiments that I have done on the correlation between adults' height and weight, I have been able to conclude that weight varies simply with the square of height.[22]

In spite of the fact that Quetelet preferred using the simple w/h index, it was the index using the square of height that was given Quetelet's name. For most of the twentieth century, and still occasionally today, this index is called "Quetelet's index" in remembrance of the statistician's suggestion that weight and the square of a person's height are, in adulthood, linearly proportional to each other. However, in 1972, the American physiologist Ancel Keys renamed (and depersonalized and denationalized) the index, calling it the "body mass index" (BMI). Such has been the dominance of American research that BMI is by far the more common term today.[23]

The third of the common indices using height and weight was suggested by an Italian physiologist, R. Livi, in 1897. Livi's index used height divided by the cube root of weight ($h/w^{0.33}$). A later version suggested by a German physiologist, Rohrer, in 1908, used weight divided by the cube of height (w/h^3). The reasoning behind using these exponents was to match the

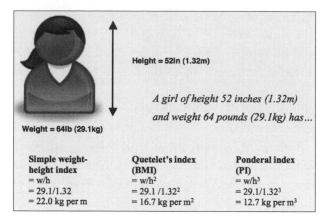

Figure 2.1 A comparison of index calculations.

dimensions of the numerator and the denominator so that the final ratio was just a number, unitless. (Weight, being related to volume, is a three-dimensional quality, while height is a linear or one-dimensional quality. The exponents used in these indices make the top of the fraction the same number of dimensions as the bottom of the fraction.) Researchers felt that an index that didn't depend on particular units was a desirable quality. The index in its form of w/h^3 is called the "Ponderal index" (PI) (more rarely, "Rohrer's index"). The theoretical elegance of the Ponderal index—the fact that the numerator and denominator of the ratio were dimensionally matched—was, for many researchers, a major point in its favor.[24]

From out of this confusing range of options, child health researchers picked and chose between the various index-based approaches to try to diagnose childhood over- and underweight more reliably. One particularly popular tool for assessing a child's body shape in school health examinations was the Wetzel grid, published by the Cleveland pediatrician and child development researcher Norman Wetzel in 1941. Wetzel wanted to develop an unequivocal, read-and-write way of using height and weight measures in school health examinations that would give a swift diagnosis of children who were too thin or too fat.[25]

To do so, he developed a special grid or chart on which teachers would plot a child's measurements. Height ran along the horizontal axis of the grid, and weight along the vertical, the latter plotted on a logarithmic scale to make the intervals equal. The grid was therefore based on a modified

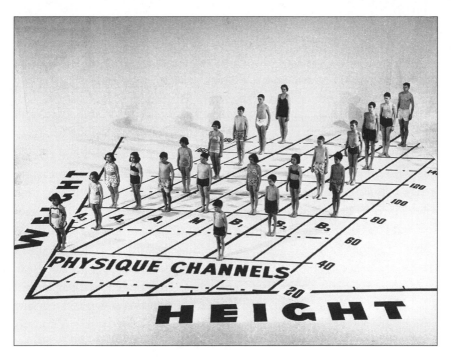

Figure 2.2 Children demonstrating the different physique channels standing on an enlarged replica of the Wetzel grid, with decreasing stockiness/chubbiness running from left to right. Note that just one child falls in the A3 band and, while plump, is hardly "obese" by modern aesthetic standards.

Source: Miller, F. "Normal Growth Illustrated by Children Standing on Enlarged Replica of Wetzel Grid." US: Time Life Images/Getty Images, 1950. Photo by Francis Miller/Time Life Pictures/Getty Images.

version of the simple w/h index. To make diagnosis easy, Wetzel drew bands, or "channels" as he termed them, onto the grid. Which channel the child's height and (log) weight fell into determined the child's "physical status" or "physique." Wetzel labeled the channels with a letter-number code and with a qualitative description. The higher "A" channels (A3, A2, A1) were described as "obese," "plump" and "husky," "stout" and "stocky." The lower "B" channels (B1, B2, B3) were "slender" or "thin," "fair" or "border-line," and "linear." In the middle of the spread was a single "good" or "medium" M channel.[26]

Wetzel's grid also included a second page where one could trace across to read off a child's basal metabolic rate and "development" level. In practice, however, people only used the first page of the grid. This was likely because Wetzel didn't explain very well how he had developed the measures on the second page, and it was very difficult to use—one commentator said that to use it, you needed to arm yourself with "courage, a magnifying glass and steady nerves."[27]

From the time it was published in 1941 through to the late 1960s, Wetzel's grid with its basis in the simple w/h index was commonly used in school health screening programs and in research into child growth and obesity rates. It was a useful tool for converting raw height and weight measurements into a diagnosis of either undernutrition or obesity. A study of high school girls in 1956 used the grid to study the incidence of childhood obesity and concluded that about 10 percent of children were obese. A much larger study of Cincinnati children, spanning ages five to sixteen, found a similar incidence of obesity, also using the Wetzel grid.[28]

At the midcentury, therefore, researchers had three principle indices available to them (and variations on them such as the Wetzel grid) for trying to get a numerical grip on a child's body shape. However, it wasn't entirely clear how the indices ought to be evaluated or, indeed, what bodily quality they were quantifying. Physiologists in the United States conducted studies comparing these three indices and discovered that the indices were not interchangeable. Children with, say, a high Ponderal index might not have a particularly high Quetelet's index. The three indices ranked bodies differently. And, unlike in adults, in growing children the average of the index varied with age. Researchers used different criteria, variously incorporating tests of meaning, utility, and ease of use, and another criterion that could best describe as "mathematical aesthetics," to evaluate the indices. On this aesthetic count, the *simplicity* of the weight-height index and the dimensional *elegance* of the Ponderal index favored these two indices. Quetelet's index, being neither as simple as the weight-height index nor as elegant as the Ponderal, was the least aesthetically pleasing.[29]

The predictable outcome of this lack of consensus on how to judge the best index was that each index attracted its own supporters and detractors across the professionals concerned with child health. Charles McCloy, a physician and physical educationalist, thought that the Ponderal index was best for "build" and "physical status"; George Wolff, a child development researcher with the National Institutes of Health, favored Quetelet's index for describing "body build" and "physical development"; Raymond Pearl, a professor of biometry and vital statistics at Johns Hopkins, suggested the simple w/h index was best for measuring "body build" or "body habitus" while Quetelet's and the Ponderal indices, he felt, had "retreated . . . into the realm of biological mysticism." Auxologists Howard Meredith and Stanley Culp at the Iowa Research Station favored the Ponderal index as a measure for children's "body form" because it decreased with age, mirroring "common observation of the transformation of the 'dumpy' toddler into the more 'lanky' schoolboy." Charles Davenport, biologist and prominent American eugenicist, didn't like the Ponderal index for this very same reason and thought Quetelet's index better at capturing children's "build" or "robustness."[30]

In 1976, the National Center for Health Statistics (NCHS, a Health Department agency) published its own charts of height-weight standards and weighed in on the issue of an index and also on the issue of who the standards ought to be based on. Since 1963, doctors and nurses had been touring the country in specially fitted-out Winnebagoes to conduct national health surveys of children for the NCHS. Called the National Health (and Nutrition) Examination Surveys (NHES and, later, NHANES), the surveys included measuring height and weight. The NHCS therefore had massed a considerable amount of data on children's body sizes and had worked with the Bureau of Census to carefully select the children to be measured so that its sample could be considered a microcosm of the United States as a whole. The 1976 height-weight charts were therefore the first such standards to be based on a group of children that was specially chosen to be representative of the racial, geographic, and socioeconomic mix in the United States.[31]

The other option open to the NHCS was to develop ethnic-specific tables, but the consensus was against that option. Although height-weight studies *had* shown racial differences in children's sizes, the NHCS's expert advisors felt that existing studies had not been designed to separate out the effects of income level from those of race. The "genetic growth potential" of the two largest racial groups at the time—"white or black"—was judged to be sufficiently similar that having a single standard covering all racial groups was "unlikely to cause serious errors." There was considerably less known about the growth of children of Latin American or East Asian descent, so the experts counseled that any standard should be used "with care" for children from these groups. Practicality and wariness of discrimination favored a racially unified standard.[32]

The NCHS's charts included a plot of weight for height (the simple w/h index) and suggested that

> Weight for length or stature greater than the 95th percentile suggests obesity although it is not diagnostic, for example, some children may be above the 95th percentile in weight-for-stature but have unusually good muscle development with little adipose tissue and are not obese.[33]

The NCHS's recommended cutoff at the 95th percentile implied that around 5 percent of the children in the United States at the time the data was collected (1963–1975) could be considered obese. That decision to make the 95th percentile the cutoff for obesity in children was an arbitrary one. (And a decision that did not take into account earlier studies of the prevalence of childhood obesity that put it at around 10 percent of the population. Had the NCHS wanted their table to be in alignment with earlier studies, they should have chosen the 90th percentile as the cutoff for obesity in children.) Although the NCHS's height-weight standards were widely used in the United States and adopted by the World Health Organization as their recommended growth standards, their suggestion of using weight for height to diagnose childhood obesity did not attract a consensus. Intriguingly, the NCHS's expert advisors had recommended *against* using a common weight-to-height ratio for all racial groups. It would be, the advisors said, "inappropriate" because "relative leg length differs systematically among ethnic groups."[34]

Researchers agreed that *some* common measure would be useful for making consistent diagnoses of obesity, but that was as far as their agreement went. For most of the twentieth century, medical opinion could not settle on a standard diagnostic measure for childhood obesity using one of the weight-height indices.

――――――

The story of the long and ongoing effort to find a quantitative method for diagnosing obesity reflects a need that is basic to modern medicine: quantifying the diagnostic criteria for a condition, like obesity, is absolutely fundamental for medicine to be able to apply its powerful research techniques. Massive epidemiological studies hoping to uncover risks of health conditions needed definitive diagnoses. Without practical ways of measuring, medicine is unable to use the major research tools at its disposal.

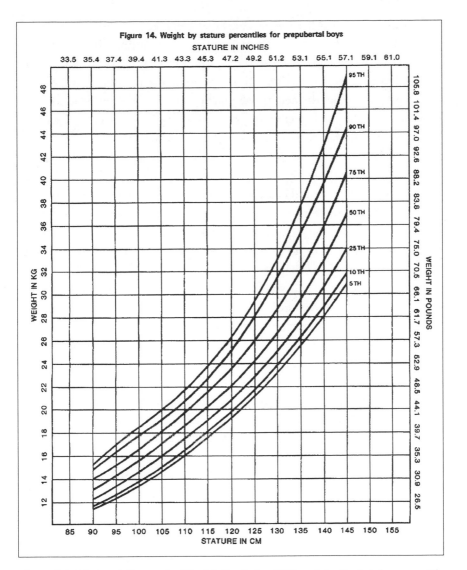

Figure 2.3 National Center for Health Statistics 1976 weight-for-height percentile chart (the Hamill standards, after the lead analyst at the NCHS, Peter Hamill) for prepubertal boys. Note the percentile lines are curved, rather than straight. That is, the w/h index varies by age in growing children.

Source: Hamill, P.V. V., T. Drizd, C. L. Johnson, R. B. Reed, and A. F. Roche. "NCHS Growth Charts, 1976." *Monthly Vital Statistics Report* 25, no. 3 (1976): 1–22, 17.

The opinion that obesity is an abnormal condition in children, found at the unhealthy extremes of the population distribution, is reflected by attempts to define and diagnose the condition using height-weight norms and indices of height and weight. This interpretation has remained the same, regardless of whether the height-weight standards were regarded as ideals to be aimed for (like the Better Babies standards) or as a snapshot of the population when the data was gathered (like the Children's Year or NCHS tables). Tables such as the popular Meredith standards of the late 1940s were based on wealthy white children—a consciously taken decision reflecting the scientific and social exigencies of that time; more recently, standards have been based on a racially and socioeconomically balanced reference group, representing the cultural and scientific exigencies of the late twentieth century through to the present. Both types of standards—standards as ideals, and standards as snapshots—raise questions about *how* they can be used to define obesity and whether it *should* be defined in that way. That debate continues today, as does the issue of whether there ought to be different standards for different ethnic groups.

None of the methods using percentage deviation of from average weight nor any of the index-based methods seemed particularly better than any other for diagnosing obesity in childhood. Nor was it even clear *what* needed to be measured or how one might go about deciding which diagnostic method for childhood obesity was "best." The result was a lack of consensus within medicine about how to routinely diagnose the condition, from when childhood obesity first became a medical concern in America in the 1920s, through to the 1970s. Developments in thinking about the dangers of obesity in childhood and technological innovations would eventually break the deadlock.

CHAPTER 3

Sugar, Spice, Frogs, Snails
The Composition of the Fat Child

> Criteria of obesity actually based on a measurement of fatness
> seem superior to criteria based on inference of fatness.
>
> Obesity researchers Carl Seltzer and Jean Mayer, 1965

For most of the twentieth century, the picture of how to measure and diagnose childhood obesity was confused. There were a few options for how to do it—making an aesthetic judgment or diagnosis-by-eyeball; choosing one of the many "standard" tables of height and weight and using some cutoff point such as 20 percent in excess of average weight; or using some criteria based on an index that captured body shape, like the Quetelet or Ponderal indices. Each method had certain advantages in certain settings where it might be used, as well as certain detractions. Consensus—that foundation stone of scientific endeavor—was nowhere to be seen.

Those options for measuring and diagnosing obesity were developed with the understanding that obesity was harmful in childhood because it made fat children stand out from their peers and be teased and unhappy, and because it was thought that the extra weight possibly strained the fat child's organs and body. While it was unclear whether this supposed strain had health effects (like the effects insurance data seemed to show that obese adults suffered), the concept of strain due to excess weight made it seemed plausible that measures of obesity should capture that degree of strain. Hence measures that used weight or bodily size and shape seemed appropriate bases for measuring and diagnosing obesity in childhood.

However, from the 1940s, medical research began to suggest that there was an alternative to that strain-based explanation of how obesity wreaked its harms. Medical attention to body size and shape was beginning to wane in favor of greater interest in body *composition* and, in particular, the role of fat itself. And there were growing indications that there was something more to the biological function of fat tissue than had previously been assumed.

At the start of the twentieth century, fat was thought to have a threefold role. Firstly, a covering of fat gave the body its particular aesthetic appearance, smoothing and beautifying the harsh outlines of bone and sinew. Secondly, fat formed a cushion, protecting the body (and especially organs) from knocks and bumps, and insulated it. And thirdly, fat was thought to be a metabolically inert energy storage site—a cache of excess fuel that the body could call upon when it needed more energy.[1]

But certain developments had raised questions over whether fat was this simple. Starvation studies carried out during World War II showed that bodies wouldn't or *couldn't* use up all their fat. With fat reserves running low, starved bodies would instead metabolize muscle rather than exhaust all bodily fat. This suggested that, contrary to what had been believed, fat was more than just a fuel. At the other end of the fat scale, epidemiological studies indicated large fat deposits were associated with a range of health problems, and some studies offered tantalizing indications that fat in different parts of the body affected health differently—location mattered. Tissue studies showed that fat was composed of specialized cells—not simply regular connective tissue—that had a considerable blood supply. And fat was responsive to some of the hormones, like insulin, that were being identified in the early twentieth century. Physiology textbook writers began to give page space to adipose tissue as an entity in its own right, rather than mentioning it only in passing when describing glucose (carbohydrate) metabolism.[2]

Taken together, these inklings suggested that, at the midcentury, medical opinion on fat was changing. Fat was becoming much more scientifically intriguing. Adipose tissue was not simply a cover, a cushion, and a cache, but was somehow more intimately involved in the body's essential functions. Although obesity had always been defined as a condition of excess adiposity, the shifting ideas about the role of fat in the body pointed out the essential mismatch between how obesity was defined, how it was measured, and how it was believed to inflict its harms. Researchers and physicians began to rethink their reasoning on why obesity was a potentially dangerous condition and what feature of the condition made it harmful. An obese person might face health problems not because they were fat—that their body was too large in some respect—but because they had too much fat: the adjective ceding to the noun.

In line with these new ideas, diagnosing obesity should therefore be based on a measure of body fat content, not of sheer body size. An above-average weight might be caused by lots of bodily fat, but diagnosing obesity using weight didn't quite get to the heart of the matter. As Carl Seltzer and Jean Mayer—prominent childhood obesity researchers—put it, "criteria of obesity actually based on a measure of fatness seem superior to criteria based on inference of fatness." Weight was therefore a poor measure to use—it was just an "inference of fatness." But how to measure what a body is composed of? How much fat, bone, and tissue are in a child's make-up? That question is the subject of this chapter.[3]

The only way to determine a person's body composition directly is to divide his or her body into its constituent parts and measure how much of each component there is. This direct analysis of body composition can therefore be done only on dead bodies. There are essentially two techniques for direct analysis of body composition, both of which read like pages out of a serial killer's handbook. The first, favored by U.S. researchers, has been to cut the cadaver up into about twelve pieces, carefully conducting this dismemberment in a big container like a bath so as to keep all the bits. Then each piece can be filleted into its different parts—fat, flesh, and bone—and by a repeated process of washing with different solvents, drying out, and eventually grinding down, the fat and water content of the body, along with its levels of sodium, potassium, calcium, zinc, iron, and so forth can be determined. The second direct analysis technique was preferred by European researchers, notably Elsie Widdowson at the University of Cambridge, a sweet-looking lady who was best known for her work on rationing in the United Kingdom during World War II and on child nutrition. Her method involved dissolving the body in hydrochloric acid. This produced a "uniform dark brown suspension," which was essentially the body in pureed form. The sludge could be chemically tested for fat, protein, and mineral content. More studies on human bodies have been carried out using the latter technique because, as one researcher explained, "manual separation of compartments is tedious at best and heroic when assayed upon mammals of more than a few kilograms body weight." (In his own research into body composition, this very practical researcher used guinea pigs.)[4]

A more recent study used a combination of both techniques—the cadaver was frozen solid (which took two days) and then sawn into cubes of about two inches. The cubes were then ground down and chemically analyzed. This method would be disputed by purists of cadaver analysis because the four hundred cuts of the buzz saw required to dice the body meant about two pounds of body matter was lost as, in the researchers' own words, "sawdust."[5]

Few direct analysis studies of human cadavers have been carried out, regardless of which technique they used. Before 1951, only five adult bodies had been analyzed for their composition, and since then, less than a handful of studies have been performed. Studies of fetuses and neonates are more common (because "they are of a more manageable size"), but, to date, only one study has analyzed the body of a child—a four-year-old boy who died of tuberculosis in 1951.[6]

There are so few direct analyses of cadavers because of enduring difficulties and dilemmas inherent in such research. The wholesale dismemberment of a corpse is a rather distasteful activity, even for anatomical researchers used to dissecting cadavers (more usually kept in larger chunks). Along with logistical issues, legal processes make obtaining "fresh" and "healthy" dead bodies difficult. And further, so few bodies are donated for medical research, both now and historically, that completely destroying a whole body for a single research project seems like a less than satisfactory use of a precious donation, although this is sometimes done. There is also the question as to whether *any* dead body—fresh or otherwise—would even have the same composition as a healthy living body. One researcher pithily summarized the dilemma: "The obvious fact that death occurred raises the distinct possibility of chemical derangement."[7]

Indirect analysis of a body's composition—that is, inferring or calculating the composition of the body from external measurements—is therefore the only option for assessing the fat content of a living subject. This chapter looks at three of the many, many efforts that researchers have made trying to find reliable ways of determining a person's body content without having to dismember him or her. The reason there have been so many attempts to do this is perhaps that all of the methods invented for measuring body fat content are, perforce, indirect estimates rather than direct measures, and so none can be "perfect." Body composition studies remind us that sometimes there are fundamental barriers to investigations of the human body—in this case, barriers to inventing an objective, easy diagnostic measure for childhood obesity. But it is also a reminder that a reasonable estimate is preferable to no measure at all because it at least may deal with the frustrations of the profession and the public, and allow research and treatment to proceed.

Technologies for studying body composition now form the basis for modern clinical definitions of obesity in both adults and children. But none of these technologies were, in fact, developed with this purpose in mind. For most of the century, worries about obesity have not been what drove physiological research. Rather, obesity research has simply been the lucky beneficiary of other research interests—notably efforts to make submarine rescue operations safer for the divers and to assess the impact of nuclear test fallout on U.S. citizens.

———————

"Dilution methods" that used the extent to which a tracer substance was diluted in the body's water had been used since the 1930s for body composition investigation. Cadaver and tissue studies had shown that the body's water makes up about 73 percent of the bones, muscle, and flesh—the "fat-free" or "lean" mass—with the waterless "fat mass" making up the remainder. Having a measure of the amount of water in a person's body therefore meant that the amounts of water, fat, and nonfat could be calculated. Although this was the first technique developed for investigating body composition in a living person, the method did not become the gold standard for body composition investigation. Rather, a technique developed in the 1940s with the aim of making navy salvage operations safer became the favored method.

Albert Behnke, a Stanford-trained doctor and physiologist who worked at the U.S. Naval Medical Service from 1929 to 1959, was charged with trying to find ways of making naval diving safer for the divers. Certain body compositions are better suited than others to navy diving, which requires diving to very deep depths for submarine rescues and salvage operations. Behnke's work led him to develop *densitometry* (also called "hydrostatic weighing," "underwater weighing," or "hydrodensitometry") as a way of determining which recruits were physiologically suited to deep diving and would therefore be likely to withstand the dangerous conditions better. Although he was a navy doctor, Behnke's work was also useful to the air force in helping select high-altitude pilots.[8]

Deep-sea diving (and high-altitude flying) involves breathing compressed air, but when the pressure is raised, ambient gases in the air are absorbed through the lungs into the blood and then into other tissues in the body. In particular, nitrogen—a normal component of air—is absorbed into the body. If the diver rapidly comes up to lower-pressure depths, the dissolved nitrogen returns to its gaseous form, making bubbles. The nitrogen bubbles trapped in the blood or in body tissues cause "the bends"—painful and potentially deadly. The bends can be avoided if the diver decompresses slowly, giving the nitrogen time to circulate back through the blood and be breathed out gradually.

Nitrogen, which causes the bends, is absorbed about five times more by fat than by other tissues, and so the more fat in a diver's body, the longer the time needed to decompress. Leaner naval recruits were therefore better suited to being divers than fatter men—they were less at risk of the bends and could decompress faster, making them physiologically safer divers. Weight alone was not a good indicator of a recruit's leanness. Exceptionally buff men, such as the "all-American" football players that Behnke had also studied, were classed as "obese" on purely weight-based definitions of obesity, but were actually extremely lean. Their dense muscles made them heavy and strong but not fat, and so Behnke reasoned that such men would probably make good divers. As a naval doctor responsible for identifying potential divers and for working out how long a diver would need to safely decompress, Behnke looked for a way of measuring a person's body fat content.[9]

Behnke's technique, described in a famous paper from 1942, was to have his naval volunteers submerse themselves in a large tank of water. He weighed them while they were breathing out so that the amount of air in their lungs would be minimized. Archimedes's principle (that of the "Eureka!" moment in the bathtub) states that an object submersed in water is buoyed up by a force that equals the weight of the water displaced. The difference in the volunteers' weight when they were weighed on dry land and their lighter weight when they were weighed in the tank gives the weight of the water displaced.[10]

The volume of the displaced water is then the same as the volume of the volunteer's body. From the volume of the person's body and his weight on dry land, Behnke calculated the density or specific gravity of his volunteer's body (weight/volume). Behnke knew from direct-analysis studies of cadavers by German physiologists that fat is less dense than the other tissues of the body, so the less dense a recruit's body was, the more fat content he had and the less suitable he would be as a navy diver.

Other physiologists derived mathematical models that would use the specific gravity of a person's body that densitometry provided and from it calculate how much fat was in that person's body. Two formulae—one derived by UC Berkeley physiologist William Siri in 1961 and the other by psychologist Joseph Brožek and his physiologic research colleagues at the University of Minnesota in 1963—have become the standards used with densitometry. Built into these equations are estimates of the density of fat and the average density of the fat-free mass from cadaver studies and biopsies of fat tissue. The equations assume that all fat in adults has the same density (an assumption that the authors felt was valid because of support from animal studies) and that the average density of the fat-free mass is also fairly constant. (The Siri and Brožek formulae differ slightly in that they use different estimates for the density of fat and of the fat-free mass.)[11]

Densitometry—Behnke's underwater weighing technique combined with the Siri or Brožek equations—became the gold standard for measuring body fat content. All other techniques for measuring body composition are calibrated against results found from densitometry. Densitometry is therefore the trunk of the tree of indirect methods for analyzing body composition. Why it should have become so primary is an interesting question. Densitometry has not been tested on cadavers—a ghastly exercise to imagine—so there is the fundamental uncertainty as to whether the figures the technique generates match a body's true fat content. The Siri and Brožek equations do, however, incorporate estimates for the densities of fat and of flesh and bone that were derived from cadaver studies, so perhaps that link to direct analysis has been a factor in making densitometry so important in body composition studies.[12]

———

By the midcentury, these new technologies for assessing a body's composition without having to dismember it gave new clarity to obesity research. In light of these developments, in 1950, leading U.S. physiologists Joseph Brožek and Ancel Keys proposed a bold new direction in obesity studies: clinical investigations of obesity should not use weight-based definitions or measures for diagnosis of the condition but should use measurements based on fat content. While weight-based definitions accorded with "popular ideas" that "a 'fat' person is thought of as a heavy, overweight individual," medical researchers needed to remember the condition was an excess of body fat and use an appropriately matched measurement tool—which the body composition technologies could now provide. Keys and Brožek were adamant: only measures that captured fat content ought to be used in studies of obesity.[13]

How might such a diagnostic basis for childhood obesity work? "The fat percentage estimate might be used to follow individual changes in body composition, and to yield an incidence of population obesity," wrote child-hood obesity researchers Rauh and Schumsky in 1968. But, they said, this "requires that a cut-off be established dividing the obese from the non-obese. We hesitate to do this since such a line must be arbitrarily drawn."[14]

Again, here was the problem—what was the difference between a "normal," chubby amount of body fat and an "abnormal," worryingly obese amount of body fat? Using body fat content to diagnose childhood obesity required a decision, one that Rauh and Schumsky were reluctant to take, as to where the dividing line would be. It was one of the same problems with the older weight-based definition of obesity (an arbitrary cutoff of 20 percent above average weight). Ideally, the decision as to the cutoff point should properly be made based on the likelihood of developing obesity-related illness, but for children no such data existed. For adults, epidemiological studies had suggested that adults were more likely to suffer health problems above a certain proportion of body fat, but this was a much harder experiment to carry out for children. Children's body fat proportions naturally change as they grow, starting high in babyhood, decreasing through toddlerhood to hit a low point called the "adiposity rebound" at around age seven or so and thereafter increasing again through puberty to reach a final, steady, adult level. The demarcation between "normal" and "obese" would therefore have to change with age (a difficulty, but not an insurmountable one). A bigger problem is that the health effects of overweight can take time to manifest, so what with the time lag, coupled with children's changing bodies, it is rather hard to draw any linkage between a child's weight and health problems at a later age.

While Rauh and Schumsky hesitated to define what percentage body fat constituted obesity in childhood, other researchers did not. Definitions differed, but commonly used figures to define obesity in children were percentage fat in excess of 20 or 25 percent of total body weight, a figure chosen perhaps partly because it chimed with the older definition of childhood obesity as a body weight 20 percent in excess of average. (The average nine-year-old boy was composed of about 13.5 percent fat; the average adult male about 15 percent.) Dilution techniques and densitometry meant that obesity in children could be defined as a condition of excess adiposity and diagnosed through measurements of body fat content.[15]

More recent techniques for finding body composition have allowed for the body to be divided up into more than just two compartments (fat and fat-free masses). These techniques can determine the proportions of fat, water, protein, and various minerals. As with densitometry, there was a military connection to a technique that was eventually called "potassium counting," invented in the midcentury. The method was not originally developed with body composition studies in mind. Indeed, until very recently, with obesity gaining in prominence, research into obesity has borrowed techniques developed for other conditions and with other investigative questions in mind. In this instance, with regular nuclear weapons testing on the U.S. mainland at the Nevada Proving Ground (starting in 1951) and the growing use of nuclear reactors (from the 1940s), government and researchers were worried about nuclear fallout.[16]

> As more and more people are potentially exposed to contamination, genetic considerations indicate lower levels for the maximum permissible exposure. There appears to be a growing need of [sic] an instrument capable of detecting radioactivity in human beings and in foodstuffs at levels well below the recommended maximum permissible concentrations.[17]

Children were an especial source of worry about radioactive contamination since they were still growing and radiation might compromise their growth. Moreover, being young, any cancers due to radiation would have a longer time to grow; children also drank more milk and played outside more, which would also increase the dose of radiation they picked up from the environment. Measuring how much radiation children in America were absorbing was therefore an important part of the radiation detection program.

Scientists at the Los Alamos Laboratory, under the auspices of the United States Atomic Energy Commission, were tasked with developing a sensitive radiation detector for determining people's exposure to nuclear fallout. What they built was called a *liquid scintillation detector*. "Scintillation" is the phenomenon in which certain substances give off a flash of light when they are hit with a radiation particle or wavelength. The number of flashes of light is therefore an indication of how much radiation is hitting the scintillating substance. In the Los Alamos detector, the radiation given off by a person's body would hit the surrounding scintillating liquid and cause a flash. The flashes would be detected by photomultiplier tubes and counted. After building a small prototype and trying it out on their boss, in 1956 the team built a larger machine, called the "human counter" (HUMCO-1) and with this machine started inviting visitors to the laboratory to be tested. Going to the Los Alamos lab and having one's radiation emissions measured was a fun day out.[18]

The human body scintillation detector was designed to be highly sensitive to radiation emissions given off by people's bodies. That feature meant that it also offered a new technique for determining body composition. People's bodies naturally contain potassium and its radioactive isotope, potassium-40 (^{40}K), mostly in their muscles. The potassium-40 in a person's muscles gives off small amounts of radiation, which a human body scintillation detector can measure. The radiation count therefore indicates how much muscle the person has. Wrote the body counter's creators:

> Since about 98 percent of body potassium is intracellular, change in potassium concentration reflects a change in the ratio of lean, oxidizing, protoplasmic mass to the mass of other body constituents containing little or no potassium (for example, skeleton and fat).[19]

The body's potassium content could therefore be used to calculate the body's lean mass and its water content, and that, as a rival research team at the University of Rochester pointed out, could be used to calculate fat content. The University of Rochester team, lead by pediatrician Gilbert Forbes, was particularly interested in applying the new technology to the issue of childhood obesity.[20]

In one study, Forbes took potassium counts on twenty-seven obese children (all over 20 percent in excess of average weight) and found that the children's total body fat ranged from twenty-four pounds up to 260 pounds per child. For some children, their weight in excess of average was entirely due to their body's fat content, but often children who had been obese since infancy also had a larger lean body mass as well as high body fat. Forbes suggested that, given this, "body weight alone loses some importance as an index" of obesity in childhood. He was a strong advocate of using body fat content, measured using techniques like potassium counting, as a better diagnostic index for childhood obesity.[21]

———————

From the 1960s, physiologists used indirect body composition technologies like dilution methods and densitometry and a number of other allied techniques to investigate how children's bodies changed as they grew and to establish norms for body composition in childhood and adolescence. However, the invention of these technologies did not resolve basic uncertainties about indirect body composition analysis. Most of the indirect technologies had never been tested against direct (cadaver) analysis, so it was not certain how close the estimates they gave for body fat content were to the actual fat content. Moreover, researchers investigating children's body content raised the question of whether it was valid to use techniques and formulae developed to assess adults' body fat content. Was adult fat of the same composition or at least of the same density as childhood fat? Was adult flesh-and-bone the same as childhood flesh-and-bone? If not, using the same equations that calculated adults' body fat would give wrong values for children's body fat.

Some researchers felt that it *was* valid to use the adult equations to calculate children's body fat. For this, they relied on evidence from a 1923 study conducted by C. R. Moulton, a biological chemist who had worked at the Institute of American Meat Packers. Moulton had gathered together cadaver data on many different types of mammals—guinea pigs, pigs, mice, rats, rabbits, cows, dogs, cats—along with the little that there was on humans (fetuses, four neonates, and a thirty-three-year-old). He was interested in how mammals' body composition changed as they grew. After birth, all the mammals lost water content as they matured, while the proportion of protein (indicative of muscle) and bone minerals increased. The changes smoothed out after a short period and thereafter held constant proportions into adulthood. Moulton described this point—when the animal's body composition reached steady adult-like levels—as achieving "chemical maturity." Mammals seemed to "reach chemical maturity at different ages, but these ages are a fairly constant relative part of the total life cycle": between 3.9 percent (for cats) and 4.6 percent (for guinea pigs and cows) of the animal's lifespan. By extrapolation, humans ought to be chemically mature by early childhood. Therefore, as body composition researchers argued, Moulton's study showed it was justifiable to use adult-derived formulae for calculating children's body fat content.[22]

Although Moulton's work was enthusiastically cited as justifying using adult equations for body fat in children, it was really not a firm foundation, and some researchers did indeed avoid using adult equations for this reason. Moulton had a crucial gap in his data—he had no information on how people grew between age four months and thirty-three years. He had simply extrapolated from what little data he had on humans and inferred the rest from other animals. And while the other animals were mammals, they were not primates. Primates, humans among them, have unusually long childhoods, so it was not a reasonable assumption that a human's maturation rate was similar to that of, say, a cow which can walk shortly after birth.[23]

By the 1980s, however, the increasing incidence of childhood obesity in the United States forced researchers to be more critical and decisive about the body fat equations. Physiologists compared children's body fat calculations made using different equations and reviewed the evidence on child body composition. The physiological evidence showed that children did not in fact reach chemical maturity at a young age—rather it was more like fifteen or even as late as eighteen, with girls maturing chemically earlier than boys. Before adolescence, children had more body water than adults, less protein, and less bone mineral. Moreover, children's body composition and the densities of each body component changed as they aged and also varied with sex. Children's fat was not the same as adults' fat, and children's flesh-and-bone was not the same as adults' flesh-and-bone, and the proportions and densities of these were different in children and adults.[24]

So applying adult body composition formulae to children was wrong. In fact, the biggest errors would be made when calculating the body fat of children six to eleven years old—an important age range in investigating the onset of obesity. Calculating body fat in children correctly would require using sex- and age-specific values for body density. With obesity in children becoming a more pressing medical concern in the 1980s, physiologists' work on developing reliable equations for calculating a child's body fat content was increasingly important.[25]

Body composition technologies like densitometry opened a view onto the inside of the obese child body. Finding out what fat children were made of without having to dissect them was a possibility by the midcentury. Technologies for indirectly assessing a child's body fat content continued to multiply: potassium counting, neutron activation analysis, bioelectrical impedance, and Dual X-ray Absorption Analysis (DEXA). All these offer investigators wanting to inquire into body fat content and obesity a choice of methods they might use to do so. More than this, researchers were approaching consensus that any diagnostic measure of obesity in childhood should be based on body fat content, not just on sheer bodily largeness or heft. But, if such a measure could be found, could it ever match the simplicity of a child stepping on a scale?[26]

CHAPTER 4

Insides Made Easy

Measuring and Diagnosing Obesity Using Body Composition

Body weight in proportion to height or to some function of height is interesting because it should indicate something about "build" or shape and about obesity or fatness . . . The body mass index seems preferable over other indices of relative weight on these grounds.

Physiologist Ancel Keys, 1972

By the 1960s, researchers had a number of technologies, including dilution methods, densitometry, and potassium counting, available to them for investigating childhood obesity. But all the technologies had a major drawback: they needed significant lab equipment, analysis time, and well-trained staff to carry them out. These were high-end laboratory techniques. None were suitable for a quick estimate carried out in the pediatrician's office, during a school health examination, or for an epidemiological survey of thousands of children. One research team investigating childhood obesity in 1968 summarized their dilemma:

> Obesity among children continues to be a major health concern. Yet accurate estimation and definition of the magnitude of this problem are still forthcoming. There are two pertinent aspects. First is that of estimating the incidence of obesity within the general population. Second is the accurate and objective identification of the individual case by the physician or health worker. Both of these aspects can best be solved by the development of a simple technique which accurately identifies the obese child.[1]

Physicians, health workers, and researchers needed a bread-and-butter test for body fat content.

Classic anthropometric techniques for measuring bodies were the obvious route to investigate: calipers, stadiometers, and scales again. Anthropometric measurements were easy and cheap to make, used techniques familiar to and well accepted by the public and the medical profession, and were easily understandable.

Although anthropometry had traditionally been used to quantify the size or shape of a person's body, could anthropometric measurements function as a "simple technique" for approximating body *composition?* Obesity researchers investigated anthropomorphic measurements afresh, testing them against body composition analysis to see if external body measurements could be used to approximate body fat content.

Taking measurements of the thickness of subcutaneous fat layers using calipers was one possible approach. Measuring a "skinfold thickness" involves the measurer pinching out the subject's flesh to form a fold. The measurer nips the calipers around the fold, and the instrument gives a reading of how far apart its two jaws are. The technique therefore measures the thickness of the subject's skin and her underlying fat layer, and can be done in different body locations to get an indication of the amount of subcutaneous fat the person has. Using calipers to measure skinfold thicknesses in this way had been done since the late nineteenth century. From the 1960s, some researchers interested in childhood obesity investigated whether skinfold thicknesses correlated with children's body fat measured using densitometry. They did. So, in theory at least, skinfold measurement offered a simple method for diagnosing childhood obesity based on body fat content.[2]

But in practice, the caliper method was yet another dead end in obesity diagnosis. There were problems with it. A person wanting to check the skinfold measurement she had taken would quite often get a significantly different number the second time (repeatability is low). For the children involved, it could be embarrassing to have their folds of skin gripped and pinched, and this became even more of a problem with teenagers. And— most damningly for a technique to be used in relation to childhood obesity—it was hard to take accurate skinfold measurements on obese people. It was (and is) difficult to set calipers around a very large skinfold. Ironically, though seemingly promising as a diagnostic measure for obesity, skinfold measurements worked most accurately on lean bodies. Skinfold measures seemed promising, but practical considerations meant that the method was never widely accepted as a simple method of judging body fat content.[3]

Another anthropometric route taken from the 1960s that *did* change the way in which childhood obesity was diagnosed was also a reinvestigation of old practices: weight-height indices. The simple w/h, Quetelet's (body mass), and Ponderal indices had earlier been used to quantify build or shape. But from the 1960s, the trio of indices was reinvestigated to see if they might say anything about body composition—and hence, as physiologist Ancel Keys pointed out, about obesity or fatness. One investigator set out what an index would have to do in order to define and diagnose obesity:

> The following criteria are commonly proposed for a "good" index of obesity: (1) it should be highly correlated with measures of relative adiposity; and (2) its distribution should be independent of height.[4]

Researchers in the 1960s and 1970s compared the various indices against body fat content (measured using indirect analysis techniques like densitometry) and used the criteria above to judge which index was the "best." A winning index emerged from the scrum.

In 1962, a British team lead by W. Z. Billewicz found that Quetelet's index correlated most highly with body fat content and was therefore the best index for adiposity. The only downside to the index, said Billewicz, was that it "is rather tedious to calculate when large numbers of cases are involved." He was having to do his calculations by hand. "Electronic computers," as he called them, were available in the 1960s, but were sufficiently rare that Billewicz did not have one. More studies by British and American researchers agreed that Quetelet's index correlated with body fat content the most highly of all the weight-height indices for most groups of people, but also grumbled about the "great deal of tedious arithmetic . . . involved in its calculation."[5]

By the early 1970s, though, the expansion of computer power reduced researchers' objections on the basis of the "tedious arithmetic" involved with an index having a squared power in it. In America, noted physiologist Ancel Keys renamed the index the "body mass index." With his clear explanatory style and step-by-step reasoning, Ancel Keys's 1972 paper was seminal in crowning the BMI as *the* index for obesity: "The body mass index seems

preferable over other indices of relative weight . . . as well as on the simplicity of the calculation and, in contrast to percentage of average weight,
the application to all populations at all times."[6] From the 1970s onward,
BMI began to be used in epidemiological studies, and as it was used, so it
continued to build consensus among researchers as the preferred practical
index of adiposity and for investigating connections between high body fat
content and illness. The Framingham Study, conducted in Massachusetts,
and the Western Collaborative Group Study, conducted in California, were
two significant longitudinal studies in which BMI was used in the analysis
as the index for obesity. Such studies helped build a general opinion that
increasing body fat content, reflected by increasing BMI, correlated positively with increasing risk of certain other illnesses or risk factors for other
illnesses, such as hypertension, high cholesterol, diabetes, certain cancers,
lowered longevity, and coronary heart disease.

Starting in 1985, a series of consensus-building conferences worked
toward establishing diagnostic criteria for obesity in adults using BMI. The
idea was to set a BMI limit beyond which corresponding risks for illness
became significant. In practice, the conferences decided on a compromise
that melded together the older definition of obesity in adults (weight in
excess of 20 percent of average) with BMI. Weight in excess of 20 percent
of average worked out as a BMI of between 26.4 and 27.2 for men and
between 25.8 and 26.9 for women, depending on which set of life insurance
tables were used to give the average weight. The old weight-based criteria for
defining obesity were recast in terms of BMI. Historical continuity was
therefore preserved, even though the new measure was now meant to be
representing body fat content rather than sheer body bulk.[7]

Although the precise BMI numbers the consensus conference arrived at
did not become the sole standard for defining obesity, the conference certainly furthered the idea that BMI ought to be the measure of choice.
Thereafter, a number of United States government publications adopted
various BMI cutoffs for defining "obesity," "overweight," "at risk for obesity," or "desirable BMI" ranges. The situation was greatly clarified in 1997
when the World Health Organization (WHO) held a conference on obesity. At that conference, the WHO adopted the standard that adults who
had a BMI of between 25 and 30 were "overweight" or "preobese" with an
"increased" risk of health complications. BMIs above 30 signified "obesity"
with moderate to very severe risks of health complications, depending on

how high the BMI was. This two-tier standard based on BMI cutoffs—a lower category described variously as "overweight," "preobese," or "at risk for obesity" and a higher category of "obesity"—has become the de facto standard for measuring population incidence of obesity.[8]

A simple Internet search for "BMI calculator" shows how dominant BMI has become over all other ways of gauging obesity. Enter your height and weight and the calculator will give you your BMI number and tell you where that places you in terms of health risk. BMI is the newest member of the range of numbers—height, weight, cholesterol, blood pressure—the health-conscious citizen of today knows about his body and its health.

————————

Using the BMI to define and diagnose obesity in children has been more contested than its use for adults. From the 1980s onward, researchers carried out numerous studies on children to compare estimates of body fat content using BMI against indirect analysis techniques. Skipping over the still-open issue of using indirect analysis on children, researchers have interpreted the results of these studies as both heartening and discouraging. Heartening, because the studies have strongly indicated that BMI does indeed seem to correlate highly with body fat content in children, but discouraging because the relationship is not one to one (two children can have the same BMI value but quite different body fat content). For one, highly athletic children tend to have high BMI because of their muscle bulk, not because they have high fat content. Once again, that "splendid young husky" who caused diagnostic headaches for obesity researchers in the 1930s is defying routine identification.[9]

Furthermore, BMI naturally changes as a child grows and matures. A child's BMI rises rapidly after birth up to about age one, and then dips down again during early childhood, reaching its lowest point between about ages four and seven. After this low point, his or her BMI begins to increase again. (There is some evidence that the younger this upswing or "adiposity rebound" happens, the more likely a child is to become obese both during childhood and later in life.) The increase plateaus by the late teens and early twenties and settles at the person's adult value.[10]

Varying BMI in childhood means that having a single, simple cutoff value of BMI that defines obesity, such as a BMI of 30 in the case of adults, is not possible for children. Cutoffs defining obesity in childhood *have* to

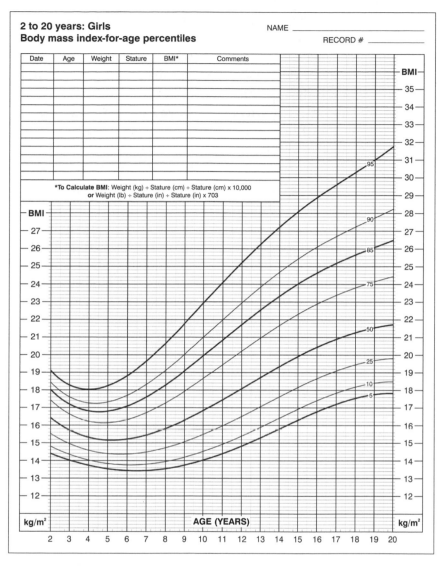

Figure 4.1 BMI changes with age in children. This chart shows the variation of BMI with age for girls, with the distribution indicated using percentile curves. The low point where BMI begins to swing upward is called the adiposity rebound. Note that heavier children (the upper percentile lines) experience their adiposity rebound younger than lighter children.

Source: Kuczmarski, R.J., C.L. Ogden, et al. "2000 CDC Growth Charts for the United States: Methods and Development." *Vital and Health Statistics* 11 (2002), 32. Published May 30, 2002; modified June 30, 2010. Developed by the National Center for Health Statistics in collaboration with the Centers for Disease Control (2000). http://www.cdc.gov/growthcharts.

vary with age and sex. Further, BMI in childhood varies with height, much more than it does in adulthood: taller children are likely to have a larger BMI than shorter children. Whether or not this should rule out using BMI to diagnose obesity in childhood is not something researchers currently agree on. Since the early twentieth century, childhood obesity investigators have remarked upon the fact that obese children tend to be both taller and sexually more mature than their slimmer peers. So, since childhood obesity itself seems to be somewhat connected with height, the fact that BMI in childhood is also connected to height is not necessarily a bad thing for an index. Researchers are divided on this point.[11]

A further complication that emerged in the late 1990s is that it appears that, for a given BMI, people of different ethnicities can have a different body fat proportion. For an equivalent BMI, Asian children have more body fat than white children, and white children have more body fat than black children. These differences may be genetic, or they may be environmental. In an echo of the history of height-weight standards (see Chapters 1 and 2), these results prompted discussion among health organizations, policy makers, and researchers as to whether there should be ethnic-specific BMI cutoffs for diagnosing obesity, especially in the case of Asian children (and adults). In 2004, the WHO considered the issue and decided against revising its standards because from the available research it was not clear what the cutoffs should be. But in 2013, Britain's National Institute for Health and Care Excellence (a government body that advises on health and care standards) issued lower BMI cutoffs for Asian adults.[12]

Despite these dilemmas and the ensuing criticism of the index particularly since the 1990s, the BMI has become widely accepted in school health surveys and epidemiological investigations (and to a certain extent in clinical practice) as the measure and basis for diagnosing obesity in children. In the 1990s, researchers published graphs of percentile distributions of BMI by age and sex for children using data already collected on children's height and weight, like the National Health and Nutrition Examination Surveys (NHANES), mentioned in chapter 1. In 2000, the Centers for Disease Control (CDC) published new height-weight charts using the national survey data collected since 1963, and included charts for BMI. The BMI charts, however, did not include the most recent data (gathered between 1988 and 1994) "to circumvent the influence of increases in body weight that occurred between [survey rounds] NHANES II and NHANES III."

That is, because levels of obesity in children had risen so much by the early 1990s, the population was no longer sufficiently "normal" to base a standard on it.[13]

Selecting BMI cutoffs to define obesity in childhood has been a point of major contention. In adults, the BMI cutoffs for "overweight" and "obesity" were selected via committee fiat on the basis of deciding when the risk of disease became "too large." Using the same reasoning to establish cutoffs in childhood is much more difficult because the conditions for which obesity is a risk factor (like cardiovascular disease and certain cancers) seem to arise from gradual bodily damage over a long period of time. It is very hard to make a connection between a childhood condition of obesity and the onset of diseases in adulthood. A number of factors may confound the relationship. Does the childhood obesity have to persist into adulthood to be dangerous? Is being obese during adolescence more risky than being obese in earlier childhood? Would findings apply equally to children of all ethnicities?

Various studies were conducted to try to quantify the risks of obesity in childhood, but the impression of clinicians and epidemiologists was that the condition was too prevalent and too risky to wait for clarification (which may not be possible anyway) on how obesity in childhood relates to morbidity and mortality either immediately in childhood or later in adulthood. Instead, organized medicine took the approach that workable definitions of childhood obesity based on BMI were needed sooner rather than later, and convened expert committees to decide on the best possible compromise definition of childhood obesity.[14]

A committee of adolescent health experts jointly convened in 1994 by the American Medical Association, the Maternal and Child Health Bureau, and the American Academy of Pediatrics was charged with finding the criteria that should be used to identify obesity in adolescents. They explained the pressing need for such metrics:

> Overweight and fatness in adolescents are significantly associated with current levels of and changes in blood pressure, blood lipids and lipoproteins, plasma insulin, and other factors known to be risks for obesity-related disease in adults. Evidence from longitudinal studies indicates that overweight and fatness, and increases in these measures during adolescence, may predict later elevated health risks and increased adult

mortality . . . The wide variation in research and practice [in the indicators used to identify overweight or obese adolescents], and the importance of identifying those at greatest risk, emphasize the need for a uniform approach to identify adolescent overweight in preventive services . . . [Our] intent was to establish a consensus based on the data available, recognizing that some recommendations would be based on insufficient data.[15]

The committee agreed that BMI was the best measure to use, and it further proposed cutoffs that would define two levels of obesity. The committee recommended using BMI percentiles, based on data from one of the National Health and Examination Surveys (NHANES I). They recommended that BMIs between the 85th and 95th percentiles be classed as "at risk of overweight." The adolescents in question should be examined further to see if they had any health complications associated with their obesity (like high cholesterol or blood pressure, prediabetic insulin abnormalities, or orthopedic problems) that would signify they needed treatment. A teen whose BMI was beyond the 95th percentile (or greater than a BMI of 30, whichever was the lower) was "obese" and needed medical intervention.[16]

The basis for choosing these particular cutoffs, said the committee, was that these levels successfully "identif[ied] adolescents with the highest percentage of body fat." Since, however, "little published information exist[ed] regarding specific degrees of overweight in adolescence and current or subsequent health-related outcomes" it was not possible to decide on the cutoffs on the basis of health risks, as was done in the case of adult obesity. Rather, the 85th and 95th percentiles had the big benefit that, as the adolescent drew toward the end of his or her childhood, the percentile cutoffs would merge with the adult cutoffs. (At age eighteen, the 85th percentile is close to the adult "overweight" BMI cutoff of 25, and the 95th percentile is close to the adult "obese" BMI cutoff of 30.) A similar expert panel convened in 1998 recommended that the same percentile cutoffs be used for obesity in younger children as well.[17]

The two expert committees' recommendations were, they said, not intended "to define or diagnose . . . obesity" but rather "to provide a protocol to identify those at greatest risk of obesity and its adverse sequelae." However, the committees' delicate distinction between "a protocol to identify" obese children and a definition or diagnosis of childhood obesity has not been maintained. In practice, the cutoffs are presented and used as defining childhood obesity and overweight.[18]

For example, when the CDC published their BMI-for-age percentile plots in 2000, they recommended:

> BMI-for-age may be used to identify children and adolescents at the upper end of the distribution who are either overweight (≥95th percentile) or at risk for overweight (≥85th, and ≤ 95th percentile).[19]

In more recent years, on the recommendation of the Institute of Medicine, the terms used to describe the two tiers have changed to "overweight" for BMI above the 85th percentile and "obese" for BMI above the 95th percentile.[20]

———————

The body mass index—renamed, denationalized, and depersonalized from being Quetelet's index—has emerged from the range of alternative methods to be widely accepted as the standard means of quantitatively diagnosing and defining childhood obesity. That BMI has borne up in this way is the result of two undercurrents.

One undercurrent was practical and technological. As the understanding of the dangers of obesity shifted from weight to body fat, medicine sought to measure fat content itself, and the technologies of body composition analysis provided the means to do so. Taking a person's BMI didn't require overly specialized equipment, the increase in computer power and availability removed the difficulties of calculation, and, critically, BMI correlated with body fat content. Moreover, BMI was a convenient device for screening large numbers of children for mass epidemiological studies or school health surveys—it was a tool suited to the modern style of medical research.[21]

The second undercurrent was historical. There was a great depth of history behind height and weight measuring—the ubiquity and familiarity of scales and stadiometers and all those surveys of children's bodies starting with Henry Bowditch's in 1877 through to the National Health Examination Surveys. This historical foundation meant that BMI measurements could be taken cheaply and reliably, and there was an archive of historical data without compare that could be drawn on to investigate how children's BMI had changed over time. An index that could take such ubiquitous measurements as height and weight and give them new significance as indicating body fat content is powerful indeed.

However, the overlying utility of BMI for defining and measuring childhood obesity conceals some major dilemmas. Technologies for measuring body fat content are, by and large, not validated against results from cadaver studies. And although the techniques incorporate tissue density constants that have been found from cadaver analysis, the cadaver values are themselves derived from just a few bodies. Moreover, BMI only *correlates* with (that is, is associated with) body fat content, and different indirect analysis techniques for determining fat content give different answers, especially in the case of children. And even further, there is a lingering question mark over whether the BMI above the 95th percentile definition does in fact capture all children whose health is at risk from the fat in their bodies. Researchers are inquiring into whether ethnicity, age, sexual maturation, and, especially, the location of a child's fat depots influence how dangerous obesity in childhood is—the location of the fat being, perhaps, more pertinent than a child's total body fat content. In other words, BMI correlates with body fat content, but this may not be what makes childhood obesity a health problem. It is possible that BMI is not *quite* capturing the essential quality of childhood obesity that makes the condition a health hazard, in the same way that the older weight-based diagnostic standards came to be regarded as missing the mark. The Centers for Disease Control's assured public pronouncements on how to use BMI to assess childhood obesity overlay a roiling controversy.

Considering another context, although BMI works quite well as an automated diagnostic test for obesity when screening huge numbers of children for large epidemiological surveys, in the doctor's office it is a different matter. The astute physician takes a child's high percentile BMI with a proverbial pinch of salt and may factor in race, maturational level, sex, and build before she decides if the child is obese or is simply one of those "splendid young huskies" who continue to make quantifying childhood obesity so difficult. The aesthetics of the child's body—the dimpled knees, the stomach rolls— also play a major role in interpreting BMI, as does how socially and emotionally debilitating that particular child finds his or her condition. In the doctor's office, BMI has not purged the diagnosis of childhood obesity of subjective elements. BMI has, therefore, like weight-based measures before it, been incorporated into a range of different metrics, some subjective, some objective, for determining whether a particular child is obese or not.

While BMI may be the current winner of that long-running competition to measure and diagnose obesity, its position at the top of the heap of indices, skinfolds, densitometric measures, scintillation counts, and so onward is by no means secure.

PART 2

Causes and Treatments

CHAPTER 5

Something Wrong Inside

Childhood Obesity as a Biological Fault, and the Hope for a Drug Treatment

It is notorious that children can eat enormous quantities of food without becoming abnormally heavy. As Mendel, the great authority on nutrition, phrased it, "No normal boy or girl can overeat."

Hans Lisser, endocrinologist, 1924

What makes a child fat? That is a question that has had different answers throughout the twentieth century. Driven by medical vogues, successes, and failures, each answer added a different way of understanding the condition and a different way of treating it. The result at the end of the century was a condition that was seen as complex and multifactorial, with a range of treatment options—each with problems.[1]

The idea that childhood obesity is caused by some kind of physical or "organic" problem *within* the obese child's body that can be corrected by drugs is a concept that has one of the longest histories of all explanations for childhood fat. How popular this explanation is has waxed and waned as other explanations and treatments have come in and out of favor. What the physical problem was, exactly, that the drugs were supposed to target, has also changed. This chapter and the one that follows considers three major episodes in this pas de deux of physical problems and their partner drug solutions: endocrine dysfunction and gland-based drugs; metabolic theories and amphetamine use; and lastly, the potential development of antiobesity drugs based on physiological and genetic studies of the body's signaling hormones, such as leptin. Each of these examples is based on a fundamental premise that obesity is a sign of a physical failing that can be rectified by drugs. But each episode also carries its own special features and says something about where fat children stand in their complex environment of scientific theories, parents' anxieties, doctors' hopes, and pharmaceutical companies' interests.

87

Prescribing a drug is one of the most powerful therapeutic interactions between a doctor and his or her patient. Historically speaking, this act draws its effectiveness from, firstly, the patient's and the doctor's beliefs about how the body and medicines work; secondly, the social authority of the physician; and, thirdly—as all involved hope—the biochemical action of the drug. Depending on the drug, the disease, and the time period in question, these three factors range in their contribution to how "effective" a treatment is, from negligible to total. Moreover, what sign or evidence a physician and his patient will use to decide whether a drug is "effective" is also historically variable. Modern pharmacy—that is, pharmacy of the later nineteenth century onward—aims to offer "rational" therapeutics: drugs for which there is scientific evidence that they work; that the mechanism of their action is known; and that the drug either targets the specific disease process (active or causal therapy) or at least works to ameliorate its symptoms (symptomatic or palliative therapy). Drugs that met these requirements (as amphetamines and organ-derived drugs were considered to do during their respective vogues as obesity treatments) have been lauded as the avant-garde of drugging, examples of the power of biochemistry.[2]

However, these same episodes in the history of childhood obesity also show that deciding whether a pill or an injection is a good drug or a quack remedy is not such a straightforward task. Both of the two earliest approaches to drug treatment for childhood obesity were popular for a time; thousands of children were treated by physicians and parents who believed they were doing good—and had evidence of it. Yet both of these treatments fell from grace. What changes make a drug that is acceptable in one decade unacceptable in the next? New experimental evidence does play a role, but it is not the only, nor even the most important, factor in these cases. Sometimes, as in the examples in this chapter, professional bodies like the American Medical Association (AMA) have delineated good and bad drugging practices and imposed controls over prescribing physicians. Federal drug regulations have, to a lesser extent, also shaped prescribing habits for obesity drugs. However, drugging practice is also complicated by the dilemma of suffering patients, anxious for a solution; the pressure on and desire of doctors to do something to help; and drug companies who operate in the world of large profits from popular medicines but who also need to cultivate and protect their reputations as purveyors of rational medicines. All of these factors combine to muddy the issue of what constitutes effective drugging practice.[3]

Childhood obesity first became a condition of medical concern in the 1910s, in part because the new field of endocrinology was a discipline looking for conditions to treat. In the late nineteenth century, two particular events had sparked a massive vogue for all things glandular. One, in the 1890s, was the successful treatment of cretins (people with myxoedema—a thyroid dysfunction) with sheep thyroid glands. The other, in 1889, was when Charles-Edouard Brown-Séquard, the seventy-two-year-old *pater patriae* of French physiology, told a Société de Biologie meeting that he had been injecting himself with extracts of dogs' testicles and found himself "radically changed." The "most troublesome miseries of advanced life" that he suffered had been cured, he thought, by the "essential nutrition" that the testicle injections had provided—"nutrition" that his own aged glands were no longer able to provide.[4]

Together, the cured cretins and the frisky old man launched massive interest in investigating the operations of the "ductless glands"—the thyroid, pituitary, renal, suprarenal, pancreas, testicles, ovaries, and other glands—and their "internal secretions." By about 1900, experimental evidence on animals and on humans showed that the internal secretions could have drug-like effects, like raising heart rate and blood pressure. This established a new view of gland secretions, not as "essential nutrition" for the body as Brown-Séquard thought, but as a chemical signaling system that operated in tandem with the electrically based nervous system to coordinate body functions. The British physiologist Ernest Starling gave internal secretions a new name and explained how they worked:

> These chemical messengers . . . or "hormones" (from ορμαω, I excite or arouse), as we might call them, have to be carried from the organ where they are produced to the organ which they affect by means of the blood stream . . . [Then] speeding from cell to cell along the blood stream, [hormones] may coordinate the activities and growth of different parts of the body.[5]

It was a hugely exciting time. The enthusiasm over things glandular extended to the general population, which offered a ready market for gland-based products of all sorts. Along with fresh breath and cavity prevention, toothpaste advertisements claimed to "keep the mouth glands young." Proprietary medicines like Glendage, Sexvitor, and Glandogen, "scientifically

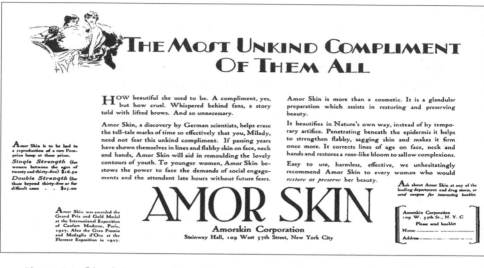

Figure 5.1 Glands became a big selling point for products of many kinds. Here, Amor Skin claimed to be "more than a cosmetic."

Source: Advertisement: "The Most Unkind Compliment of Them All" (Amor Skin, by Amorskin Corporation). *New York Times,* 13 May 1928, 92.

prepared" from "the glands of healthy animals," were advertised in newspapers and magazines as restoring "pep, vigor, [and] virility." Nor were the miraculous effects of glands confined to products for the human species: Burnett's tropical fish food, Glandex, which consisted of "endocrine gland elements," would "heighten colors, increase fertility, produce bigger spawns, [and] build firm bodies" in pet fish.[6]

In the medical realm, it seemed to many physicians that their profession was about to enter an exhilarating "new era in therapeutics": gland-derived drugs hinted at a "land of vast promise." What was needed were conditions that might be caused by malfunctioning glands so that this thrilling new era of treatments could begin. Since one of the characteristics of gland-based disorders like gigantism and cretinism was that the sufferer's body was of an unusual size and shape, obesity was an obvious candidate to include under the glandular banner.[7]

That obesity, especially in children, might be glandular also helped explain a feature that troubled some physicians: "cases [of obesity] only too frequently occur in individuals who are innocent of all dietary excesses; indeed, they may be spare eaters and of a vigorous habit." In 1900, German physiologist Karl von Noorden had proposed a highly influential theory that aimed to capture this distinction in obesity cases. The gluttonously fat, caused by too much food and too little exercise, he called *exogenous* obesity. Von Noorden called the frugally fat *endogenous* obesity, and it was this sort he suggested was caused by a malfunction in the person's endocrine system. Mothers apparently often told their physicians that their husky son "keeps fat with very little food" or that their chubby daughter was "a poor eater." This maternal claim was sufficiently common—and sufficiently accepted by physicians—to give the idea that obesity in childhood was of the endogenous or glandular kind.[8]

The president of the Association for the Study of Internal Secretions (later the Endocrine Society), Hans Lisser, also weighed in on whether obesity in childhood was exogenous or endogenous. Lisser, who had a clear professional stake in expanding the conditions his specialty was expert on, felt that it was simply impossible for children's natural eating instincts to be so distorted that they could become fat. Children were unsullied and innocent, he reasoned—and this included their appetites. A normal, healthy child, according to Lisser, could not be a glutton. (Adults might be gluttons, however, because their naturally moderate instincts had had a longer time to be corrupted.) And, Lisser said, this view had support from influential quarters: "As Mendel, the great authority on nutrition, phrased it, 'No normal boy or girl can overeat.'" Fat boys and fat girls were, therefore, not normal. Consequently, Lisser reasoned, childhood obesity was almost always of the endogenous variety. "The 'fat boy' or 'fat girl'," he said, "demands careful study of their ductless glands, and proper glandular therapy prior to and during adolescence is very important for their future."[9]

The "future" that Lisser was referring to was the proper sexual maturation of the child. Since medical research had shown that glands affected sexual maturation, fat children with malfunctioning glands might not sexually mature properly. Their gland problem (and therefore their obesity) ought, therefore, to be addressed before puberty.

For fat boys (although not girls), the connection between fatness and sexual mal-development was captured in the diagnosis of "Fröhlich's syndrome" (sometimes Froehlich's syndrome). The syndrome was named after Alfred Fröhlich, the endocrinologist who, in 1901, described a case of a twelve-year-old boy who suffered from headaches, vomiting, progressive weight gain, hair loss, and dry skin, who had small genitals and who failed to enter puberty even by his twenties. The boy was diagnosed as having a pituitary disorder. When his doctors removed a tumor from his pituitary gland, his strange symptom complex—including his obesity—seemed to improve. The diagnosis of Fröhlich's syndrome was, however, extended beyond the original symptom complex to a simpler combination of fatness, small genitals, and delayed onset of puberty. It was especially applied to boys (perhaps because the original case had been of a boy), although there was no particular medical reason that this should be so. Fröhlich's syndrome became a common and popular diagnosis in the 1920s and 1930s, and was used as a catch-all diagnosis of fat boys.

While some physicians treating childhood obesity concurred with Lisser's position that obesity in children necessarily meant an endocrine disorder ("endocrine therapy is indicated in every case of obesity in childhood"), others felt this was gross overenthusiasm for things glandular. One obesity specialist remarked:

> It is remarkable how general is the idea even among physicians that the usual cause of obesity [in children] is some abnormality of the glands. Such abnormalities do occur, but with the exception of the thyroid, are so rare that this cause may be disregarded except in large hospital clinics where such cases may be considered medical curiosities. The use of thyroid extract in the treatment of obesity is a short cut attended with danger to the growing tissues and is seldom, if ever, necessary.[10]

Between these two ends of opinion were those American physicians who took a moderate stance on the issue. This middle line of reasoning was that ascribing all cases of childhood obesity to a glandular cause was going too far, but glandular conditions causing fatness in children were not especially rare either. Wrote one St. Louis doctor, Borden Veeder, who conducted a study in 1924 on overweight in schoolboys:

> To show how far this [gland-blaming] can be carried, one has only to quote a recent statement that every baby weighing more than 8 pounds (3.6kg) at birth is a subject of endocrine disorder. I do not agree at all with the view of some endocrinologists that every obese child is the subject of an endocrine disorder . . . about 50 per cent of the children in our [study] were obviously endocrine cases, but in the other 50 per cent. we feel very positive that there was nothing that could be attributed to the ductless glands.[11]

Veeder, like many medical authorities of his time, instructed that it was possible to tell the difference between children who were fat because of an endocrine problem and those who were fat for other reasons by looking at the distribution of their fat and how developed their genitals were. Fat located in certain body parts was considered symptomatic of a particular gland malfunctioning. A "definite pelvic girdle adiposity" was considered characteristic of pituitary dysfunction; upper-body fat suggested hypothyroidism; fat about the hips suggested hypogonadism (dysfunction of testes or ovaries). The idea was to look, localize, and treat with the relevant gland extract. Children who had "a generalized distribution of the excess fat tissue and . . . no other [genital] abnormalities" had "ordinary obesity," which was just the result of overeating. Journal articles and textbooks giving instructions on how to diagnose endogenous obesity were often illustrated with photos of nude children, sometimes with their eyes blanked out (to preserve anonymity), turning their bodies into objects to be assessed and judged.[12]

However, when it came to actually prescribing gland drugs to treat a child's obesity, the professionally pleasing hips-means-gonads/shoulders-means-thyroid diagnostic criteria were very often thrown out of the window in favor of trying various gland extracts and seeing which ones would have a result. Thyroid and pituitary extracts were the two most commonly prescribed glandular treatments for children—thyroid because of its effectiveness in treating cretinism and myxoedema, and pituitary because Fröhlich's syndrome was connected with pituitary dysfunction. Fat children were also treated with combination therapies of both thyroid and pituitary glands, along with more exotic gland cocktails, like ovarian extracts (in the case of girls), testicular extracts (in the case of boys), and renal extracts. Precisely targeting which gland was allegedly malfunctioning, and targeting only that gland with therapy, was not always a priority.[13]

Fueling the "gland-ridden world" was a thriving industry producing gland-based drugs. In the early years of the vogue, physicians had limited options. Feeding patients the fresh gland was one option, although a rather distasteful one. Alternatively, physicians could make their own gland drugs by following helpful instructions in scientific journals: "To the slaughterhouses we must go for our raw material." Having obtained some glands from the local abattoir or butcher, the instructions recommended cleaning and macerating the glands into a pink pulp. The pulped glands could either be juiced and injected, or dried and made into tablets or powders. The dried preparations, unfortunately, had a "sickly, disagreeable taste, [and] an objectionable odor." And injections, in spite of the "most rigid antiseptic precautions" that physicians were advised to take with their macerated glands, often had the unfortunate side effect of the injection site becoming infected, hot, itchy, and pus-filled.[14]

Established pharmaceutical companies such as Eli Lilly, Squibb, and Parke, Davis and Company all added organ-based compounds to their drug lists from the 1890s onward, and certain enterprising physicians also set up their own companies to serve the enthusiasm for gland-based drugs. Notable physician entrepreneurs included a Civil War doctor and former surgeon general of the U.S. Army, William Hammond, and Harry Harrower, one of the founders of the Association for the Study of Internal Secretions and first editor of their *Endocrinology* journal. Under pressure from the AMA to "combat the present influence toward commercializing the subject of endocrinology," Harrower was run out of the endocrine association. But he had his retribution, making a considerable living from selling proprietary medicines, promotional textbooks, and guides. Harrower's huge gland-drug business made him the largest employer in Glendale, California, in the 1920s. Looking back, there was considerable fuzziness about who was selling "rational" and supposedly effective gland therapies and who was selling more dubious concoctions. Harrower, shunned by mainstream medicine, manufactured an effective thyroid preparation; Parke Davis, the sophisticated laboratory-based pharmaceutical company, sold the nostrum of mammary gland extract.[15]

For the meat-packing industry, the new medical interest in animal organs was a boon. Animal glands had previously just been rendered down with the scraps and made into fertilizer; but as medicines they were worth much more. And, because of the low concentrations of hormones in the glands, and the nature of preparation methods, a *lot* of glands were needed—fifty sheep produced one pound of fresh thyroid or three-sixteenths of an ounce when dried. One thousand cattle were needed to produce one pound of dried pituitary gland.[16]

Meat-packing companies made money by supplying raw glands to pharmaceutical companies and to firms like Harrower's, but some also saw the chance to diversify into new market sectors. Armour and Wilson meat-packing (two of Chicago's "Big Five" meat-packers) established their own pharmaceutical subsidiaries, specializing in gland- and other animal-based medicines. (Wilson also created the now-famous sporting goods subsidiary, making the most of its access to cheap leather and gut for balls and racquet strings.) Of the meat-packing pharmaceutical spin-offs, Armour's desiccated thyroid in particular was well regarded by physicians and became the major brand of thyroid preparation used in the United States. The product is still manufactured today, although not by a company associated with the meat-packing branch of Armour. The unofficial motto of the meat-packing industry—a "use for everything but the squeal"—was bringing home the bacon.[17]

Fat children were treated with this extensive range of gland products, from single-gland extracts to "pluriglandular" cocktails. Synthetic thyroid hormone (not extracted from animal glands) was commercially available from the late 1920s. Two physicians, writing in 1937 in the *Journal of the American Medical Association,* reported great successes in treating eight cases of obesity in children with a combination of injected pituitary extract and thyroid tablets. The therapy was a success, said the physicians, because most of the children lost weight *and* their sexual organs began to develop. Another feature that the investigators said was evidence of the gland therapy's effectiveness was that some children's fat depots became more evenly spread over their bodies, rather than localized in one spot, which the authors interpreted as the "endogenous" obesity becoming a simple, "exogenous" one.

Through the 1910s to the 1930s a significant segment of medical practitioners thought obesity in children was due to sluggish or malfunctioning glands and favored treating fat children with gland products—an opinion shared by the general population. By the late 1930s, however, the balance of opinion within academic medicine, and some segments of clinical medicine as well, was shifting away from endocrine explanations and turning against gland-based drugs for children. Physicians questioned whether gland extracts (especially pituitary gland extract, which had not been demonstrated to be effective in the way that thyroid extract had been) were worthwhile. One report noted that "among conservative clinicians there exists a widespread skepticism as to their value." The indiscriminate treatment of multiple glands with "pluriglandular therapy" was also increasingly seen as a dubious practice and merely an excuse for poor diagnosis and medieval drugging practices. "I suggest that the administration of a mixture of the above nature [a pluriglandular cocktail]," wrote one critic, "is as far removed from rational therapy as is the writing out of a charm on a piece of paper and giving that to the patient to swallow." Most of the major pharmaceutical

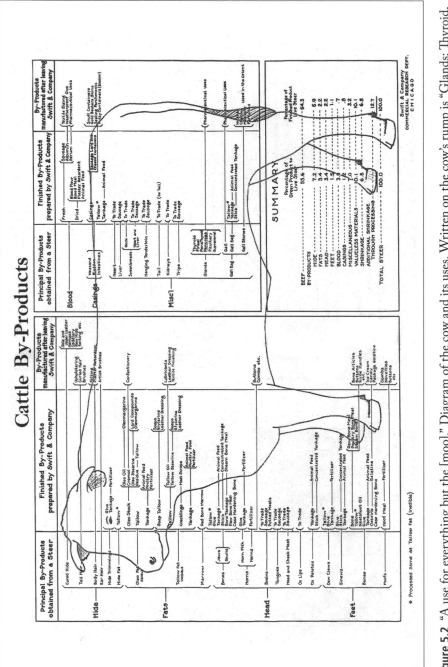

Figure 5.2 "A use for everything but the [moo]." Diagram of the cow and its uses. Written on the cow's rump is "Glands: Thyroid, Pineal, ParaThyroid, Pancreas, Pituitary, Suprarenal—Pharmaceutical uses."

Source: Swift and Company Year Book. Chicago: Swift, 1923, center panel.

houses pulled out of manufacturing gland cocktails, leaving that diminishing segment of the market to the fringe operators.[18]

Furthermore, evidence against the glandular explanation for obesity in childhood was mounting. Studies of fat children's basal metabolic rate (a measure of how much energy a person's body is using for basic maintenance and operations, and therefore used as a measure of gland function) were showing that, contrary to what had been expected, fat children did not have a low metabolic rate. If anything, it was slightly raised. Fat children's glands were working properly. Why, then, was there evidence that gland drugs and especially thyroid treated childhood obesity?[19]

Yes, giving thyroid to fat children did slim them down, but not because the fat children's own thyroid was not working properly. Rather, thyroid worked as a slimming agent because it caused a state of hyperthyroidism and essentially poisoned the child. "In our experience," said authors of one paper on childhood obesity,

> thyroid therapy has usually caused toxic symptoms in obese children and has rarely been beneficial. There is no good evidence that thyroid deficiency is present in obese children unless its clinical signs and symptoms accompany the obesity.[20]

In most cases of obesity, then, thyroid was not a *causal* treatment, but a *symptomatic* one. Although adult slimming remedies continued to contain thyroid for some decades after this insight, giving thyroid to children for weight loss was seen as improper. Adults might be allowed to take a "diet pill," but children were not. The fact that thyroid was not (in most cases) treating an organic disturbance made such remedies seem inappropriate for children.

Physicians had also become much more wary and distrustful of what their child patients (or their patients' parents) reported to them. They were less likely to accept wide-eyed assurances that a fat child "hardly ate anything at all." One physician recounted a story of a very obese high school girl called Selma who had told him "that she never ate breakfast or lunch and that her evening meal consisted only of a small piece of fish, tomato salad, apple sauce and a glass of milk." Her obesity was therefore diagnosed as gland based. But when a dietician gained her confidence, she revealed that she ate oatmeal or cornflakes for breakfast with scrambled or fried eggs, oranges, bananas, and devil's food cake or butter cake, sugar biscuits, fresh bread rolls, and milk. She had nothing for lunch but candy and then had milk and strudel when she got home. Dinner was "chicken soup with rice or barley; gefilte fish cooked with carrots and celery; mashed potatoes; lettuce and tomatoes; bread with butter (three slices); apple sauce, a glass of milk, apple strudel, devilsfood or butter cake, and rice pudding." Her doctor thus concluded, "There is no specific metabolic abnormality in obesity."[21]

The common diagnosis of Fröhlich's syndrome for fat boys was also coming under fire as being used indiscriminately and for cases that did not match the original symptom complex that Fröhlich had described. It wasn't that a fat boy had small sex organs: rather, his sporran of stomach fat was hiding his genitals, making the boy seem less sexually developed than he was. That organotherapy seemed to initiate puberty was simply a happy coincidence:

> The sweeping claims of the remarkable effects of glandular injections on the pubertal development of obese children say actually no more than that puberty takes place, an event which will occur just as impressively if the patients are not subjected to long-continued, and exceedingly expensive, glandular treatment.[22]

The glandular explanation of the cause of obesity in childhood was defunct in academic circles by about 1945. Obesity in children was by then sufficiently common that it seemed unlikely that so many children could have bad glands; fat children had normal metabolic rates and sexually matured on time or even earlier than thin children; and thyroid treatment thinned a child not because his or her thyroid wasn't working but because the extra thyroid hormones poisoned the child. While certain glandular disorders were known to cause obesity, these were rare cases. In popular opinion, however, the gland explanation continued to be common well into the 1960s. Ask adults in their fifties or sixties today, and they will remember that when they were young, Husky John or Chubby Jane was suffering from a "gland problem."

———

This episode in the history of childhood obesity and the fact that the gland explanation continued to be popular long after academic medicine had turned against it shows that the idea that obesity is caused by a biological failing has long been highly appealing to patients. Medical historians have observed that biological and drug-treatable conditions are (usually, but not always) exempt from the moral stigma—the patient-blaming—of lifestyle-related diseases. Taking a drug to correct a condition also seems more convenient, and, with the notable successes of modern drugs in the twentieth century, more reliable than other, less scientific-seeming responses. In the case of treating fat children with drugs, it is likely to be much easier to give a child a pill than it is to change the child's or the family's behavior.[23]

But the case of organotherapy for childhood obesity shows that not only are the patients or their parents sometimes enthusiastic about drugging, but so too are many physicians. This is a more rounded view of the doctor-patient relationship when it comes to making treatment choices: doctors have been as keen and hopeful to take action and offer their patients a solution as the patients have been to receive it. Childhood obesity has been no exception to this pattern. Doctors, patients, and drug manufacturers alike have long been enthusiastic about the prospect of a pill for childhood obesity. The endocrine vogue of the 1920s to the 1940s was but the first of an ongoing attraction with that alluring possibility.

CHAPTER 6

The Enduring Promise
The Continued Search for a Pharmaceutical Remedy

> When it is considered desirable to reduce the child's weight, a low-calorie dietary régime may be supported by the administration of small doses of dextro-amphetamine sulphate with complete safety.
>
> Medical textbook *Amphetamine in Clinical Medicine*, 1955

Organotherapy or gland treatment for childhood obesity, popular from the 1920s through to the 1940s, was just the first episode in an ongoing courtship with potential drug treatments for fatness in childhood. Its *rise* was buoyed by the bubble of enthusiasm for things endocrine and supported by a theoretical model of childhood obesity that ascribed the condition to failure of various glands. Its *fall* was due to that model breaking down and the realization that the apparently successful thyroid treatment was, in fact, poisoning children to make them thin, rather than dealing with any root cause of their fatness. Its *persistence* in the popular mind and in suburban doctors' offices for twenty years beyond its demise within academic medicine showed the powerful allure of a drug treatment, for both patients and physicians, and the convenience of drugs within modern medical practice with its short appointment times.

Over the course of the twentieth century, new elements have been added to explain what causes childhood obesity, and some of those elements have offered potential drug treatment options. The highs and lows in such drug treatments illustrate the complexities of developing responses to childhood health conditions. Our decision to give a child a pill or to hold off from doing so is backed by an intricate support structure of beliefs—beliefs about the nature of the medical condition to be treated, the nature of childhood, the practicable aspects of drug therapy—as well as the matter of the drug's effectiveness. Those considerations are well illustrated in the case of one drug used to treat obesity—a drug that has had a roller-coaster history from modern marvel to problem narcotic.

100

When amphetamine was first developed for clinical uses in the 1930s, the drug was heralded as one of the good (that is, demonstrably effective) modern medicines. The pharmaceutical company Smith, Kline and French introduced their Benzedrine inhaler (amphetamine in a volatile form) in 1934 to be used as a nasal decongestant. Subsequent investigations of the drug showed that it, and its sulfate, had a number of physiological effects that could be therapeutically useful—or potentially dangerous: it raised heart rate and blood pressure, it promoted a feeling of well-being, it made a person wakeful, it constricted blood vessels when applied topically, and the effects lasted a comparatively long time after taking the drug. The wide range of these effects suggested that the drug was acting both on the central nervous system (the brain and spinal nerves) and peripherally in different parts of the body. Its earliest uses were in the treatment of symptoms of narcolepsy, fatigue, and depression, conditions where its ability to convey wakefulness, uplift the spirits, and give "pep" seemed very useful, at least in the short term.[1]

Amphetamine's association with obesity started when, in one 1937 study of the effects of Benzedrine on exhaustion, the investigator noted a further "rather striking physical and mental reaction": one-quarter of the patients being given the drug lost weight. "The loss of weight," speculated the researcher, "can probably be explained by the lessened appetite and increased physical activity" that the patients felt the drug caused. The following year, physician Abraham Myerson and his research associate Mark Lesses at the Boston State Hospital carried out a study specifically to test the potential use of Benzedrine in treating obesity. They thought the drug produced results: used in conjunction with a low-calorie diet, the drug helped the seventeen trial patients lose one to two pounds a week—not a spectacular rate of weight loss, but a solid one. (A modern interpretation of these results would be less positive about the drug than Myerson and Lesses were—diet alone could achieve a similar, moderate rate of weight loss in the short term.) Nevertheless, word about the new drug began to circulate in the popular press. Benzedrine started to accrue a reputation for giving a person "lift," for helping to treat alcoholism (wives were, however, cautioned not to slip it in their husband's coffee, however tempting this might be), and, because of Myerson and Lesses' work, as a weight-loss aid.[2]

For the next two decades, the number of amphetamine-derived and related drugs marketed for weight-loss purposes steadily increased. Amphetamine and its sulfate (Benzedrine and Benzedrine Sulfate) were joined by chemical variants: dextroamphetamine (trade named Dexedrine), methamphetamine (trade named Desoxyn, Methedrine), phenmetrazine (Preludin), phentermine (Fastin, Ionamin), benzphetamine (Didrex), and fenfluramine (Ponimin). Each new product was a slight pharmacological tweak of the basic chemical to produce a patentable—and therefore lucrative—new drug for the pharmaceutical companies manufacturing the drugs.[3]

Using amphetamine to treat obesity in childhood followed closely on its application to obesity in adults. In spite of the American Medical Association (AMA) cautioning in 1938 against using amphetamines as an obesity treatment without better understanding of the drug's effects, from the 1940s to the 1960s a number of American and European researchers conducted studies of amphetamine treatment for childhood obesity. All the studies found that amphetamines did in fact produce weight loss and seemed to achieve this by their anorexigenic (appetite suppressant) effect. In one instance, children on the drug lost one pound a week while the control group on placebo gained about a pound. All studies reported that the children taking the drugs experienced very few, if any, side effects: "so slight and transitory as to be negligible," described a team of Danish childhood obesity specialists. However, all the researchers also noted that the *first* treatment a fat child received—whether it was diet, amphetamines, or a placebo pill—was always the most effective. The children "eagerly confirm[ed] the fact that the pills had helped to curtail their craving for food" for both placebo and amphetamine alike. The first flush of attention and hope helped the children lose weight regardless of the specific treatment they were receiving, and, since the studies were all of short duration (the longest was just five months) the studies were really insufficient to tell whether amphetamines would work in the long term once novelty and anticipation had worn off.[4]

Although none of the experiments provided rousing evidence for amphetamines as an effective treatment, amphetamine sulfate did become a part of the standard therapeutic armamentarium for treating childhood obesity in the 1950s and, to a lesser extent, the 1960s. These years were the high-water mark of prescribing amphetamines to obese children. The drug was used in conjunction with a reducing diet and was usually recommended for short periods of time, to help children adopt their newly reduced eating habits. As one medical textbook of the mid-century counseled, when a child needed to

lose weight "a low-calorie dietary régime may be supported by the administration of small doses of dextro-amphetamine sulphate with complete
safety."[5] The dosage used could vary widely, between 2.5 milligrams of
amphetamine per day up to 32.5 milligrams per day. (Adults' doses recommended in the AMA's *New and Non-Official Remedies* handbook were
between 15 to 30 milligrams per day, which also recommended that "in no
instance should it exceed 30mg daily." In practice, both adult and child dosages could—and did—exceed the recommended maximum.) Child dosages
were determined by being set at about half the adult dose.[6]

How was this new "wonder drug" meant to help someone lose weight?
Amphetamine's advocates speculated that amphetamine might have a
number of different actions, inferred from physiological effects that could be
measured or observed and from patients' own reports of what they felt. One
theory was that the drug produced a "marked loss of appetite" by acting on
some "hunger center" in the brain. Animal studies showed the remarkable
fact that, given a high enough dose of amphetamine, a dog would starve to
death rather than eat—apparently because its "hunger center" had been
completely shut down by the drug.[7]

A second theory held that the changed appetite wasn't due to physical
changes but mental ones. What the drug was really doing (so the theory
went) was affecting a person's mood. Myerson, who had carried out the first
studies of Benzedrine and obesity in the 1930s, theorized that obese people
suffered from a depressive condition called *anhedonia*. Unable to find joy in
life, the person simply ate, and ate, and ate—"a restless seeking for stimula-
tion in order to secure the longed-for satisfaction"—with the result that he
or she became obese. Myerson's position was that amphetamines treated the
obese person's anhedonia, restoring his appreciation of life's nongustatory
pleasures. Amphetamines worked as weight-loss pills, according to this
theory, because they made one happy. On amphetamines, pleasure didn't
have to be found on a plate.[8]

A third theory also posited that the drug worked through mood effects
but in a completely different way from Myerson's anhedonia idea. It wasn't
that obese people *couldn't* find any joy or satisfaction in life—lack of bon-
homie was not the problem. The trouble was that they couldn't steel themselves to endure hunger or temptation. Amphetamines made a person
wakeful, energetic, highly motivated, and active—they helped a person
endure, and that included enduring dieting. Indeed, amphetamine-derived

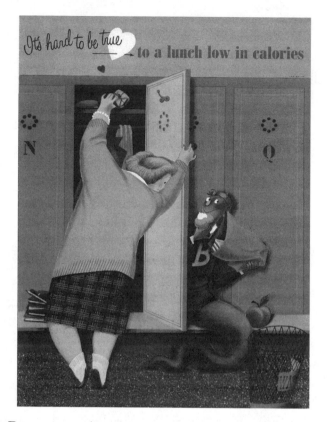

Figure 6.1 Desoxyn, a methamphetamine marketed to teenage girls wanting to lose weight, as in this 1951 advertisement. Note the girl in the advertisement is opening locker "O"—perhaps "O" for "obesity" or "overweight."

Source: Abbott Laboratories. "It's Hard to Be True to a Lunch Low in Calories . . . When Her Heart Belongs to Dagwoods." "Advertisement for Desoxyn (Methamphetamine Hydrochloride) Weight Loss Pills." In *Papers of Hilde Bruch.* Houston: Texas Medical Center Archive, 1951, inside panel.

weight-loss pills become popularly known during the 1950s as "diet pills." Amphetamines, wrote one New York health journalist and doctor, "give the person—at least for the time being—a sense of power and the desire to take on" the calories. Amphetamines worked as diet pills, said this theory, because they gave one backbone.[9]

In addition to the possible appetite and mood effects of amphetamines, some clinicians and researchers felt there were particular aspects of amphetamine treatment that made it especially suitable for children. The idea was that amphetamines could, to a certain extent, make up for social and familial failures that were considered to have contributed to the child becoming obese in the first place. Drugs could be a way for fat children from a poor family or with incompetent parents to lose weight. For example, John Lorber, a British physician who conducted a series of trials into the use of amphetamines compared with dietary treatment of childhood obesity, concluded that while diet was the most appropriate treatment for children, some child patients needed additional pharmaceutical support. "There are," he wrote, "many children who are so grossly overweight and under such poor parental control, that to expect sustained good results from advice and dietary treatment alone is unrealistic."[10]

Successful dieting, Lorber argued, required the "full enthusiastic support" of the parents. If the parents were insufficiently engaged with or concerned about their child's health, the drugs could help ameliorate this poor parenting. Amphetamines "treated" a fat child's less than ideal family environment. Similarly, the authors of a study conducted with poor inner-city Chicago adolescents in 1967 concluded that drug treatment of obesity could be useful for poor, fat children:

> Adolescents in a low socio-economic population, when frustrated by deprivation of poverty and further disturbed emotionally by the problems of obesity, seem more prone to avail themselves of between-meal snacking . . . This double-blind study has shown that an anorectic drug can be helpful in the management of obesity in underprivileged children.[11]

By making dieting easier and lessening the need for parents to take a role in the child's well-being, amphetamines were seen as a way to treat poverty-induced childhood obesity.

Lorber's study and the Chicago youth study showed that, by the later 1960s, enthusiasm about amphetamine treatment for childhood obesity was tempered. There was a growing sense that amphetamines were not an ideal response to the condition—that diet was more appropriate and drugs should only be used in the short term and only in very severe cases of obesity, or in patients whose parents wouldn't support their dieting. Physicians suggested amphetamine treatment for childhood obesity only with considerable qualifications. The peak of interest in prescribing amphetamines for child weight loss in the 1950s and early 1960s had passed. The next few decades saw a further chilling of opinion regarding the usefulness of drugging children to treat their fatness.

This turn against diet drugs for children was partly a symptom of a wider backlash against diet pills in general in the 1960s and 1970s. Contributing to the waning fortunes of amphetamine treatment were several studies, in both children and adults, that had found that amphetamines became ineffective for weight loss after only a short period of use, sometimes as little as a few weeks. Moreover, although some researchers in the 1930s and 1940s had warned that the drug was addictive, most researchers displayed a breezy confidence that amphetamines had negligible side effects and were not habit-forming: "There are no reports in the literature to suggest that use of Benzedrine leads to formation of a habit" was the opinion of one researcher in the late 1930s. But in the 1960s and especially in the 1970s, this feeling was giving way to a sense that the drug was indeed addictive. Further investigations into amphetamines found that a person who had been taking them could experience withdrawal symptoms—anxiety, agitation, depression, or tiredness—when he or she stopped the drug.[12]

After the Kefauver-Harris Amendment to the Food, Drug and Cosmetic Act was passed in 1962, the Food and Drug Administration (FDA) required diet pill manufacturers to demonstrate that they had more rigorous evidence of the effectiveness of their products. Based on this new data, the FDA concluded in 1972 that amphetamine-based diet drugs were effective, but that they were also addictive. Increased controls and labeling requirements further dulled enthusiasm for the drugs. And Aminorex, an American-manufactured weight-loss drug, was withdrawn from sale in 1968 when it was discovered to significantly increase the risk of a person developing primary pulmonary hypertension, a very serious lung disease. *Life* magazine devoted its January edition in 1968 to "the dangerous diet pills." That same year, the AMA entered the fray with an editorial suggesting that weight-loss drugs were "blandishments" used by "those who promote allegedly quick, simple weight reduction" to sway "obese patients weary of the prolonged effort necessary to readjust to a sensible dietary way of life." Amphetamines were still sometimes prescribed to overweight children, but by the late 1960s, their sheen as effective, safe drugs had worn off.[13]

By the early 1970s, the mainstream medical position on prescribing diet pills to children became even more hostile. Diet pills, wrote one physician in a book of weight-loss advice for children, "are *dangerous* and contraindicated in children. Besides, they don't work." In the same year that President Nixon declared the "war on drugs," the American Academy of Pediatrics (AAP) instructed its Committee on Drugs to conduct a review of the medical indications for the use of amphetamines in children. The committee recommended that amphetamines could be useful for narcolepsy and hyperactivity, but that there was no evidence that the drugs had anything more than a "generally evanescent" effect on childhood obesity. Pediatricians, the committee maintained, had had "unduly optimistic expectations of therapeutic responses [to amphetamines] for . . . the overweight child." The committee was also wary of how this prescribing practice might relate to the growing drug problem in the United States. The AAP concluded: "Pediatricians must reflect on their role in introducing patients to these agents; they must not unwittingly contribute to the current problem of overuse, misuse, and abuse [of drugs]." The AMA followed suit. Reversing its position of thirty years earlier, the AMA was, from 1973, against amphetamine treatment for childhood obesity.[14]

Physicians who continued to prescribe amphetamine diet pills to children—and some did in spite of the AAP and AMA's recommendations to the contrary—were regarded as dangerously on the fringe of practice. "If you want to send a roomful of doctors into orbit, just mention giving diet pills to teen-agers," wrote Dr. Barbara Edelstein, the author of a best-selling diet book for adults in her companion book on teen dieting. Dr. Edelstein was one of the few remaining pro-diet pill physicians in the 1980s. "It's too bad," that doctors had turned against prescribing amphetamines to children for weight loss, she wrote,

> because I feel they have a definite place in the treatment of obesity in well-selected, well-motivated patients who must bring their daily calorie requirement down to hardship levels (below 1,000 calories) for very long periods of time.[15]

Edelstein suggested that if teens couldn't persuade their physicians to prescribe them weight-loss drugs, then they could take over-the-counter antihistamine and cold medication containing the amphetamine-related drug propanolamine. She noted that, "unfortunately" for teens who might want to try her rather troubling recommendation, there were indications that the drug might soon be banned. She was right—eventually. The FDA issued a public health advisory against propanolamine in 2000 because of its effect in increasing the risk of stroke—even in young people—and asked drug manufacturers to remove the ingredient from their products. In 2005, the FDA started taking steps to have the drug banned as an over-the-counter medication. Edelstein's support for amphetamines in the 1980s was not, therefore, the only aspect of her weight-loss prescription that was medically worrying.[16]

Although amphetamine-derived diet pills continued to be sold for adults, by the later 1970s and into the 1980s the use of diet pills for weight loss in children was generally considered deeply unsuitable. This was a considerable change of heart from the height of amphetamine treatment in the 1950s and 1960s. Why such a change? In part this was due to the growing dominance of the diet-and-exercise theory of childhood obesity from the 1960s onward (see Chapters 8 and 9), and a decline in the idea that childhood obesity had some drug-treatable biological basis.[17]

But also the climate of attitudes about prescribing drugs to children had changed considerably—a concern that continues to this day. Especially since the 1960s, with the rising incidence of drug abuse, people in both medical and lay circles have become more worried about medicating children. Do the possible effects of the drug outweigh the dangers of the condition? Does pill-giving initiate children into a culture of drug use? Is there really a physical problem to be fixed, or should blame lie with the child's or parent's behavior? Does medicating "send the right message" to the child that a drug can solve his or her problems? Will a pill treat the underlying cause or just fix a symptom? Since the 1960s, physicians and parents have been more likely to consider and weigh these ethical and practical aspects when it comes to treating a child with drugs. This has considerable implications for any possible future drug treatments of childhood obesity.

Can and should a fat child be given a drug for his or her obesity? A key determinant in this history of drug treatments for childhood obesity has been changes in the thinking about what caused the condition. When obesity in a child was interpreted as a sign of physical dysfunction, as in the glandular explanation, drugging to correct that dysfunction was considered appropriate. But when the prevailing opinion about the causes of childhood obesity shifted to emphasize emotions, behavior, or environmental causes (as was the case in the 1960s), drug treatments for childhood obesity became viewed as purely symptomatic—a Band-Aid measure that didn't get to the heart of the matter. From this perspective, drugging a fat child becomes regarded as inappropriate and incompatible with the idea of childhood as a time for character development through personal effort and engaged parenting. Drugs are then seen as the "easy option" and as supplanting proper parenting. The *appropriateness* of drugging children, and *parents'* role in their child's condition, are two closely intertwined historical themes in this part of the story of childhood obesity.[18]

The past gland-based and amphetamine drug treatments for obesity were both products of times of great enthusiasm for certain medical developments. The current search for a future drug treatment for obesity is no different, being part of that most dominant discipline in contemporary medical research: genetics. Indeed, one of the most talked-about developments in obesity genetics in the last few decades has been connected to finding an answer to some of physiology's big questions: what makes people feel hungry and what makes them stop eating? How much of one's body shape is determined by genes, and how much by environment? How does a person's body "know" when to store fat and when to metabolize it?

By the 1940s, results from animal experiments suggested that there was some sort of "hunger center" located in the brain, specifically in the hypothalamus (a small area located deep in the middle of the brain, just above the brain stem, neighboring the pituitary gland). This "hunger center" would delicately orchestrate feeding, fat storage, and energy mobilization, keeping the animal's weight within a fairly narrow range of variation, and maintaining a regular supply of energy for the animal's cells so that it could continue to function and respond to its environment. (The finely regulated equilibrium that most healthy people's bodies maintain in their internal metabolic processes, including appetite regulation and energy metabolism, was called *homeostasis* by American physiologist Walter Cannon in 1912.) How did the "hunger center," the hypothalamus, "know" what state the animal's body was in and whether, say, it should metabolize fat stores or add to them? The theory was that the hunger center received updates from other parts of the body as to its energy needs, but what was the nature of the signal that the hypothalamus received? By the 1950s, physiologists had suggested two possible candidates that fit the requirements for the signal: blood sugar content (the "glucostatic theory") and some sort of signal sent by the body's fat stores ("lipostatic theory").[19]

And there things remained—glucostatic theory or lipostatic theory?—

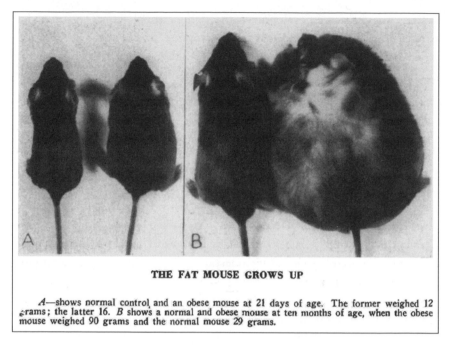

THE FAT MOUSE GROWS UP

A—shows normal control and an obese mouse at 21 days of age. The former weighed 12 grams; the latter 16. *B* shows a normal and obese mouse at ten months of age, when the obese mouse weighed 90 grams and the normal mouse 29 grams.

Figure 6.2 Photographs from the original paper announcing the discovery of the *ob/ob* mouse.

Source: Ingalls, A. M., M. M. Dickie, and G. D. Snell. "Obese, a New Mutation in the House Mouse." *Journal of Heredity* 41, no. 12 (1950): 317–318, 317. By permission of Oxford University Press on behalf of the American Genetic Association.

until 1991 when a team of geneticists led by Jeffrey Friedman at the Howard Hughes Medical Institute at the Rockefeller University (New York) reported on their work with a particular type of genetically obese mouse. The *ob/ob* mouse had been discovered back in 1949 when a worker at a laboratory mouse-breeding facility noticed "some very plump young mice . . . in the V [breeding] stock." The mice were recognizably obese from four to six weeks of age, and, the ensuing report observed, "at that time they appear to have a slightly shorter body, are rather square and have expansive hind quarters." The mice would eat constantly, almost never stopping, and continued to gain weight until they were between three to five times a normal mouse's weight. They were so obese that they looked like furry softballs with tails. Subsequent experiments breeding the fat mice suggested that the obesity was likely due to the mouse having two copies of a recessive genetic mutation. The mouse breeders gave the genetic mutation the name *ob*, standing for *obese*, so the fat mouse with two recessive copies of the gene was designated the *ob/ob* mouse.[20]

With modern genetic mapping tools, Friedman's team in 1991 located the *ob* gene on the sixth mouse chromosome and also found that other vertebrates seemed to have homologue (that is, similarly functioning) genes. Friedman's team showed that in normal mice the *ob* gene coded for making a protein. Since the gene was expressed in fat cells, this suggested the *ob* protein was made in the animal's fat stores. "Our results," wrote Friedman and his team, "particularly the evidence that the *ob* protein is secreted, suggested that *ob* may encode [the] circulating factor" that regulates energy homeostasis.[21]

Friedman was suggesting that the lipostatic theory was correct: fat secreted the *ob* gene's protein and that protein signaled the hypothalamus to regulate eating and fat storage. Unable to manufacture the *ob* protein because of its genetic mutation, the *ob/ob* mouse's body was unable to signal its hypothalamus that it had enough stored fat and could stop eating. The team proposed that the *ob* protein be called "leptin," derived from the Greek *leptos*, meaning thin.

Leptin seemed to hold enormous promise. When *ob/ob* mice were injected with the missing protein, they slimmed down dramatically. The added leptin had signaled to the hypothalamus that fat stores were sufficient and that the mouse could stop eating. Maybe obese humans carried a genetic mutation, homologous to the *ob* gene in the fat mice. Maybe obesity in humans was also due to their bodies not producing leptin, or enough leptin, to correctly regulate eating and fat storage. Perhaps leptin could be the wonder drug for obesity that gland-based drugs and amphetamines had not been?[22]

Certainly, pharmaceutical companies were willing to wager on that promise. A number of biotech companies bid for the rights to make drugs from Friedman and his team's discovery. The average cost of rights to drug research developed in university laboratories is usually around $30,000. Such was the enthusiasm about leptin's potential as an obesity drug that in 1995 the winning bidder, a Californian biotech company called Amgen, offered $20 million up front with unspecified "milestone payments" to follow.[23]

However, mice are not men, and in particular, *ob/ob* mice are not obese humans. Although the mouse *ob* gene does have a human homologue, further investigation showed that by far the vast majority of obese people did not have a mutation in their *ob* gene. Fat people with *ob* gene mutations are, in fact, incredibly rare. The first humans to be identified as having *ob* gene–related obesity were two children who were cousins and whose parents were also cousins; that is, the family was "highly consanguineous," or, less politely, inbred. (Over the next few years, a handful more cases were identified, all in closely interrelated families.) Obesity in humans attributable to *ob* gene mutation therefore seemed to be extremely rare. (Indeed, although research has discovered more genes like *ob* that cause obesity, these single-gene mutations appear to account for a tiny minority of cases of obesity in humans.) So would leptin still work as an obesity drug?[24]

Further studies showed that mice made fat by their diet (a so-called "supermarket" or "cafeteria" diet that mimics the sort of high-fat, high-sugar diet on offer in the processed-foods areas of supermarkets) *could* be slimmed by injecting them with leptin. And normal-sized mice could even become skinny when injected with leptin. These results suggested that leptin would still work as an antiobesity drug even when an *ob* mutation wasn't the cause of the obesity. Leptin appeared not only to cut appetite but also to increase metabolic activity. The results kept the promise of leptin as an anti-obesity drug alive.[25]

But not for long. Endocrinologist Robert Considine and his research team in Philadelphia showed in 1996 that not only was obesity in humans generally not a consequence of an *ob* gene mutation, but that "serum leptin concentrations [in obese people's blood] are correlated with the percentage of body fat, suggesting that most obese persons are insensitive to endogenous leptin production." In other words, most obese people were *resistant* to leptin. The fat in an obese human's body was correctly signaling the hypothalamus by secreting leptin, but for some reason their body failed to respond properly to the leptin signal. The implication was that treating an obese person with *more* leptin would probably not work.[26]

When the first clinical trials of Amgen's $20 million hope were carried out, the results were, perhaps predictably, disappointing. On average, the human test subjects did lose weight, but the average amount they lost was small. Amgen damned the results with faint praise, characterizing their subjects' weight loss as "fairly moderate." The subjects also found it difficult to keep going with the leptin injections because the injection site became painful and irritated. (Leptin, being a protein, cannot be made into a tablet because it would simply be digested—broken down into amino acids.)[27]

Friedman reviewed the unhappy outcome of the clinical trials in a sanguine light:

> Whether leptin finds its way into general usage as an anti-obesity drug,
> [which was looking increasingly unlikely] the use of modern methods to
> identify and target the component of the leptin signaling pathway will
> form the basis for new pharmacological approaches to the treatment of
> obesity and other nutritional disorders.[28]

And indeed, this does seem to have been the case. The major contributions
of the *ob/ob* mouse and other animal models of obesity to date have not been
in leptin-based drug development, much as that has been desired. A brief
reprisal of hopes that leptin might work in combination with other signaling
hormones also seems to have been abandoned. Given the rarity of obesity in
humans resulting from single-gene mutations (at most recent report, only
176 cases of single-gene obesity have been identified in humans, corresponding to mutations in one of eleven genes), leptin-based therapy itself
appears then to have reached a dead end. Rather, it is the *implications* of the
leptin research—the insights into the body's signaling mechanisms and
pathways, homeostatic control, and the influence of behavior on these
mechanisms—that now hold the most promise. Genetic studies of obesity
suggest that the majority of cases of obesity are likely to be due to combinations of genes that make certain people more susceptible to fatness, given an
encouraging environment.[29]

For researchers and pharmaceutical companies hoping to find an antiobesity drug that will target some physical failing of the body that is causing the
obesity, findings from animal experiments are both exciting and depressing.
On the upside for drug prospects, mouse experiments show that the homeostatic signaling system involves multiple hormones of which leptin is just
one, albeit a very important one. Each hormone link in the signaling chain
might fail, and in failing cause obesity. So each one of these hormones could
potentially be an antiobesity drug—as, indeed, could be finding drugs that
could restore leptin sensitivity. The sheer complexity of the signaling system
offers many possible targets for drug interventions.[30]

However, on the downside, animal experiments have also shown that
there are fallback circuits or redundant pathways in the hormone signaling
system and that hormones work in concert with each other, which complicates

matters. Possibly only a combination of hormones might work, but it might be difficult to obtain FDA approval for such a treatment, since the FDA requires that each component of a drug cocktail should be at least partially effective in its own right.[31] The other issue is (as has been found with leptin) that simply increasing the amount of the hormone in a person's blood may not work either, especially if the person has become resistant to its effects. The question then becomes: how does one become resistant to a hormone? Research within the past decade has suggested that a person's overeating leads him or her to become leptin resistant. What the genetic research has done is—ironically—emphasize the role of behavior.[32]

As favorable as the mouse evidence seemed to be for leptin to become the new, rational drug for treating childhood obesity, "the best laid schemes o' mice an' men, gang aft agley." Disappointed with the results of clinical trials for leptin, Amgen sold its rights to the technology for an undisclosed sum in 2006. The buyer, Amylin Pharmaceutical Company, after its own disappointing experience with leptin-related drugs, has decided to "explore [the] potential of other assets to address [the] obesity epidemic." But the medical profession is still cautiously sanguine that some sort of drug—perhaps not leptin itself, but some other class of drugs that the leptin research and genetics of obesity help guide—will be developed that could treat obesity in adults and in children. Drugging optimism continues to spring eternal.[33]

CHAPTER 7

Feeling Fat

Emotions and Family as Factors in Childhood Obesity

I ate Grammy's fried chicken and Grammy's cobbler because they tasted good and because I was trying to fill up the grave my father and mother had dug for me.

"Fat girl" Judith Moore, 2005

By 1930, the endocrine theory of childhood obesity was fast unraveling. There was a growing and somewhat sheepish sense in pediatric research circles that, as one pediatrician described, "when all is said on the score of the endocrine glands, it leaves one with the impression that their role in the production of obesity has been astonishingly overestimated." Cases of childhood obesity that could be definitively attributed to underperforming glands were the small, rare minority. Once those rare endocrine cases had been identified, researchers looking at obesity in childhood were still left with what one researcher described as "this huge group of fat children" for whom glands, it seemed, were not the answer.[1]

The 1940s, in fact, saw a general turning away from biological approaches to childhood obesity, at least in medical circles. Researchers and clinicians increasingly inclined toward the idea that there was nothing *organically* wrong with fat children's bodies. Instead, new theories that suggested the condition was due to *behavior, emotions,* and the influence of *family* became popular. And that meant that childhood obesity could also come under the umbrellas of psychology and sociology, rather than just medicine. Not only were there new explanations for the condition but also new specialties offering insights and treatments.

The two behemoths of American psychology—Freudianism (psychoanalysis) and behaviorism—both entered the picture of childhood obesity in the middle decades of the twentieth century and contributed new elements to the increasingly multifactorial nature of the condition. In neither case, however, was childhood obesity originally a core concern or application of that psychological perspective. Neither Sigmund Freud nor John Watson and Burrhus Skinner—the respective founders and figureheads of these psychological ideologies—concerned themselves or their theories with fat children. Rather, it was the acolytes, the adherents and followers of these approaches, working in hospitals and clinics, who sought to apply Freudian and behaviorist insights to childhood obesity, and who sometimes wandered far from the theoretical origins of their discipline in doing so.

An émigré physician, Hilde Bruch, working at the Babies Hospital in New York, began to apply psychological insights to childhood obesity in the 1940s. Bruch was first a pediatrician—not a psychologist—and only later trained in psychoanalysis. Running a clinic for fat children at the Babies Hospital, Bruch gathered data showing that the glandular explanation of childhood obesity was, in most cases, incorrect. Hers was one of the most sustained and systematic attacks on the glandular theory and was a significant contribution to its decline. Instead of glands, Bruch suggested a new, psychological interpretation of what made children fat. Her earliest theories about what caused obesity in childhood were Freudian, involving the particular dynamic of the mother-child connection and the emotional symbolism and function of food in that relationship.

The Freudian particulars of Bruch's theories and treatment of childhood obesity were not widely adopted by mainstream medicine, but where her work was influential was in the broader insights she brought to the condition. Families—and mothers, especially—could play a role in childhood obesity. Emotions, social dynamics, and behavior were important. This brought a new and growing complexity to the understanding of childhood obesity: biology would be joined with mind and behavior.

———————

After spending her early life and professional career in pediatrics in Germany, Hilde Bruch came to the United States in 1934 to escape Nazi persecution. On the boat to the United States, she was fortunate to strike up a friendship with a doctor who helped her secure a position at the Babies Hospital in New York, running a pediatric endocrine clinic. The clinic was an outpatient service that saw children from the local area—mostly the children of immigrants—who were brought to the hospital or referred by school nurses for supposed "glandular problems." The most conspicuous symptom that many of these child patients displayed was that they were fat.[2]

It was, however, apparent to Bruch from her measurements of the fat children's metabolic rates that glands were usually not the problem. What was?[3]

Bruch felt that there were certain features about the families of the fat children she was seeing that were striking and odd. Most especially, the way the mothers behaved toward their child struck her as strange:

> In the pediatric department the examining rooms are very small. Here would be the examining table and here would be a little table—your desk and here would be a chair. And the common procedure is the mother sits down in the chair next to the desk while the child either stands or leans against the bench, the table or sits up on it. With fat children, invariably, the child sat on mother's chair . . . [W]hen I noticed this mother says it is all right let him sit and that the mothers were overprotective and subservient to their children. [T]hey dressed and undressed them and I recorded that that can't be the glands.[4]

Bruch hypothesized that this unusual family interaction—overprotective mothers who cosseted their fat children—might be associated with the child's obesity. The family environment of the child therefore warranted further investigation. She was familiar with Freudianism and psychoanalysis from her early career in Germany and, having suffered a nervous breakdown shortly after her arrival in the United States, Bruch had sought psychoanalysis as treatment. She was also friendly with a young colleague at the Babies Hospital, Janet Rioch, who was training in psychoanalysis. From chats in the lunchroom at the hospital and accompanying Janet to her psychoanalysis classes, Bruch had learned about both classic Freudian thinking and about how some American psychoanalysts considered certain medical conditions, like asthma and diabetes, to have a psychological cause.[5]

Bruch and a social worker visited the homes of forty of her two-hundred-odd fat children at the endocrine clinic, interviewing the parents and noting how the parents and children interacted. There was, she said, a consistent set of features in fat children's families: what she called the "family frame" of childhood obesity. Fathers were weak or absent. In contrast, the mothers dominated the family environment and were controlling, but, Bruch thought, were ambivalent toward their fat children. Freudian theories, said Bruch, could explain how this "family frame" caused childhood obesity: mothers of fat children hadn't wanted the child and didn't love them, but they felt guilty about this. Incapable of offering authentic love, the mother

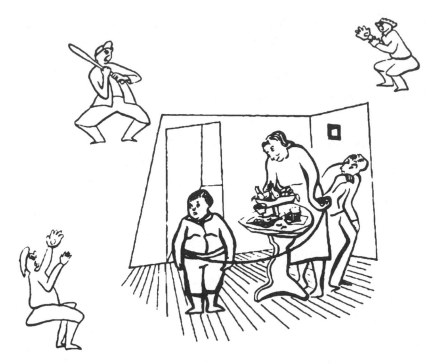

Figure 7.1 A cartoon representation that Bruch used to illustrate her model of the obesity-causing family frame. The father cowers in the background, while the mother ties the fat child to her with offerings of food, keeping him away from playing with his peers.

Source: Bruch, H. "Transformation of Oral Impulses: A Conceptual Approach." *Psychiatric Quarterly* 35, no. 3 (1961): 458–481, 463. With kind permission from Springer Science+Business Media.

instead offered ersatz love: food.[6] "Food had been charged with a high emotional value," wrote Bruch "and stood for love, security and satisfaction and represented in all instances an important tie in the relationship between parents and children." Food stood in for the love that the mother could not give. Denied real love, the child developed a craving for this fake love. Striving for emotional satisfaction and loving recognition the only way he or she could, the child overate—and became fat.[7]

In fact, Bruch's private clinical notes on her interviews show that the family frame that she described was not a consistent picture. Rather, she had selected different features from different children and different families, and combined them. Some mothers interviewed had desperately wanted their children, so it would have been possible, in these cases, to interpret their over-feeding as expressing *a lot* of love for the fat child, not its absence. But instead, Bruch selectively stressed the cases in which the child had been unwanted, choosing instances and examples to assemble her loveless "family frame."[8]

And not only did the family frame shape the child's body; it molded personality as well, said Bruch. Fat children were shy, withdrawn, and lacking in self-reliance and self-confidence. They were the "butt and laughing stock" of their peers, and they were "ashamed" of their bodies and their inability to take part in active play as did slim, less dominated children. Bruch's suggestion that fat children were unhappy and that obesity in children was a troubling social handicap was a striking contrast with majority opinion at that time that fat children were satisfied, contented, and jolly.[9]

Interestingly, Bruch's first attempts to treat childhood obesity made very little effort to address the family frame that was supposedly causing the fatness. She suggested simply putting the children on a diet, curbing some of the starchy or fatty foods traditionally eaten by the ethnic groups she saw at the Babies Hospital clinic. Italians should cut back on "spaghetti and macaroni"; Jews should reduce sour cream; bread, cakes and sweets were out. But gradually Bruch's treatment approach evolved to be more in line with her psychological theory. Dieting a fat child who was made fat by his or her family circumstances, she said, would just be cruelly taking away whatever assurance and love the child gained from food. Dieting alone would produce, in Bruch's terms, a "thin fat person"—someone whose *body* was thin but whose *mind* and personality were still immaturely dependent on his or her mother. Instead, successful therapy needed to have a psychological component as well. The pediatrician had to help her child patient loosen those too-tight maternal apron strings, find new outlets for expression, and try to get the parents to reduce their nagging and let the child mature. Giving the child personal responsibility for dieting might work, but, ventured Bruch, "probably the most important therapeutic tool which the pediatrician has to offer to an obese child is a respectful and understanding approach to his problems." Along with diet, the clinician herself was an important part of the therapy.[10]

Bruch's fat child patients did lose weight under her treatment, whether it was diet, psychological support, or, later, psychoanalytical therapy. But very often, the losses were temporary. While the majority of patients lost weight in the first year or so of therapy, her patients struggled to maintain their weight once they stopped dieting or coming to therapy sessions. In a follow-up study of her patients when they had reached their teens and twenties, Bruch found 40 percent had been able to achieve a normal weight, although more than half of these she considered "maladjusted"—they were "thin fat people" who still struggled with food and maintaining their weight.[11]

Indeed, one of the features of childhood obesity that Bruch thought supported her theory that fatness perversely benefited the fat child and lubricated the dysfunctional family relationship was the great difficulty in treating the condition. Fat children and their families were "notoriously poor" in cooperating with her dietary recommendations. They "loudly bemoaned" the child's fatness but showed a "seeming unwillingness or inability to do something about it." Although she used cruel and condemning language, Bruch interpreted this difficulty and the common failure of dieting as significant in the psychological aspects of obesity—that there were important, protective barriers that made dieting difficult for fat children and their families. The next chapter investigates how other obesity researchers interpreted the frequent failure of dietary treatment in a quite different way.[12]

In the face of criticism of her loveless family portrait, in the 1950s and 1960s Bruch reversed her idea that mothers didn't love their fat children. Rather, she said, parents of fat children treated their child as an object or a doll—*much* prized, *much* loved. But Bruch's failure to find a consistently successful treatment for childhood obesity led her later in her career to reevaluate her family frame idea once more. In the early 1960s, and now having formally trained in psychoanalysis with the famous analyst and schizophrenia expert Frieda Fromm-Reichmann, Bruch believed she saw similarities between the obese patients she was familiar with and the schizophrenic patients that her mentor Fromm-Reichmann dealt with. Both types of patients would often say things like they "did not know how they felt" or that "their body was not their own." Fat patients and schizophrenic patients, Bruch hypothesized, shared a common feature: neither of them had learned to correctly interpret signals from their bodies or from the world and people around them. In particular, fat patients couldn't tell when they felt hungry and when they felt satiated. Bruch felt her older ideas had been on the wrong track: the important question was not what eating or food symbolized for the patient but how someone could fail to understand when their bodies spoke to them.[13]

What caused this deafness to bodily signals? Bruch thought the answer lay in how mothers shaped their children's early experiences and trained them in the proper response. When a baby cries, the mother has to interpret whether this is a cry for food, or a cry for a diaper change, or a cry because of tiredness, and then she has to respond appropriately with feeding, or diaper changing, or putting to bed as needed. In this way, said Bruch, the baby learns to discriminate between the different types of discomforts and associate them with the appropriate response. What went wrong for both schizophrenics and obese patients, Bruch maintained, was that the mothers didn't respond appropriately. The mother of the future fat child would consistently respond to her baby's cries by feeding him—regardless of whether he was hungry or not—so the baby would wrongly learn that eating was the response to all discomforts. Once this wrong learning had happened in infancy it could be continued right through life and the person would eat, eat, eat in response to every discomfort. The wrongly taught baby would become a fat child and then a fat adult.[14]

Bruch's theory was striking—and criticized, especially by classic Freudians—because it suggested that a person had to *learn* to respond appropriately to hunger rather than such behavior being instinctual. Moreover, the idea that hunger could be distorted in such a way as to cause obesity or anorexia was also revolutionary. (Classic Freudian thought held that only the sex drive was capable of being distorted in such a way as to produce profound effects on the body.) When Bruch outlined her new theory to a meeting of the American Psychoanalytic Society in 1962, some members of her audience responded angrily that the paper was incompatible with Freud's views and was dangerously close to that challenger to the psychological crown—behaviorism—with its emphasis on learned habits rather than symbolically expressed emotional conflicts.[15]

Bruch, ever the iconoclast, was undeterred by the reaction and continued to explore the role of learned response in obesity and other eating disorders into the 1970s. Other obesity researchers tested Bruch's theories, trying to find evidence of the family frame or connections with schizophrenia, but without success. This was understandable, given Bruch's habit of picking and choosing certain features of her patients to create a cohesive clinical picture. The details of her theories—the unloving mother, the overloving mother, the schizophrenic connection—none of these became widely accepted ideas about childhood obesity.[16]

But what Bruch's work had done was point out potential new pathways of investigation, new targets of inquiry, and new methods to workers interested in obesity. What role did families play in a child's obesity? How did a child's emotional state figure in his or her fatness? Why did dieting often fail? How were habits and attitudes to eating formed? In particular, Bruch's work opened the door for disciplines beyond medicine—psychology prominent among them—to investigate and treat childhood obesity. Childhood obesity, said Bruch, was about more than metabolism.

––––––––

In the 1960s, two varieties of psychology vied for top spot in treating Americans' neuroses and hang-ups. A Freudian-derived approach, like Bruch's, was one of them, and behaviorism was the other. While Freudian psychoanalysis stressed the role of conscious and unconscious mental processes affecting a person, behaviorism explicitly rejected relying on such unmeasurables. Behaviorism's founder in America, John Broadus Watson, explained his approach in his 1913 manifesto "Psychology as the Behaviorist Views It":

> Psychology as the behaviorist views it is a purely objective experimental branch of natural science. Its theoretical goal is the production and control of behavior. Introspection forms no essential part of its methods, nor is the scientific value of its data dependent upon the readiness with which they lend themselves to interpretation in terms of consciousness.[17]

"Introspection"—such as Bruch's hypothesis about the fat child's relationship with his mother—was out. Measurable, observable *behavior* was in.

Behaviorism is most famous for its early experiments—Ivan Pavlov's demonstration of classical conditioning showing that a dog could be trained or *conditioned* to salivate at the sound of a bell, or John Watson's experiment with baby "Little Albert" conditioning him to be afraid of a white rat. It is also famous for its association with utopian and dystopian visionary worlds: B. F. Skinner's ideal society described in his book in *Walden Two*, or Aldous Huxley's *Brave New World* and Anthony Burgess's *A Clockwork Orange*, dystopic novels in which conditioning is used to control and punish people. Beyond dribbling dogs, rats running mazes, and visionary novels, however, there existed a far bigger world of applying behaviorist ideas to therapy and to social control. Behaviorism was used in mental hospitals to smooth the running of the wards and (arguably) to treat patients' psychoses; it was used in schools to promote learning and manage classroom behavior; and it was used in prisons and youth centers to address delinquency and to prepare inmates for release. Outside of institutions, behaviorist principles were applied to treat a range of supposedly "habit"-related conditions, like homosexuality, phobias, and . . . obesity.[18]

The problem of obesity lent itself well to the behaviorist approach. Behaviorists posited that obesity was caused by eating too much (a behavioral cause), and so the treatment was to get people to reduce their eating (a behavioral treatment). And the condition also provided an in-built, scientific measuring device that was suited to assessing whether the fat person's behavior was changing: their weight.

Several early attempts to use behaviorist ideas for treating obesity in adults used conditioning methods—in this case *aversive conditioning*—to turn people's habits away from eating. The idea was that the person would be punished for thinking about eating and so they would change their associations with eating from pleasurable to undesirable—indeed, painful. In one study, the therapists placed tempting food in front of their obese subjects. When the subject reached for the food, they would be given a "punishing electric shock" of eighty to ninety volts "sufficiently painful to inhibit their immediate behavior." The size of the shock had cruelly been set to "*slightly above the levels tested by the patient as being unpleasant but tolerable.*" The patients lost weight.[19]

In a similar experiment, patients were shown flash cards of words that "symbolically represented" the behavior that they wished to extinguish. For example, the obese patient was shown the word "overeating"; a homosexual patient wanting to be rid of his homosexuality was shown the words "sodomy" and "flapping wrists." Each time an evocative word was shown, the patient was given an electric shock of between 120 to 150 volts delivered "through specially prepared shoes which the subject wears." During each "treatment session," a patient would be shocked sixty times. By her fourth session, one obese patient undergoing this process reported that she was no longer overeating and was stopping the sessions.[20]

Aversive conditioning with its cruelly creative methods of breaking habits was not (reportedly) used on obese children, only adults. The studies found that, as with other weight-loss treatments, subjects lost weight in the short term but gradually reverted to their original weight in the months following the end of treatment.

In the 1970s, however, a different offshoot of behaviorist approaches was tried for treating obesity in children. Called *behavioral modification therapy* (also *experimental analysis of behavior*), the therapeutic strategy involved not only changing a person's behavior but also changing the environmental triggers or antecedents that sparked the behavior in the first place. Again the therapy, when applied to obesity, used control of eating as the therapeutic mechanism. Later studies also added activity and exercise.

Behavioral modification therapy assumed that obesity was a behavioral disorder, characterized by excessive eating and other bad eating habits. However, these eating behaviors were "not symptomatic of underlying pathology, but [were] learned coping responses that occur within a complex social and cognitive environment." Behavioral therapy aimed to undo the "learned coping responses" and swap them for more appropriate, better-adjusted ones. First tried by a researcher at the Indiana University Medical Center on a group of nurses wanting to lose weight, other experimenters also had some success in the 1960s with adults, and in 1972 the approach was widely publicized in the popular diet book *Slim Chance in a Fat World*, written by psychologists Richard Stuart and Barbara Davis. Researchers tried the method on obese children from the mid-1970s. Behavioral modification therapists hoped for greater success with children because children were less set in their habits and therefore should be more easily "modifiable."[21]

The basic process had a number of steps. The first was to have the child and parents make a "food intake record"—a diary of what the child ate, when, where, and for what reasons. This record provided a baseline description of the child's normal habits and helped "call attention to parents of behavior that may not have been previously noted." Then, together, the parent, child, and therapist would look at the food intake record and start identifying ways in which eating habits could be changed through slight changes to the eating environment and to what was eaten. It was particularly important that the child be involved in determining the changes in order to assume personal responsibility for his own behavior.[22]

There was a whole range of strategies for change that therapists might suggest. A child who "ate on the run" or constantly grazed from the refrigerator might be asked to eat only when sitting at the dining table. Parents of a child who pinched cookies from the cookie jar would be told not to buy cookies or to put the jar on a high shelf. Children who liked oranges would be encouraged to eat them as snacks in preference to candy. In the belief that fast eating and insufficient chewing might be contributory factors, children might be asked to put their cutlery down between bites or to take regular sips of water. The idea was that certain behaviors should be increased, some decreased, some totally eliminated, and some new behaviors instituted to shape the child's behavior into a more appropriate response: "The behavioral treatment program, then, is composed of a wide variety of techniques, each providing a partial change in the maladaptive habits."[23]

Behavioral therapy was sometimes joined with other standard behaviorist approaches, such as the giving of rewards for success. (Children would be rewarded with special food treats for good eating behavior or for hitting certain weight-loss goals; in another study, parents had to lodge a deposit with the researchers that would be refunded to them if the child followed the program and attended regular checkups.) Researchers also recommended trying a "token economy"—a classic behaviorist technique. For good eating behavior or for weight loss, the child would earn "tokens"—credits—that could be saved and then exchanged for desirable things like a trip to the movies or getting out of chores.

While psychologists trained in behaviorist approaches were the earliest to experiment with behavioral treatments for childhood obesity, medical practitioners heard about the method through journal articles published by specialists in obesity. The approach looked "encouraging," offering "new promise" to the clinician treating fat children. Most previous therapies had suffered from high drop-out rates, limited weight loss, high relapse rates, and negative side effects (especially with the weight-loss drugs). In addition, they tended to make people very unhappy, angry, or resentful. This dismal status had "produced a favorable climate for the introduction of new measures," and behaviorism seemed full of possibility—no side effects, fewer dropouts, and it was easily understood as well as cheap. And early studies with children seemed to suggest that the method might produce better weight-loss results than other approaches.[24]

For the modern reader, this approach of changing the tempting environment, trying to break habits, and rewarding incremental improvements seems totally obvious. Behavioral modification techniques, used to provoke dietary change and, to a lesser extent, exercise change, have become an assumed part of the response to obesity, so much so that something like putting the cookie jar out of reach is now seen as simple common sense rather than a specifically behaviorist treatment. It is a sign of just how much American society has absorbed the tenets of behaviorism and how subtly dominant behaviorism became. (Dog owners will also recognize the behaviorist credentials of dog training programs that aim to "shape" a dog's behavior—say, to do a trick—by successively approximating and rewarding small steps that together make the whole trick.) In terms of obesity treatment, we are all behaviorists now, even without knowing it.

This is a rather strange outcome, since it was apparent within a decade of trying behaviorist techniques to treat obesity in children that the approach was not as impressive as it first seemed to be. Noted one researcher:

> Although behavior therapy has advanced the treatment of obesity, its results are still of limited clinical significance. Weight losses have been modest and the variability in results large and unexplained. Even long-term maintenance of weight loss, which, it was originally hoped, would be a particular benefit of the behavioral approach, has not yet been established.[25]

Now four decades old, behavioral modification treatment of obesity has shown that weight-loss results vary widely—some children lose weight and keep it off, and others do not—and there seem to be few common patterns indicating why this might be the case. In most cases it is only moderately effective, which is, perhaps, better than not effective at all.[26]

The behaviorist approach seems to have survived—and indeed flourished, particularly in the world of popular dietary advice (see Chapter 8) and common opinion—not because it is especially effective but because it *seems* like it ought to be effective. It has a plausible mechanism for lowering weight and it *seems* like an appropriate response to childhood obesity. It uses highly valued cultural concepts like self-improvement, character formation, personal responsibility, and rewards. And seeming plausible to both patients and physicians is, of course, one of the most fundamental reasons that a particular treatment is used in medicine.[27]

One of the elements of childhood obesity that Bruch, for one, had emphasized was the role of family. The fact that obesity "runs in families" had been noted as something of a truism in obesity research since its very earliest investigations, with the upshot being that researchers deduced it could be genetic (hereditary) or the result of cultural eating patterns passed down within the family group. Bruch's work helped sharpen these questions by showing that family connections could be closely investigated. However, this inquiry has taken a biological turn away from Bruch's interest in emotional dynamics.

Elaborating the family-centered theme, in the late 1960s large epidemiological studies investigated the similarity of body size between biologically related family members and non-biologically related family members. The results showed that children's body shapes were closely connected to those of their biological parents—fat parents tended to have fat children, and lean parents tended to have lean children. And the fatter the parents, the fatter the child. Siblings, and especially twins, also shared similar body shapes and degrees of obesity. This suggested to the researchers that a strong genetic component was involved in determining body shape and that therefore genetics would also be involved in childhood obesity.[28]

But, intriguingly, husbands and wives (who, one hopes, are not closely genetically related), also shared the same degree of fatness. While this might simply be the result of *homogamy* (like marrying like), researchers also examined diet and exercise data and concluded that there was something about people sharing the same family environment that influenced body shape. Some studies also found that adopted children shared similar levels of fatness with their adopted parents. The researchers concluded that "it is clear that fatness and obesity are both acquired in the family context" since both biologically and non-biologically related family members shared similar body sizes. The upshot was that "while fatness follows family lines, it does so in a way that implicated living together rather than simple genetic inheritance." Both nature and nurture—genetics and family environment—seemed to have a role in childhood obesity.[29]

Instead of looking at correlations between family members' weights, researchers now have changed their focus to looking at the particular genes that account for why obesity can run in families. Since the 1990s, geneticists have compiled lists of genes that are known to cause obesity in both mice and humans. The first cases of obesity in humans being caused by a single gene were identified in 1997: a two-year-old boy and his eight-year-old cousin, and a forty-three-year-old woman. The children had a mutation in the gene that is the human equivalent of the mouse *ob* gene, mentioned in Chapter 6 in connection with leptin. The woman had a mutation in a gene called CPE (carboxypeptidase E), which is also involved in hormone production.[30]

From this initial count of just two single genes that caused obesity, the count has now grown considerably with, at latest reckoning, over seventy genes causing obesity. Some of these genes affect hunger and satiety signaling; others determine fat cell growth; still others involve how fat is metabolized and used for energy. However, the number of people whose obesity is due to one of these single gene variations ("monogenic obesity") is only a small proportion—perhaps 5 percent or so—of all obesity. Instead, it is far more likely that most cases of obesity are due to a combination of genes ("polygenic obesity"), and whether or not that combination of genes causes obesity will also depend on the environment and behavior of the person. So while the target of inquiry has moved from macromeasures of weight or body fat to genes, the research is continuing to indicate that the role of family in producing obesity includes both biological and environmental connections. In most cases, a person's genetic make-up may make him or her susceptible to obesity, but it is the person's environment and behavior that determine whether that susceptibility becomes actuality.[31]

How far might the influence of family environment extend? A study carried out in 1970 found that obese pet-owners tended to have obese *pets*. The adage that "obesity runs in families" could be extended to the nonhuman members of the family as well. Most recently, Nicholas Christakis, a sociologist and physician at the Harvard Medical School, and his colleague James Fowler at the University of San Diego found that obese people tend to have obese *friends*. Christakis and Fowler interpreted this as evidence that obesity can, in some ways, be considered as an infectious condition, being transmitted through social networks in the same way as a common cold.[32]

Researchers have pondered further on the role that mothers play in their child's fatness, exploring both what mothers do (how they behave) and their biological ties to their children. Since investigations during the 1970s when formula-feeding had reached its height, formula- or bottle-feeding has been found to be a risk factor in causing childhood obesity, while breast-feeding seems to be associated with lower likelihood of being fat in childhood. This was just one factor that led to public health advisories encouraging a return to more breast-feeding. It is not entirely clear why breast-feeding seems to lower the risk of obesity—perhaps it is because a breast-fed child can control how much it eats more than when it must finish the bottle. Perhaps it is because formula can be mixed to be more calorie-dense than breast milk, or perhaps there is some quality to breast milk that affects the child's development or metabolism and protects against obesity. Researchers have also considered whether the developmental stage in which solid foods are introduced might be a factor in later obesity, with some evidence suggesting that early introduction of solid foods is a risk factor—the longer the breast-feeding, and that alone, the better.[33]

Other studies have taken a sociological approach to the question of how mothers might shape their child's body. As Hilde Bruch did in the 1940s, sociologically minded researchers of the 2000s noted that some mothers did not notice that their child was obese and resisted suggestions for treatment. Taking a different line from Bruch, these researchers suggested that cultural factors (such as ethnic-specific aesthetic standards and beliefs about the healthiness of childhood chubbiness), educational levels, and socioeconomic status all play roles in determining how concerned a mother is about her child's obesity, and how willing and able she is to follow medical advice.[34]

Studies have also extended the period of inquiry into the mother's role much earlier by investigating how *her* nutrition and *her* fatness during pregnancy might affect her fetus's postnatal development. Animal studies have shown that changing maternal nutrition levels can affect the offspring's body. Epidemiological studies have shown similar effects in humans. Most famously, a 1976 study of Dutch men who had been *conceived* during World War II—when Holland was suffering from great food shortages so that mothers were underfed—found that the children, who were of low birth weight, were more likely to be obese when they grew up. Studies investigating the other end of the spectrum have found that children of mothers who put on a lot of weight during pregnancy were also more likely to become obese. (High birth-weight babies are also at greater risk of developing obesity when they grow into children.) The relation between maternal nutrition and a child's later obesity therefore may be "U"-shaped with both low and high levels of maternal nutrition being associated with childhood obesity.[35]

One theory that was put forward to explain the connection at the upper end of the nutritional scale was the "fat cell hypothesis," first proposed in 1967 by researchers who were investigating how early nutrition would affect the number of fat cells in baby rats. They found that baby rats in small litters (that is, pups who were getting a lot of milk) were significantly heavier and had more fat cells than pups from larger litters (who were raised on less milk). When the baby rats grew up, the rats with more fat cells got even fatter because their fat cells grew in size. When the rats were put on a restricted diet, the rats with more fat cells lost weight because their fat cells shrank in size, but they kept the same number of fat cells. The study suggested that the number of fat cells an animal has is set in early life. If an animal is overfed in infancy, the animal would have more fat cells and would therefore be able to get fatter when they grew up.[36]

Support for the fat cell hypothesis has waxed and waned over time, but its underlying assumption that there may be "critical periods" in a person's growth during which physiological features become set or "programmed" has received ongoing interest. (And there may be more critical periods than just the prenatal one—researchers have suggested that early childhood and adolescence are also times during which physiological features that might determine obesity are set. This theory has been enjoying renewed popularity since about 2000.) It is, however, difficult to precisely delineate how much a mother's nutrition during pregnancy determines her child's later obesity because so many factors influence the connection between mother and child. This makes it hard to separate in utero nutritional effects from genetic and postnatal effects.[37]

There has been considerably less inquiry into the potential role of the father in contributing to his child's obesity, both because mothers carry the child and then, historically, have been primarily responsible for the child's care and feeding. As one researcher put it, "the mother tends to be the keeper of the calories and the pusher of provender in most households."[38] (One earlier exception to this lack of interest in a father's contribution was in studies of the hereditary nature of obesity conducted in the 1970s. Researchers hypothesized that children would be more likely to be affected if their mother was obese than if their father was obese because of gestational effects and feeding habits, but this assumption was confounded: both maternal and paternal fatness appeared similarly to affect the child's chances of becoming obese.) More recent research has begun to suggest tantalizing indications that a father's genes and his dietary habits when a child is conceived may affect the child's likelihood of becoming obese. Fathers and mothers may therefore affect their children's susceptibility to obesity through their genes and from their diet both before and after the child is born.[39]

Further investigations into the family environment of the fat child, particularly since the later 1990s, have suggested that parenting style affects a child's likelihood of developing obesity. A consistent finding has been that children whose parents are most controlling about their eating—restricting how much they can eat and insisting that they "clean their plate"—are more likely to be obese than children whose parents take a more laissez-faire attitude to their children's eating. That is, "authoritarian" parenting styles are most highly associated with obesity in children; "authoritative" styles where the parent is a firm, fair leader and allows the child appropriate autonomy is the parenting style associated with the lowest rates of childhood obesity.[40]

———

From Hilde Bruch's opening forays into the emotional and familial aspects of childhood obesity, the approach to these factors took a distinctly physical turn, helped along by behaviorism's emphasis on eating habits and the strictly biological formulations of in utero and genetic effects. Feelings, philia, and frustrations do, however, live on, not in the medical mainstream, but in the world of "common knowledge" and, especially, in popular dieting advice. That eating can have a symbolic purpose and food can have a symbolic meaning has reached the status of "obvious fact"—the zenith of popularization. For example, in a 1980 diet book for teenage girls, the author says,

> the most important emotional reason for eating is the idea that
> $$mood = food.$$
> Moods like boredom, frustration, anger, and nervousness create tension, and often people eat to relieve this tension. Pretty soon it becomes automatic: "I'm bored, so I'll eat."; "I'm angry, so I'll eat."[41]

Around this time in the 1980s, the pithy phrase of "emotional eating" (referring to eating in response to emotional cues rather than hunger) entered the vernacular.[42]

In recent years, a subgenre of autobiographies (and the occasional biography) concerning what could be called "the secret lives of fat people" has achieved a new level of popularity.[43] These books are written by people who are fat, or who were fat, and the book uses the person's weight struggles as the central motif in their life story. Such stories tell of the origins of the author's obesity, which are usually in childhood and which the author often attributes to family factors and especially relationships. "Fat girl" Judith Moore, for example, felt she "ate Grammy's fried chicken and Grammy's cobbler" because she was "trying to fill up the grave [her] father and mother had dug for" her.[44] Biographies such as Moore's and others like it approach the question of weight in different ways, however. Some are stories of triumph—either of successful weight loss or of coming to accept being overweight and proudly defying conventions of thinness. The finale is the author's achieving contentment with (usually) her, but occasionally his, body. Others are stories of an Oprah-esque continuing struggle: a postmodern approach to biography that emphasizes ongoing existential tussles rather than a resolved story arc.[45]

In every case, however, the writer's struggle from childhood with weight is presented as not simply a medical issue but as a personal battle. These are stories of "the triumph of the human spirit" and are, more than anything, intensely emotional tales. They speak to the lived experience of being a fat child, the enduring psychological and emotional factors in childhood obesity, the hurt and judgment that fat children feel, and the complex family dynamics in fostering the condition. They encapsulate the involvedness of childhood obesity with its intricate interlacing of biology, psychology, family, and emotion.

CHAPTER 8

Kalorie Kids

Energy Balance and the Turn to Child Responsibility

> It stands to reason: every normal human being wants to look fit, feel fit and fit tidily into the proper-size clothes. And why not? If you're happy, healthy, and comfortable to look at, you're an easy person to love.
>
> Ruth West's *The Teen-Age Diet Book*, 1959

Dieting and, to a lesser extent, exercising have been a part of the treatment for childhood obesity for the entire twentieth century. Diet and exercise were, for example, sometimes part of the prescription even in the 1920s and 1930s when the cause of childhood obesity was believed to be glandular. The rationale for manipulating food intake or physical activity to influence the shape of the body was the idea that the body was an engine that needed to be kept in "energy balance." Out of balance, it would get fat or thin.[1]

The concept of the body as a machine that ran on caloric energy—taking in food as fuel and using it up for maintenance and activity—owed much to the work of American chemist Wilbur Atwater. In the late nineteenth century, Atwater developed techniques for measuring the energy content of food. In explaining to a popular audience how the body used caloric energy and needed to be kept in energy balance, scientists have used metaphors of bank accounts, car engines, and balance beams:

> Your body is like a bank. You put calories in; you take out energy. When you deposit and withdraw equal amounts of money, your bank account remains as it is. When you deposit calorie food [sic] and withdraw an equal amount of calorie energy [sic], your weight remains as it is.[2]

Dieting would alter the intake side of the energy equation; exercising would alter the output side. "Put in more [energy] than you take out, and both your

133

bank account and your figure grow fat. Take out more than you put in, and both slim down."[3]

In theory, either dieting or exercise might be prescribed to balance a fat person's "energy equation," but in practice, fat *adults* have more often just been prescribed diets—and, indeed, have enthusiastically followed dieting advice—whereas *children* have been prescribed both diet and exercise for weight loss. This seeming discrepancy was because, before about the midcentury, physicians felt exercise would make their fat adult patients hungry and therefore make them eat more. In contrast, childhood was meant to be an active time, so instructing children to get out and about was simply telling them to be like children ought to be anyway. It was the dieting part of the prescription for obesity in childhood that raised many more questions.

Should a fat child diet? Such a simple five-word question is paradoxically the subject of a continuing controversy in the history of childhood obesity. There are strong cultural pressures against restricting a child's eating—as Hilde Bruch, for one, had pointed out, feeding a child well is a way parents show care and love. On another level it is a medical issue, as one school physician pointed out in 1924:

> The question of the limitation of diet raises a very nice theoretical problem as well as a practical one. How far can the diet of a growing developing child be cut down without the danger of injury?[4]

And should a fat child's weight be reduced by dieting, or should the physician simply try to keep the fat child's weight constant so the child could "grow into" his or her weight? While there has been a broad trend over the course of the century's worth of dieting advice away from recommending reducing a fat child's weight in favor of keeping it constant, this was by no means consistent or absolute. The age of the child and degree of overweight might be factored into decisions. There have also been national differences in practice on this point: American physicians have been more likely to put a child on a reducing diet than British physicians.[5] When physicians did give dieting advice for treating childhood obesity, the content of that advice has been quite consistent over the past century: cut down on candy, cakes, pastry, bread (especially white bread), and potatoes; eat more fruit and vegetables; and drink moderate amounts of milk.[6]

While clinicians argued back and forth about the merits of child dieting as a treatment for obesity, children themselves had taken matters into their own hands. There is evidence from letters written by children that, even though dieting books and magazine columns in the 1920s were not directed at them, some girls and boys followed these expert prescriptions to lose weight just as avidly as adults did. Teenage dieting became an acceptable element in girls' serial novels catering to middle- and upper-class girls— sweet, chubby, sidekick Bess Marvin in the Nancy Drew books published from 1931 onward was a dieter. However, this sort of self-initiated child dieting was not always—or even often—done because the child was fat. In fact, when the first studies of the prevalence of child dieting were carried out in the 1960s, researchers were shocked that so many children (high-school age girls in particular) had dieted when their heights and weights implied they didn't need to for health reasons. Rather, youth culture and most especially girl culture of the twentieth century embraced ideals of slimness and dieting as a means of achieving that happy state. Eating disorders—anorexia, bulimia—shadowed the dieting enthusiasm. Studies in the 1980s showed that children were also embracing another dangerous habit if they were anxious about their weight—smoking. Both fat children and children who were not especially fat dieted (and also sometimes smoked) to look good and, they believed, become socially successful.[7]

In the late 1950s, the market awoke to the commercial opportunities presented by eager young dieters—both obese and otherwise. The subject of this and the next chapter, the first diet books directed at children were published and the first fat camps were established in the late 1950s. Dieticians, pediatricians, physical education teachers, psychologists, cookery book writers, and former fat children entered the roll call of authorities offering advice and commercial products and services to fat children in the second half of the twentieth century.[8]

This new turn in the energy balance approach to weight loss in children was much more elaborate and involved than the simple prescriptions parents had previously been given on cutting candy and cake. Eight-week summer camps and two-hundred-page diet books fetishized the mechanics of child weight loss.

From the 1960s onward, eating control was *the* dominant element in the mélange of treatment approaches to childhood obesity, pushing endocrine, family-based, and psychological treatments into the minority. Results from investigations of the condition and new ways of thinking about the harms of obesity in childhood favored early interventions along diet-and-exercise lines.

That shift in emphasis in the understanding and treatment of childhood obesity was a significant one and had ramifications for what it was like to be a fat child. The energy balance approach to obesity emphasized personal responsibility and personal action. *Your* eating, *your* lack of exercise causes *your* obesity. And, conversely *you* can make yourself slim again. The premise—that personal action can change your body shape—is highly appealing in a society like the United States that values personal responsibility and individual freedom. (This partly accounts for why diet-and-exercise advice in general is so popular as a commercial product.) The upshot of the energy-balance approach becoming dominant in the picture of childhood obesity was that fat children were increasingly required to take personal control of treating their condition—and take personal blame if they failed. It is no coincidence that the first formal investigations of how fat children were stigmatized by their peers also date from the 1960s. The cruelty of the condition increased with the increasing emphasis on diet and exercise.[9]

The weight-loss prescriptions that child dieting books and fat camps offered worked with the social value of slimness and with medical understanding of childhood obesity as it had been built up by the midcentury. Writers of children's dieting guides and owners of summer fat camps enthusiastically endorsed the idea that the remedy for childhood obesity would be found in the realm of personal behavior. Do what they advised, they suggested, and fat children would slim down, become happy, and achieve more in their lives than they would if they stayed fat. Diet books and fat camps sold more than just diet-and-exercise advice: they were purveyors of personal transformations, fairy godmothers who said, "Slim down, and you *shall* go to the ball." In dieting books and at fat camps, balancing the energy equation through diet and exercise was elevated into an art form and a way of life: to be happy, healthy, and slim, children needed to become expert at managing their body's balance.

One of the most vocal and commercially successful early recommenders of weight-loss diets for fat children was Lulu Hunt Peters. Hunt Peters was influenced by her own experience as an unhappy fat child and her subsequent happiness after successfully dieting as an adult. She was a former teacher who took her MD from the University of Northern California in 1909, and spent her early medical career teaching pathology and infant feeding at hospitals in Los Angeles and New York. But it was in her lecturing duties for her role as chairman of public health for the California Federation of Women's Clubs that she developed the material for her best-selling adults' diet book, *Diet and Health with Key to the Calories* (1918). The title ironically echoed that of the founding text of the Christian Science movement—Mary Baker Eddy's *Science and Health with Key to the Scriptures*—and set the playful, humorous tone of the book.[10]

Hunt Peters preached a secular faith in the midst of World War I—that fatness was akin to hoarding food and that thinness was a happy state, much to be desired. There was no greater joy, she said, than taking in one's clothes. Huge satisfaction could be gained "when you find your corset coming closer and closer together (I advise a front lace, so this can be watched), and then the day you realize that you will have to stitch in a tuck or get a new one!"[11]

The secret to weight loss, Hunt Peters said, was in counting calories. For her followers, the concept of the calorie—a unit for the energy value of food—was likely a new one. Hunt Peters taught readers how to say the word ("pronounced Kal'-o-ri"), told people how many calories were in staple foods, and gave formulae for calculating how many calories one should eat to lose weight. People could eat anything they wanted, provided they watched their calories, she said. She took her own advice in this regard—when she put on weight while serving with the Red Cross in World War I, she lost it again by having coffee for breakfast, a full meal at lunch, and only dessert for dinner, much to her colleagues' amusement.[12]

When Lulu Hunt Peters came back from her war service, she found her diet book had become the first best-selling weight-loss book in the United States. *Diet and Health* reached the *Publisher's Weekly* best-seller lists for five years (1922–1926), holding the top spot for 1924 and 1925. A newspaper syndicate, the George Matthew Adams Service, contracted her to write a daily column on "Diet and Health," published nationwide. Lulu Hunt Peters became a household name.[13]

From letters Hunt Peters received via the newspaper, it was clear that not just adults, but children and teens, too, were following dieting advice from "America's best-loved woman physician." Mary, aged sixteen, wrote,

Dearest Dr. Lulu: I . . . formerly belonged to the F.F.F. [the Friendly Fat Fraternity], but becoming wearied of them, I followed your instructions and left the bunch. You know they are so unpleasant to look at! After a reduction of eighteen pounds I can now march along with those girls with the 'wonderful' figures without a bit of envy in my heart.[14]

Dr Lulu wrote back saying, "You should be proud of yourself, Mary, because you have shown that you have strength of purpose and character." A boy who said his mother read the column each day wrote to Hunt Peters asking for advice on how to reduce:

Most young men have no abdomen, and as my companions tease me when I go swimming, I would like to reduce what they call my "Provision" and my thighs, and as I am very fastidious I wear the latest style in suits which have very narrow pants, and with my fat thighs I split my pants.[15]

Hunt Peters did not intend for children to follow her column—she wrote it with adults in mind—but children were nevertheless reading her advice over the shoulders of their parents and following it for themselves.

In 1924, Hunt Peters published a special two-part series addressing the topic of "the Fat Child" and issued a stern warning to parents using what she described as "rough language":

Your child is not fat, mother, because you are fat or because his father is fat or someone else in the family is fat. Your child, if he is fat—and healthy—is fat because he eats too much.[16]

This was quite a contrast to the idea popular at the time that fat children had a gland problem. Dr Lulu prescribed weight-*loss* diets for fat children, not simply weight-maintenance diets, but she did counsel that calorie cuts not be made by cutting milk, protein, fresh vegetables, or fruit. Instead, she advised that cuts ought to be made in reducing sweets, candy, sugar, desserts, and in the amount of bread and butter the child ate.[17]

Hunt Peters's readers sent her "exceedingly numerous" letters responding to her child-related advice columns, so she revised and combined some of her columns and made a book out of them. It was published as *Diet for Children (and Adults) and the Kalorie Kids* in 1924. Along with general nutritional advice, Hunt Peters also had a special chapter on "The Fat Child" in which she advised parents—a first in parental advice guides—to rigorously diet fat children by cutting their calories.

Children who were more than 15–20 percent above their average weight for height (and she gave a table of height-weight standards in the book) ought to be placed on a reducing diet, she recommended. The method was to calculate how many calories the child ought to be eating for his or her age and height and cut this amount by five hundred to one thousand calories per day. Milk, however, should not be cut—all children, fat and thin, needed a good two to three glasses of milk a day—because, she said, it contained complete protein and "wonderful calcium," phosphorus, and vitamins. Weekly weights were to be recorded on a chart. Parents were advised to encourage activities, and could enroll their child in a gym if they could afford it—not because the exercise would burn fat, she said, but to keep the body in tone. The doctor's prescription also strictly limited candy and desserts.

> Get the child, if old enough, interested in counting his calories himself and make a game of it . . . Have a little reward for each week when he loses [weight]. *Insist on very thorough mastication* as that helps to control the appetite and is beneficial in other ways, as you know.[18]

In contrast to her *Diet and Health* book for adults, with its playful names like Mrs. Sheesasite and Mrs. Knott Little, Dr. Lulu said that diet in childhood was too serious to "lend itself to any funny treatment" and that childhood obesity held "real danger."[19] Fat children were more at risk for pneumonia and respiratory infections and diabetes, but for Hunt Peters, the real damage of childhood obesity was caused by its emotional pain. Hunt Peters quoted letters she had received from children, ranging in age from eleven years up to eighteen, recounting stories of being teased, and of being lonely and without friends:

> Oh, Doctor, please have pity on me and answer this as soon as possible as I am getting so fat that I shall be ridiculous. Any boy that I shall meet will say, "Gee, but you're fat!" And I cannot bear to hear that from a boy.[20]

She contrasted this with how happy the children were when they wrote of their dieting successes. Moreover, Hunt Peters implied, children who succeeded at weight loss would succeed in other areas of life as well. One eleven-year-old wrote that she had lost eleven and a half pounds, and then got "As" in penmanship and gym. The fat child was a deeply unhappy child, thought Hunt Peters. Dieting could lead a fat child back to the right path for life success. With the fate of the unslimmed child in mind, she gravely warned her readers, "I am sure you will do your best to prevent and to remedy excessive overweight in your children."[21]

————————

Lulu's *Kalorie Kids* was unusual in suggesting that parents rigorously diet their fat child so that he or she *lost* weight. Few parental advice manuals before 1960 even covered overweight in children, and those that did generally advised mild measures such as encouraging exercise and cutting back on bread and candy. After her death in 1935 at age fifty-six from pneumonia— possibly made worse by going on a crash diet ahead of a public speaking engagement—Lulu Hunt Peters was succeeded as queen of the diet column by Ida Jean Kain. From 1937 to her retirement in 1969, Ida Jean Kain wrote "Your figure Madam!" (later "Keep in Trim!") for a newspaper syndicate that was a rival of Hunt Peters's.[22]

Ida Jean was a home economist, who, although she wrote and spoke on a range of health-and-beauty topics like vitamins, posture, and skin care, was most famous for her weight-loss advice. Her weight-loss prescription was to cut fat from the diet, avoid dessert, eat small meals, and do sports for general exercise and more targeted exercises for certain body parts. ("To beautify the legs, 'strut.'") Readers could write in to ask for copies of pamphlets with titles like "Reducer's Recipes," "Hip, Hip Away," and "Exercises for Twin Chins."[23]

Like Lulu Hunt Peters, Kain herself had been fat as a child and teenager. Her interest in writing about dieting was motivated by her own success at reducing before she started college. But Ida Jean's style was quite different from Lulu's—Kain favored gossipy references to Hollywood stars and their dietary regimes. ("Hollywood Director Cuts down Weight by Diet and Swimming"; "Olivia de Haviland Avoids Dessert When her Scales Warn.") For Lulu Hunt Peters, dieting was humdrum but necessary and rewarding; for Ida Jean Kain, it was the portal to a glamorous, beautiful life. And one should prepare for that glamorous life by staying slim in childhood.[24]

A moderate degree of overweight in children and teens was, Kain said, a good thing as it provided "some insurance against tuberculosis" and "makes you prettier, too." "Curves and a round face go with youth." But children needed to watch their weight the same as adults did. (Or at least have their weight watched for them by their parents.) To reassure parents that their concerns about childhood overweight were justified—and, she implied, all the *best* parents were concerned—Kain noted that Shirley Temple, then aged eleven, had her weight watched, and the famous Dionne Quintuplets had recently gone on a diet—aged five. (The Dionne quintuplets, who were born in 1934 in Ontario, were the first quintuplets known to survive infancy. They were a major tourist attraction in the 1930s and early 1940s—one could go and watch them in their play enclosure. Their images were used to advertise many products, including Carnation Evaporated Milk and Palmolive Soap.)[25]

A "wise mother," said Kain, would not be complacent about her child's fatness, but would take action early and not allow "subteen laziness" to "lure fat." Age ten was the perfect time for a mother to suggest dieting to her fat son: he would have been teased at school by this age and so would be more willing to cooperate. Good parents, Kain implied, controlled and guided their children, and Kain conveyed the expectation that this could be easily achieved. There were no complicating factors to the family dietary arrangements in Kain's presentation of the family.[26]

For older children and teens, Kain also used the same appeal to Hollywood glamour as she did with adults. The dieting, exercise, and beauty rituals of Hollywood starlets and ice skaters were Kain's models for teens to emulate:

> What teen agers [sic] need is more beauty advice from movie stars their own age if they're anywhere near as cute as Shirley Temple. The first tip she gave me was, "tell them not to eat chocolate bars!"[27]

Shirley, who Ida Jean mentioned a number of times in her column over the years and who was seventeen when Ida Jean interviewed her in that instance, advised that she "hardly ever" ate desserts, but did drink milk, and ate "good wholesome food" at proper mealtimes. (She also recommended never going to bed with one's face dirty, standing up straight—especially if one "tends to be sort of plump"—and putting on lipstick with a brush.) Teens could be as attractive as movie stars, implied Kain, if they only followed her secret "tips" for slimming and grooming. Losing weight and looking pretty was simply a matter of following her instructions.

———————

While enthusiastic about the prospects of child and teen dieting, commercially successful columnists like Ida Jean Kain and Lulu Hunt Peters of the 1920s, 1930s, and 1940s also needed to reassure parents. Their message for parents was that young overweight people could diet without harm and that good parents would cut their children's food. By the late 1950s, however, these ideas that a young person might diet and a parent might withhold food were much less contentious than they had been at the start of the century. Writers no longer included such reassurances for parents about child dieting, although they continued to caution against putting a child on too low a diet. Child dieting was no longer strange: it had become normal. Normalized, the diet-and-exercise response to childhood obesity—and the commercial opportunities it offered—flourished in the latter half of the twentieth century. The parent was increasingly cut out of the loop as would-be diet-and-exercise advisers turned to speaking directly to children.

On the medical front, two developments moved diet and exercise into center place of the agglomeration of theories concerning the condition. One development was that, by the latter half of the century, other theories such as the glandular hypothesis and psychosomatic causes had declined in popularity and moved to the periphery of how childhood obesity was understood and treated. These were now subsidiary elements in the mélange of theories that explained the condition. Instead, in the dominant orthodoxy of the 1950s onward, diet and exercise were centrally involved in obesity as both the cause and the remedy. The deep complexities of the glandular hypothesis and the psychosomatic model of childhood obesity ceded to a mechanical explanation and a mechanical response—energy in, energy out through diet and exercise.

The second development that gave a huge boost to child dieting for overweight concerned the assumption that "baby fat" was transient and, therefore, more benign than adult fat. Up until about 1950, both popular and medical belief was that "there is a general impression, with no figures to support or refute it, that most people who are fat in childhood and early youth become thin later." The majority belief was that childhood fat would clear up with puberty. However, in the 1950s, new evidence from longitudinal studies showed that childhood obesity was likely to persist into adulthood.[28]

The new scrutiny of the connection between child and adult obesity was partly due to a novel way of thinking about certain noninfectious medical conditions. Diseases such as cardiovascular disease and type 2 ("adult-onset") diabetes had come to be understood as having very long gestational periods and were related to what would become known as "lifestyle" factors. The new concept of the "risk factor"—a behavior (like smoking) or a physical measurement (like high blood pressure) that was correlated with greater statistical likelihood of illness—offered a way of noting associated factors without having to know the precise mechanism of illness causation. (Risk factors are *correlated with* an increased risk of illness, but are not necessarily *causes,* although they may point toward possible causes.)[29]

The risk factor concept was accompanied by a new research methodology: the mass cohort, long-term, epidemiological study. Given titles like "The Framingham Study" and "The Build and Blood Pressure Study," and involving large teams of different specialists to collect and analyze the data, such studies brought statistical likelihood tests to bear on the question of what risk factors were associated with diseases like cardiovascular disease and diabetes. These mass studies became the gold standard for researchers investigating epidemiological patterns, and the results they generated have become central to orthodox medical understanding. While insurance data from the early twentieth century had shown overweight in adulthood to be associated with a higher mortality rate, midcentury epidemiological studies refined the understanding of why adult obesity was dangerous. A number of studies suggested overweight in adulthood (especially in combination with high blood pressure) was a risk factor for a range of health problems, including heart attacks, stroke, and diabetes.[30]

Importantly, the risk factor concept implied that a long-range perspective was needed when thinking about how and when certain diseases developed. The cause or causes of an obese woman's type 2 diabetes might be found throughout the whole course of her life, not just in the few days or months before her blood sugar started to rise. So did being obese in childhood affect adult health? Was the popular assumption that childhood obesity usually "went away" correct? In the new reckoning of longitudinal epidemiological studies, a clinician's impression "with no figures to support or refute it" was not considered a persuasive answer to these questions.

Studies in the 1950s—particularly a 1958 British study and a 1960 American study—provided epidemiological data on the issue of whether childhood obesity persisted into adulthood. The results were a major contradiction of the idea that puberty would resolve childhood fatness: the great majority of fat children remained fat into adulthood. After infancy, the fatter a child was, and the older they were, the more likely the fatness would persist into adulthood. An analysis by researchers of twenty years of U.S. Public Health Service data contributed one of the most widely quoted statistics: fully 80 to 85 percent of overweight children would grow up to become overweight adults.[31]

By the late 1950s, then, the thinking about childhood obesity had changed considerably from just a few decades earlier. A number of physicians, including Lulu Hunt Peters and Hilde Bruch, had suggested there were social and emotional harms to being fat in childhood. And although there was little evidence that fat children were physically harmed by their size, there was now evidence that childhood obesity persisted in adulthood. Since obesity in adulthood was known to be dangerous, this created renewed pressure to treat the condition in childhood. The result was a fetishization of the mechanics of reducing. Child dieting—manipulating children's eating as a way of treating overweight—and to a lesser extent exercise reached new heights of popularity and elaboration from the midcentury.

———————

In the late 1950s, the dieting manual market noticed that fat teens and occasionally younger children were dieting without much guidance or, generally, medical supervision. American publishers had produced a number of best-selling dieting books for adults in the early and mid-twentieth century, including Lulu Hunt Peter's *Diet and Health* (1918), Victor H. Lindlahr's *You Are What You Eat* (1940), Gaylord Hauser's *Look Younger, Live Longer* (1950), and Adelle Davis's *Let's Eat Right to Keep Fit* (1954), showing that dieting advice could be one of the most profitable subcategories in the United States of the ever-popular self-help genre. With dieting for children and teens increasingly being seen as a normal and acceptable response to child overweight by the late 1950s, the market was well positioned—and well experienced—to exploit this new, younger clientele. Magazine writer and diet authority Ruth West's *The Teen-Age Diet Book*, released in 1959, tapped into this richly prepared publishing niche. The author of the first diet book directed at overweight child and teen readers, West would also later work with controversial diet book author Dr. Robert Atkins on his famous high-protein diet, the "Atkins Diet."[32]

"Child diet book" refers to any advice guide that recommends manipulating a child's eating in some way as a means of dealing with fatness. Here "diet" is used in its older meaning of a shaped eating regimen rather than food restriction. Although child diet books do intend to speak to overweight children, they may, of course, be read and followed by children who are not overweight. For that reason, child diet books inhabit an uneasy cultural position. Medical advice guide? Or prop for an eating disorder? Indeed, when medical researchers have studied child dieting they have mainly investigated the connection between increased child dieting and pathological behavior: dieting was established in the 1980s as a risk factor for developing an eating disorder. In contrast, there is a comparative dearth of research looking at the effectiveness of dieting as treatment for childhood obesity.[33]

In fact, not all authors of books that fit the category of "child diet book" would be happy with the term "diet." Because of the lettuce-and-water overtones of the word and the connection with eating disorders, some child diet book authors vociferously denied that *their* eating program was a "diet." ("This isn't a 'diet book.' It's a kind of way-of-life book.") The genre of the child diet book is split between books suggesting short-term weight cures and whose authors tend to accept the term "diet," like *The Fast and Easy Teenage Diet* (1973) or *The Doctor's Quick Teenage Diet* (1971) ("I can assure you that with my speedy reducing methods, you'll lose many pounds and inches in a hurry   you won't be on the diet 'forever'") and books recommending longer-term "healthy living" measures, like the approach taken by the *Teenage Sure Fire Diet Cookbook* (1979): "It is not merely a diet that you are learning, but a new way of eating that can keep you thin and healthy all your life."[34]

While the healthy-living style of prescription became more common in children's dieting books towards the end of the twentieth century, "spot" diets (short-term, highly restrictive diets) for children declined in popularity—but they still remain a part of the genre. The history of the child diet book therefore runs the gamut from commonsense instruction to what orthodox medicine would consider dubious advice, sometimes, ironically, given by qualified health practitioners. Although with some connection to medicine, or at least to health, the child diet book and its contribution to the history of childhood obesity is therefore best thought of as a commercial and pop culture phenomenon.

Common to all diet books for children is that they are commercial products and therefore try to persuade readers to buy them and follow their prescriptions. The methods publishers and authors have used to do this are wide-ranging. Some strategies that have been employed are similar across the fifty years that child diet books have been published, while others have changed to appeal to changing perceptions of what the diet book audience wants.

One lasting advertising strategy has been to use prior commercial success. Some children's diet books were spin-offs from successful dieting books published for adults, and they echo their pedigree in their title, such as the *Hilton Head Diet Book for Children and Teenagers* (from *The Hilton Head Metabolism Diet*), and *The Doctor's Quick Teenage Diet* ("by the authors of the 5-million-copy best seller 'The Doctor's Quick Weight Loss Diet'").

The author him- or herself has also commonly been used as a big advertising point. Scientific expertise—sometimes burnished with advertising gold dust—features prominently. "Approved by the American Medical Association" noted the cover of *Slimming for Teenagers,* while "Dr Susan," author of *Dr. Susan's Girls-Only Weight Loss Guide* (2006) turns out not to be an MD as one might assume but a PhD in psychology. Indeed, the genre of child diet book is marked by the wide range of authors claiming authority to speak on the topic of childhood overweight. Medical and allied health professionals like nutritionists, medical doctors, and psychologists like Dr. Susan have been joined by cookbook authors, weight-loss camp directors, and successful dieters to form the ranks of people involved in writing child diet books. The *"New York Times'* Bestselling Author of 'Life Strategies for Teens,'" Jay McGraw, was in fact a law student when he wrote his child diet book, *The Ultimate Weight Solution for Teens* (2003). McGraw is, however, the son of Dr. Phil McGraw (of Oprah fame), and has appeared on the *Dr. Phil* spin-off program as the "teen expert": "As a young person, I know how hard it is to get people to take us seriously." Diet book authors often have referred to their personal history, like Jay McGraw referring to being himself "a young person," as their platform for giving advice. Often, the writer uses his or her own experience as a successful child dieter or mother of a successful child dieter as evidence of his or her qualifications to write the book. Diet-and-exercise expertise was, in the later twentieth century, a broad and democratic field. A number of acceptable pathways lead to that position of diet book author.[35]

Beyond some form of expertise, the diet book author has also typically offered his or her child readers more subtle attractions to buy and read the book. One attraction is that the book sought to serve as the child's friend, guide, and confidant. In the case of medical authors, like Dr. Stillman, coauthor with self-help writer Samm Sinclair Baker of *The Doctor's Quick Teenage Diet* (1971), the book was crafted to read as a take-home consultation—one's personal weight-loss doctor, always on call.[36]

The diet book's tone was often intimate; the author was personally interested in and dedicated to helping the reader. Both a commercial strategy and a (presumably) true declaration of the author's intent, the diet book commonly reached out to the reader to build a personal relationship using no-nonsense straight talk or youth-speak:

Before we go on, let's make sure we understand each other. First, *you can't eat everything you want and lose weight.* Second, *you will be hungry.*[37]

Being fat is a bummer.[38]

The diet book author therefore aimed to establish a relationship with his or her child reader, even to the point of speaking the child's language. (Or perhaps *trying* to speak might be a more apt description, in some try-hard cases. It is easy to imagine young eyes being rolled at one author's reference to "punkers." "Punkers"?) As Hilde Bruch had pointed out in the 1940s, the relationship between the fat child and the therapist—in this case the book standing in for the author—was an important part of the therapeutic approach.[39]

The major attraction that the diet book offered the fat child reader, was, of course, the promise of transformation—a metamorphosis from fat to thin. The author contrasts the fat child's presumed current status—"Do kids tease you at school? Do you envy Brooke Shields, Marie Osmond, Barbie dolls, and all of Charlie's Angels for being thin?"—and suggests all that can change by following the book's prescriptions. The diet book offers a vision: a vision of what childhood ought to be like, of what girls and boys ought to be like, and of what being a fat child is like. Children's diet books are, however, deeply conservative in the social roles that they portray and advocate.[40]

Consider, for example, the vision of what girls and boys ought to be like suggested by this 1959 discussion of the rewards of dieting:

> A girl might buy herself a fresh pink carnation to wear to school the day after the scales tell her she's lost an even five pounds. For the big final reward, our girl might promise herself the dress she's never been able to wear—in the tiny size she's aiming for. A boy might wrangle the family into letting him have the car for a weekend hunting trip with a couple of friends.[41]

Here, the successfully dieting girl will celebrate by drawing attention to her new appearance; the dieting boy will celebrate his newfound virility with a group of friends. Dieting books for children commonly reflect and reinforce the conservative gender roles of the time period in which they are written: girls are worried about their looks and boys are worried about their strength.

The conservative stance of the diet book also extends to the fashion and personal grooming advice that children are given. Dee Matthews, herself a former overweight child and who later ran a dieting business, rapped her teen readers over the knuckles:

> Sharpen your appearance. Some of the young people who show up at my classes for the first time look as if they came straight from the ragpickers' convention in Skuz City . . . Uncombed, greasy hair. Stained, untucked shirts. Too tight, zipper-busted shirts.[42]

Matthews told fat teens to get a haircut, throw out their old clothes in favor of new, clean, ironed ones, and to stand up straight. Child dieting books promote certain aspects of stereotypical social roles—aspects that serve the diet book's purpose—such as the 1959 girlish longing for a dress in a "tiny size." Overweight children were invited to become average in more than just their weight.

Along with physical transformation, diet books for children tempted and encouraged their readers with less measurable rewards. Earlier dieting books, especially those published before about 1980, often plainly stated that a fat child who lost weight would be rewarded with happiness, attractiveness, and, in the case of older dieters, a date. Ruth West, for example, suggested in her 1959 diet book that a slim person was "comfortable to look at" and "an easy person to love." Readers of Stillman and Sinclair Baker's

Doctor's Quick Teenage Diet (1971) were advised that following their prescription would "help you stay slim for the rest of your more attractive, happier, healthier life . . . Wonderful things can happen for you."[43]

However, since the 1980s, with rising concern about eating disorders and also the early sexualization of children, diet books for children became increasingly wary of blatantly suggesting that children diet for reasons of appearance or popularity. Some recent dieting books have been openly critical of their forebears for drawing such implications. But diet books for children since the 1980s did not abandon the tactic of appealing to such insecurities—instead, they handled it in more subtle ways. For example, one recent book, *Weighing In* (2006), cautions that children ought not expect dramatic transformations in personality and likeability just because of losing weight:

> You might be fantasizing about becoming the new class heartthrob, or about how awestruck all of your friends are going to be at your incredible transformation. Just so as you're not disappointed, keep in mind that it might not turn out exactly like that.[44]

But the illustrations contradict the writing: the final picture in the book is a drawing of a cartoon boy and girl, slim and cool-looking, eying each other with salacious interest. The pictures—not the words—imply that successfully dieting children could expect to be become interesting to the opposite sex.

Weighing In illustrates the conundrum that diet books, as commercial products, have faced since the 1980s: when children are asked *why* they diet, their reasons are often to do with wanting to be attractive and, they believe, to be more likeable and popular. From a sales perspective, diet books are well advised to appeal to their readers' motivations. However, the adult world is against stressing the benefits of appearance for children, worried that this sexualizes children too young and potentially places them at risk for eating disorders. The child diet book, and especially the diet book that is written for children to read, is therefore in a difficult position. Children want to diet for appearance reasons, and commercially it makes sense to appeal to this desire, but social opinion holds it irresponsible to do so.[45]

The compromise that post-1980s diet books reached was to first acknowledge the social discrimination that fat children face, and then imply that dieting will, indirectly, fix this. Consider the following paragraphs from *The*

You Can Do It! Kids' Diet (1985). The first acknowledges the social problems of being a fat child:

> Sometimes you want to cry or scream because you are so angry and frustrated. Sometimes you lock yourself in your room and never want to come out. Sometimes you feel so awful you just want to die . . . Like it or not, we live in a "thin-is-in" society that has no room for fat people. As a result, you are treated like a second-class citizen . . . You have been wounded so much by snide comments in school, at home, and in public that you avoid contact with others as much as possible. You don't even bother joining in all the activities that bring excitement and fun to young people . . . You begin to feel like a spectator in life rather than a participant.[46]

But once you have successfully dieted, says the book,

> you have changed physically. Your body is lean and primed with energy. Your hair shines, your skin glows. But the most important change is the one that takes place inside your head. Your dieting success has inspired you with a dynamic feeling of accomplishment that carries over into all facets of your life: at school, at home, at play, and in public. You have won! And just knowing that fact can give you the edge you need to reach whatever other goals you have set for yourself in life.[47]

Post-1980s dieting books are therefore operating in a difficult world where they try to please child consumers but also offer advice that is sound and responsible from an adult point of view. The "success breeds success" tactic or the implication that dieting produces mental improvement were two strategies that allowed dieting books to gesture toward social rewards for thinness without appearing to condone children focusing on their looks.

Studies of child dieting have confirmed the popular impression that girls diet much more frequently than boys and at rates that do not match those of obesity in children—that is, girls diet when they don't need to. In studies of girl and boy dieters, girl dieters appear more likely to use books as their source of dieting advice than boy dieters. Boy dieters, who have been formally studied only in the limited context of dieting for wrestling competitions, appear to get their weight-loss advice mainly from other boys and their sports coaches. This gender difference in dieting therefore puts the diet book in a troubling position as a response to childhood obesity: it makes commercial "good sense" to specifically target girls as the audience for a child diet book, but childhood obesity makes no such gender distinction. The tracked rise in childhood obesity since the 1960s has affected both girls and boys, so although boys are not typical dieters, there may be a growing market of boys interested in losing weight.[48]

Many of the earlier child diet books in the 1960s and 1970s were not explicitly written for either sex—for example, *Slimming for Teens* (1973) by Lester David and Ruth West's *Teenage Diet Book* (1959)—contain advice and examples for both boys and girls. This is in keeping with both authors' insistence that their books are for children who are actually fat and that losing weight will benefit their health. However, both of these books have pictures of girls on the front cover, implying that the publisher (who made the decision about cover art) saw the market as being the girl dieter. Since the 1980s, child diet books have become even more gender-specific—pink doodles, pink blurbs in handwriting font, and dot points for calorie counts in the shape of pink love hearts have all been used in diet books to give them the feel of a girls' journal. Such girl-only dieting books work to reinforce the expectation that dieting is a "girl thing," creating a self-fulfilling circle of advertising appeal and girlish buyers.

Sociological and medical commentary on the increasing numbers of girls dieting has seen this as a bad thing. Girls focusing on and worrying about their bodies was not the sort of preoccupation feminism hoped young women would choose, given alternatives. Medicine's investigation into child dieting has generally been in connection with eating disorders like anorexia nervosa or bulimia—with a comparative dearth of formal investigation into dieting as an obesity treatment in children. Authors of diet books for girls in 1980s and 1990s have responded to the backlash to girlish dieting by presenting dieting in a different way, not as a sign of bodily adolescent angst but a symptom of burgeoning "girl power":

You have a right to feel good about your body and yourself. You also have a right to information and knowledge that will give you the *power* to make intelligent changes so you can become healthier and feel happier with your body. Most importantly, you deserve the right to have *control in* [*sic*] *your own life.*[49]

Dieting and feeling happy about one's body, as Dr. Susan of *Dr. Susan's Girls-Only Weight Loss Guide* says here, is a right that all girls have. It is, she suggests, their destiny. Dieting gives a girl power and control. Anthropological studies of girls confirm that girls themselves have taken on dieting as an integral part of *girl culture*. Girls use "fat talk" (conversations revolving around the opening gambit of "I'm so fat," inviting their friends to jump in and contradict them) as ways of solidifying their friendship group. Dieting has become a form of girlish bonding that publishers of child diet books have increasingly appealed to. Ironically for the socially excluded fat child, becoming a dieter could offer links within their peer group.[50]

But with childhood obesity increasing in both sexes since at least the 1970s, gendering child dieting raises more issues. The dominance of the energy balance idea in understanding childhood obesity at the close of the twentieth century meant that dietary regulation is seen as a critical element in addressing the increasing rates of the condition. But would fat boys be willing to regulate their eating habits when dieting is considered a "girl thing"?

The worry that obese boys may not want to regulate their eating because they see dieting as effeminate may explain why some recent child diet books have been written to target an audience of boys. Cullen Meyer, author of *I was a Teenage Loser (You Can be One, Too)* (2007) tells of how he was obese, but successfully changed his eating pattern and exercised to slim down because he wanted to further his acting ambitions. As a newly slim, attractive, cool teen, he has been signed with a talent agency, does modeling, and has performed in music videos. Similarly, Jonathan Scott, formerly fat author of *Off the Scales: A Battle to Beat Teenage Obesity* (2009), dieted, exercised, and muscled up to become a bodybuilding champion and fitness instructor. Both strongly reject the girly "diet" book moniker: "I never went on a diet. I simply chose to make an eating lifestyle change."[51]

Girls might diet, but boys like Meyer and Scott "make eating lifestyle changes." The rationales for weight loss that Meyer and Scott present to boys—looking more attractive, being more popular, and being empowered to achieve life goals—are the same appeals being made to girls in recent girl diet books. But these boy diet books also feature before-and-after pictures of the author, which is *never* the case with recent girl diet books. Publishers are much more wary in an eating-disorder conscious world of suggesting that girls ought to study pictures of models and aim to look like them, but this reticence appears not to apply with the same force to the budding variety of boy diet books.

———————

Where do parents fit in the prescriptions of child diet books? By dealing with the issue of family meals and activities, child diet books involved themselves in the complex interaction within the family. But the assumptions that such books made about how the parent related to their fat child, and vice versa, changed over the fifty years of child dieting, as did how the diet book author sought to talk to parents. Some earlier child dieting books directly addressed parents and suggested that parents would need to take charge of the child's weight loss. Fat camp director Gussie Mason in her 1975 book, *Help Your Child Lose Weight and Keep it Off*, suggested that a child might not have noticed his or her weight, so parents had to subtly impel their teen toward wanting to diet, using the parents' control over the household and over money:

> Hang a few full-length mirrors around the house. There's nothing like a good hard look at themselves to convince children that it's time to take off weight. The girl who tells herself she's just "pleasingly plump" and the boy who thinks that he's just a little "huskier" than his friends can get a rude shock when they are confronted by their mirror image.[52]

Or . . .

> Go for a little shopping trip. The pleasingly plump girl who tries to buy a bathing suit will discover faster than words can convey that there's nothing pleasant about being overweight. The young man who pictures himself in a pair of dungarees and then discovers that the only pants that fit him would look better on his grandfather will be ready and eager to lose weight.[53]

In contrast to the view Mason took that parents would be the ones to initiate their teen's weight loss, other diet books of the same era advocated a less interventionist, more supportive role for parents. Lester David in *Slimming for Teens* (1966), which was also based on the program at a fat camp, advised parents of overweight teens that "they [the children] need *Love*. They need *Listening* to their problems. They need sensible *Limits*. And they need to be *Let Go*—that is, they must not be treated like babies." Still other diet books were far harsher about the parents' responsibility in having caused the child's obesity in the first place, and expressed frustrations over what they saw as excessively permissive parenting. "Stick to your guns and your healthy habits," remonstrated pediatrician and diet book author Alvin Eden, "and remember that parents who truly love their children *do not* demonstrate their love by overfeeding them . . . It's time for the parents to assume their responsibilities." Early child diet books therefore suggested different parenting styles to accompany their dietary recommendations, from Mason's knowing authoritarian, to Lester's companionate supporter, to Eden's firmly authoritative parent.[54]

Not all child diet books delivered their advice to parents directly to the parent, however. While some books did write directly for the parent, either because the whole book was meant to be read by parents or because there was a special section for parents to read, other books left the task of educating the parents up to the child dieter, and gave tips on how she could handle this. The child might, for example, sit down with her mother and go through the dietary recommendations together. She could even help out with the shopping and the cooking. If this was too threatening for the child to do, Dr. Susan, for example, recommended young dieters write down what they needed to tell their parents:

> I know it can be tough to talk to your mom (or dad or grandparent) about making changes, but you really need to do your best to speak to them directly. If you're not sure what to say, write it out and even read it to them. However, if it really is too difficult to describe what you need, below is a "fill in the blank" letter you can rewrite (by hand or on the computer) and then give to your parents to help them understand the changes you'd like to make in your eating.[55]

"Dear Mom/Dad," went the letter. "Lately I have been thinking about the eating patterns in our family. I realize now that our family has a 'clean the plate' approach to eating . . ."[56]

In all child diet books until recently, the authors—like Dr. Susan or Ruth West or David Lester or Gussie Mason or Alvin Eden—assumed that parents were potentially willing and able to help, but simply did not know how to do so. Together, the child and the diet book would educate the parents, with child and parents happily becoming partners in improving the child's health. Since about 2000, however, diet books addressed to children have suggested that there may be complications with this ideal child-parent conversation. Parents may not infallibly "come to the party" and help a child diet, these books suggest. Children may need to acknowledge that their parents have been culpable in causing their fatness and may not be happy to change family habits. The diet book tries to prepare children for this disappointing assessment of their parents:

> Pretend that I'm whispering this to you so your parents and teachers won't hear: you've grown up with bad nutrition, and now that's all you know. A lot of what you've been taught at home and at school is misleading, incorrect, and making you fat or, in a lot of cases, obsessed with dieting and getting thin.[57]

That adult figures can be disappointments and the partnership model of parental cooperation may not be possible has become increasingly part of the dieting book lexicon in the past two decades. The books counsel that, if co-opting parents as allies has failed, then children may have to take charge of their dieting and health for themselves:

> If your parents become angry or hurt by your request, you won't be able to get them to support the changes you want to make. This is part of growing up—sometimes you have to rely only on yourself to become a healthier person—physically and even emotionally. This is true in all areas; it's not just about eating and it's not just about your body. Sometimes your parents can help you, and sometimes they can't. Ultimately, it is up to you to make sure you are happy and healthy.[58]

Dieting books from about 2000 onward have therefore reflected a less optimistic view of parenting than earlier dieting books and a less supportive interaction between the parent and the fat child. In keeping with broader trends toward seeing childhood obesity as a sign of societal failure (see Part III), parenting failure has been increasingly regarded as a contributor that diet books have aimed to deal with. Children, such recent diet books suggest, need to become personally responsible for their health from a younger age.

The growing sense that adults, while powerful, could not always be relied upon is not just a phenomenon in dieting books for children, but appears in other areas of children's popular culture as well. Consider, for example, the Harry Potter novels or the Percy Jackson series—both best-selling series for preteens and teens by British and American authors, respectively.[59] In these books, the adult characters are hugely influential, sometimes caring, although not demonstratively so, sometimes petty and punitive, but unable or unwilling to protect the child characters. With little advice from the grown-ups, the children—Harry, Hermione, Ron, Percy, Grover, Annabeth—are thrown back on their own devices to save the day. In children's pop culture of the new century, from literature to dieting books, adults may not help the children they are ostensibly responsible for. Parents, say children's novels and diet books, can be a disappointment and will not always help in the battle against monsters—or fat.[60]

———————

Child diet book writers currently find themselves dealing with complex public sentiments about their offerings. Working in favor of diet books are factors such as the media attention being paid to increasing rates of childhood obesity and the continuing negative social valence of the condition. However, there is a growing backlash against dieting as a means of losing weight. Dieters' own experience, supported by studies, suggests that dieting can help people lose weight in the short term, but that it does not work consistently in the long term. Along with psychological and behavioral factors, there may also be physical aspects that constrain a person's ability to successfully lose weight in the longer term through diet and exercise, such as the "fat cell hypothesis," discussed in Chapter 7. Moreover, dieting fat children may just start them on an endless path of "yo-yo dieting" and weight cycling that is potentially more dangerous to their health than maintaining a steady, even if somewhat heavier, weight. And as a medical response to childhood obesity, diet and exercise have the problem that the results are highly idiosyncratic: some children lose a lot of weight, and others do not. Chalking the difference up to concepts like "motivation" or "drive" or "compliance" is dissatisfying for the medical profession that seeks dependable, scientific cures, and frustrating and angering to people trying to lose weight. Indeed, for the fat acceptance movement—the activist and advocacy movement that, since the late 1960s, has been urging greater social acceptance of fatness—dieting and the dietary industry have been particular flashpoints of contention. The movement's mantra "Health at Every Size" (HAES) is a pointed rejection of dieting.[61]

Dietary doubt and disappointment is also connected with another, quite different response. Since the 1990s, with more children suffering the most extreme degrees of obesity, there has been an increase in one of the most aggressive, most radical medical treatments for the condition: bariatric surgery. Bariatric surgery refers to a number of different surgical procedures, including gastric bypass surgery and gastric banding, that aim to limit a person's caloric intake, either by curbing stomach capacity or by physically limiting the body's opportunity to ingest food. In 1991, the National Institutes of Health advised against performing bariatric surgery on adolescents due to inadequate data from which to assess the safety and efficacy of the procedures and has not since revised that position; nor does the Food and Drug Administration approve the use of gastric banding devices in young people. But in spite of official reserve, rates of bariatric surgery in adolescents have increased since the mid-1990s, with pediatric surgeons and surgical departments developing their own guidelines on when, and how, to perform these procedures on young people. (Bariatric surgery on teens nevertheless forms only a tiny fraction—0.7 percent—of the total number of bariatric surgeries performed each year in the United States.) Concerns about a young person's ability to understand the nature and implications of the operation and worries about restricting nutrient intake in people who are still growing have meant that the various guidelines tend to recommend the operation be only for teens—not younger children—and only when the child's body mass index is over 40. One of the commonly used criteria for when bariatric surgery may be considered for children is when the teen has tried over a period of time to diet and exercise to lose weight and failed. The irregularity of diet-and-exercise success is therefore also tied both to a rejection of obesity as a health issue, and, conversely, to the increase in aggressive medical responses to obesity.[62]

Diet book authors have responded to this difficult situation of dietary ambivalence by increasingly saying that they do not offer child "diets" but rather offer education about healthy lifestyles for the whole family. "Dieting," indeed, advises one children's weight-loss guide, "is a significant risk factor for obesity." The exercise side of the energy equation has also grown in prominence, supported by research studies that emphasize the role of inactivity in childhood obesity. Diet books of the last two decades have increased the proportion of the prescription they dedicate to physical activity alongside food regulation, suggesting a treatment that modifies *both* the intake and the expenditure size of the energy balance equation. Although there is considerable ambivalence about diet books' recommendations as treatments for childhood obesity, the essential energy-balance motivation and the emphasis on individual accountability are strongly upheld. Public sentiment seems to currently favor treatment based on children taking personal responsibility and individual action though both dieting and exercise.[63]

CHAPTER 9

Summer Slimming

Fat Camps as a Diet-and-Exercise Obesity Treatment

> Overweight—slight or quite? America's first weight control camp, Seascape—exclusively for girls 9–18—offers a program proven effective for lasting weight control through a fun-filled summer on a Cape Cod oceanfront estate. Beautiful accommodations on 35-acre estate complete with private beach and pool.
>
> Advertisement for Camp Seascape, *New York Times,* 1975

The apogee of dieting-and-exercise treatment regimes in commercial life and youth culture is undoubtedly the "fat camp." These are summer residential camps that combine controlled diet and dietary education with a program of physical activities to help children and adolescents lose weight. A more polite term is "weight-loss camp," but "fat camp" is the popular culture term, and what children who attend them today call them.[1]

The first fat camp was Camp Seascape, a camp for girls established in 1959 in Brewster, Cape Cod. It was owned and directed by a nutritionist, Penny Peckos, and a pediatrician, John Spargo. Spargo and Peckos formed their business partnership while working at Massachusetts General Hospital in Boston. Peckos herself had been a fat child and teenager and felt that her college education in home economics had helped her slim down in her early twenties. Peckos wanted to start a camp to teach overweight girls the principles of nutrition and exercise that had helped her lose weight. Camp Seascape ran until Peckos's retirement in the late 1970s. Spargo continued to run a different camp in Rhode Island until his retirement in 1983.[2]

Camp Seascape is easily the best documented of all the early fat camps because of the directors' academic and hospital affiliations. In the 1960s and 1970s, Peckos and Spargo arranged with researchers from Harvard's School of Public Health that the campers could be subjects for research looking at childhood obesity. As a consequence, studies on the camp's results were

159

published in medical journals; Peckos herself wrote about the camp. In addition, the Seascape program was used as the model for the diet book *Slimming for Teen-agers*, a 1966 diet book that was, notably, approved by the American Medical Association.[3]

However, the reasons that Camp Seascape is more accessible to historical inquiry than most fat camps of the 1960s and 1970s also made it unusual among fat camps: most fat camps had very little to do with organized medicine. Although some early fat camps were owned and directed by physicians, and all fat camps accredited by the American Camping Association needed a nurse on staff, most directors of fat camps were not (and are not) medically trained. Indeed, the people who founded and ran fat camps represented a similar range of professions as the writers of diet books: a mixture of physicians, allied health professionals, and business people, who often had their own story of successful childhood weight loss to recommend their camp. Gussie Mason, who with her husband Irving ran Camps Stanley and Tahoe, said, that

> she got the idea for a slim-down camp because she was once a fatty (size 16) herself. After months of exercise and eating low-calorie foods—the principles on which she runs her camps—she finally dropped 30 pounds and now fits into a size 10.[4]

Mason, like other former successful dieters who went on to direct fat camps, offered her own slim physique as an advertisement for the success of her program. Like diet books, fat camps have historically been closer to commercial enterprises than medical treatment facilities.[5]

Following Camp Seascape's lead in 1959, a number of fat camps were established in the 1960s in the New England area, such as Clover Lodge (1960), Camp Tahoe (1960), Camp Lakehurst (1963), Camp Stanley (1967), Camp Shane (1968), all in New York state; Camp Camelot (1969) in Pennsylvania; Camp Napanoch (1963) in Wisconsin; and Camp Macabee (1966) in Virginia.[6] New England was where summer camps had originated, being close to the major metropolises and having the sort of woodsy, outdoors environment suited to camping. Directors of fat camps bought former summer camp facilities, country clubs, and inns with large grounds to house the campers and provide activities. Camp Napanoch, for example, took over the former Napanoch Country Club; Clover Lodge was in a skiing inn. A second wave of camps opened in the 1970s; these were more often housed in temporarily rented college dorms than in traditional rural camp locations. Weight Watchers started four camps in the United States in the early 1970s, growing to twelve camps at the height of their camping involvement in the 1980s. Weight Watchers camps offered neighboring but separate facilities for boys and girls. The company withdrew from offering children's summer camps in the 1990s. Most camps took campers from age eight or so up to age eighteen, although some, like Camp Napanoch and Clover Lodge, would take children as young as six.[7]

Of the early camps, Camp Shane, Camp Camelot, Camp La Jolla, and Camp Kingsmont are all still in business. They are run by the original founders, or, in the case of Camp Kingsmont, former campers. Camp directing can also run in families. For example, Tony Sparber, director of New Image Camps, which he established in 1991, is the son of a camping director for Weight Watchers, Mike Sparber. Fat camps are examples of small, often family-run businesses—that ideal of American commercial ingenuity. The high point of weight-loss camps was in the late 1980s, with eighty-eight accredited camps offering weight-loss programs. The number has since declined, due both to the competitive camping environment and the cultural backlash against weight loss camps that took place in the 1980s and 1990s. In 2013, the American Camping Association listed twelve accredited camps offering weight-loss programs.[8]

In organization and philosophy, fat camps drew on two established institutions: the organized summer camp and, to a slightly lesser extent, the finishing school. From each of these institutions, fat camps borrowed administrative and business techniques, physical structure, location, organizational features, and, critically, a philosophy of transformation.

The tradition of summer camps began in the 1860s as a social response to anxieties about urbanization and its effects on children's health and character development. With economic life increasingly centered in the cities and child labor laws in effect, children were no longer released from the school term to work on farms or in factories over the summer and so looked forward to a delightfully long, unoccupied summer vacation. Parents and communities were less keen on this prospect of unstructured leisure: a child might become a delinquent in these long, idle summer months. Summer camps met parental anxieties and ideals for their children on many levels. Campers would have the experience of a small, intimate community of their peers that was increasingly difficult to achieve in city life. Campers would be kept busy with activities that were age-appropriate and innocent amusements. Moreover camping activities were in keeping with the popular vision of idealized childhood—and specifically *American* childhood—as a time in which children should enjoy outdoor play in a natural setting. And parents would also have a welcome respite from what was becoming an increasingly intensive and exhausting role.[9]

There was also a particular health aim to summer camping. For boys in particular, the time spent in the wilderness was considered beneficial—huntin', shootin', and fishin' as an antidote to the softening wiles of modernity. Sending boys camping removed them from the supposed coddling of their mothers at home, bucked them up in the company of other boys and male counselors, and gave them the backbone needed for modern manliness. Camping also was thought to improve children's physical health. For summer camps before about 1940, one of the signs of the healthfulness of the camping experience was that children would come home having gained weight. One camper, reflecting on how camp had changed him, wrote, "I am now a healthy boy who gained a lot of weight and looks very brown."[10]

Although starting a century after the first organized summer camps, fat camps drew on the camping tradition of virile healthfulness. While there were more fat camps established for girls, camps catering to overweight boys, like Camps Macabee, Tahoe, and Kingsmont, were set up from the mid-1960s onward. But while summer camps of the earlier twentieth century had helped thin city children put *on* weight, fat camps used the same healthful rural environment to take weight *off* fat city children. Both types of camps were based on the idea that the child's normal, modern urban environment was unhealthy and that the proper environment for children was outdoors. (That children properly "belonged" outside was based on the eighteenth-century belief that children were natural and innocent—a belief illustrated in saccharin Enlightenment, Romantic, and Victorian sentimental art showing children in gardens with baby animals or flowers.) Camping—both fat and otherwise—drew on the belief that placing the child in the wilderness would restore the child to a harmonious, healthful state. The location of the camp (rural, often next to a lake that could be used for water sports) and the activities done at camp therefore functioned as medicine.[11]

So while the first fat camps of the 1950s and 1960s were a new type of summer camp in the sense that they offered a weight-loss program, in another sense they were a pure expression of organized camping's essential motivation—to take a child and improve him or her in health, character, and appearance. Children had long been expected to go to summer camp and come home a different person from the one who had left eight weeks earlier: healthier and with a more mature, robust character. Fat camps epitomized the transformative promise of summer camp. As one camp's slogan put it: "Become a new girl at Camp Murietta."[12]

––––––––––

Fat camps achieved the level of popularity that they did because they seemed to offer a solution to all the different aspects of childhood obesity that had developed by the mid- to later twentieth century. Fat camps incorporated the diet-and-exercise energy-balance model *and* also the psychological and environmental ideas of obesity causation that had become part of the obesity picture since the 1940s. Notably, taking the fat child away from his or her family environment was part of the weight-loss prescription.

Significantly, fat camps also introduced the idea that fatness in a child was a problem caused by modern life: cities, suburbs, and fast food. The fat camp's implied treatment was to put the fat child in a rustic, less tantalizing environment. This element of childhood obesity that fat camps introduced—childhood obesity as modern malaise—is one that would go on to become increasingly prominent and referred to in the epidemic of childhood obesity in recent decades (see Chapter 10.)

On the diet front, calorie-restricted diets were standard features of early fat camps, along with nutrition education sessions, often conducted by nutritionists employed by the camp. The details of the camps' approach to diet varied, though. Some offered menus of 1,200 calories per day—about 1,000 calories less than a maintenance diet, and which, in theory, should result in a weight loss of two pounds per week. Others followed a dietary program in which some foods were "allowed" and other foods were "restricted"—essentially a form of portion control or calorie counting. Camp Seascape, for one, made a point of having occasional candy treats so that the campers could learn to include these in moderation in their usual routines. The directors Peckos and Spargo were aware, however, that the girls at the camp were smuggling in extra candy, and the housekeeping staff would find wrappers tucked into the bed frames. When the house where the camp had been held was renovated in the 1990s, a cache of old candy wrappers was found underneath the floorboards of one of the upstairs bedrooms.[13]

For exercise, swimming, archery, horseback riding, boating, wrestling, badminton, baseball, tennis, football, fencing, dance, golf, volleyball, walking, gym, and racquetball were some of the activities offered at fat camps. The sheer range of activities on offer was a major selling point in the camps' advertisements. Peckos and Spargo, for example, advertised the fact that Camp Seascape was within walking distance to the sea and so offered premium activities like waterskiing and deep-sea diving. The activities were intended to provide unstructured exercise for the campers. In the 1980s, some girls' camps added aerobics to the offerings—Camp Shane used Jane Fonda's workout tapes. At Camp Tahoe for boys, Gussie Mason had the campers do the "Tahoe Trot" (that is, jog) between activities. (At the sister camp, Camp Stanley, they did the "Stanley Trot.") Gussie had also patented her "secret weapon" in her "war on fat"—the "beautiboot." These were "isometric exercise boots," which were essentially small beanbags enclosing two pounds of dried peas, tied onto a person's ankles using ribbons and worn for doing leg exercises. Gussie had thought of the idea from noticing that ice-skaters had, as she described, "beautiful legs." Campers could be exercising or doing physical activities for up to six hours a day. Rest periods, meal breaks, and occasional cultural excursions filled out the highly structured routine.[14]

On the psychological treatment front, taking the child out of his or her home environment—the "family frame" as Hilde Bruch would have called it, or, as Gussie Mason referred to it, the "fat environment"—and putting them into an environment that was conducive to losing weight was also an essential part of the fat camp approach. Fat camps of the 1950s through to the 1970s did not offer day camp options—staying at the camp for the full eight-week season was part of the program. In additional, the camps claimed to offer children a supportive community:

The psychology behind a slim-down camp, Mrs. Mason said, is that it allows fat children who are generally poor in sports and self-conscious about their appearance in play clothes and bathing suits to be with others who are in the same boat. As a result, she said, they tend to gain self-confidence when they realize that no one is laughing at them.[15]

Overweights rarely plunge into contact sports. Horsing around in the pool, wrestling and ball games with other boys in the same fat fix give youngster new self-confidence—in addition to good exercise.[16]

Camp directors reasoned that fat children were more likely to enjoy physical activities if they were in an environment where they didn't have to compete with slimmer, more athletic children. They therefore presented their fat camp as a psychologically "safe zone" for fat children. John Spargo of Camp Seascape expressed a crueler interpretation: "misery likes company, it's that type of thing."[17]

In the 1970s and 1980s, directors of fat camps added counseling sessions—both group and individual—to the programming as a way of helping campers investigate the "deeper roots" of their obesity, and added sessions teaching behavioral modification techniques to address snacking, binge eating, using food as a reward, and emotional responses to food. (Camp Shane calls its group counseling sessions "rap sessions.") The combination of diet, exercise, environment, and counseling allowed fat camps to address many of the factors that by midcentury were widely regarded as aspects of childhood obesity.[18]

––––––––––

Along with organized camps, fat camps drew on another established institution—the finishing school—for elements of their program. This was particularly the case for girls' fat camps of the 1960s and 1970s that leveraged campers' desire to look more attractive as part of their program. Camp Seascape used dress size instead of pounds as a way of tracking a girl's weight loss. The facilities at the camp were also specially chosen to be "therapeutic." Penny Peckos explained:

> We didn't want them [the girls] in huts. You don't take a nice big fat girl and put her in the forest and say put on your dungarees and we'll walk and now we're gonna lose weight. You don't do that. We had to find a facility that made her want to look beautiful.[19]

What they settled on was Crosby Mansion—a jewel of late Victorian splendor. Three stories high, it has a portico verandah, seventeen fireplaces, a French salon, and marble-finished bathrooms. With its "beautiful accommodations on 35-acre estate complete with private beach and pool"—ran the advertisement—it was "the perfect place" in which "a fat girl [would] want to look beautiful." At their "season" at Camp Seascape, the girls were required to dress for dinner and were taught grooming skills. Campers were taken for shopping trips in the larger Cape towns, like Hyannis, and visited

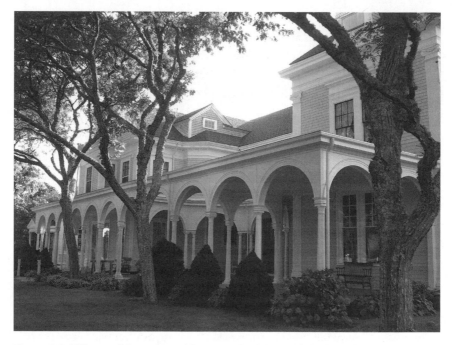

Figure 9.1 Where a "fat girl would want to look beautiful": Crosby Mansion, Brewster, Cape Cod.

historical sites. In the evenings, outings to the theatre in Dennis were some of the entertainment options, along with musical groups who were invited to the camp to give performances, and visiting speakers to give lectures. Although other girls' camps did go the hut-and-tent route, they also offered programming that emphasized weight loss for appearance's sake: "charm workshops" in which girls would "discuss makeup, poise, posture, voice and wardrobe planning," and "Glamour Week" climaxing in a shopping trip for new clothes "a few sizes smaller, they hope," a hairdo, and a fashion show for which the girls were the models.[20]

The effects of camps' weight loss programs on campers' weight were closely monitored, with at least once-weekly weigh-ins. Camp director Gussie Mason referred to the Sunday weighing-in session as "meeting the monster." For camps, the weighing-in functioned as an incentive and reward, and could also cause keen disappointment. One camp director recalled seeing girls dancing and cheering if their weigh-in showed they had lost weight—and girls crying when they had not lost weight or had not lost as much as they had hoped. Many summer camps used rituals of camp life, such as badges or certificates for achievement, to mark a camper's passage through the camp and their growth as a person. For fat camps, the weigh-in served a similar purpose of marking out the camper's transformation.[21]

Fat camps are a highly affecting topic. Attending camp, both now and in the past, can be something that the child really wants to do, in which case it can offer great hope, but it can also cause great unhappiness, especially when attending is solely the parents' idea or when the program is harsh. The contrast between the Arcadian fantasy of summer camp and the idea that a child would go (or be sent) to a camp to lose weight, combined with social discomfort about fatness made (and makes) fat camps enthralling. Popular culture is fascinated with the fat camp.[22]

The image fat camps have is of a boot camp, where fat children who don't want to be there are starved of decent food and made to run by order-barking drill sergeants. *South Park* and *The Simpsons* cartoon series have shown celebrated episodes in which the main characters attend boot camp–like fat camps and lampoon well-recognized and nostalgic characteristics of summer camps—the cheery camp director, the poetic camp name ("Camp Hopeful Hills," "Serenity Ranch"), camp food, and campfire singing. *Heavyweights*, a 1995 movie, shows campers fighting against having to exercise and wanting to keep the camp as a protected place for fat kids. *Fat Camp Commandoes*, a children's novel, is narrated by Ralph Nebula who along with his sister Sylvia is sent to Camp Noo Yoo when his parents are seduced by a motivational speaker. The camp is run by Richard "Dick" Tator, so you can see where the author is going with this:

> Noo Yoo is a fat camp. The campers wear three layers of sweatsuits when they play softball, to sweat off those pounds. There are compulsory aerobics three times a day. There are Creative Abuse and Motivation classes three nights a week. There are special diet meals—(remember those shredded carrots and raisins?) The idea is that Mommy and Daddy's pudgy darling goes off to camp a little butterball, and comes back a fashion model. This has never happened once, but people send their kids anyway.[23]

These angry leitmotifs of the fat camp are partly based on criticisms of the camps that arose especially from the 1980s onward. Fat camps were criticized for emphasizing appearance too heavily and contributing to children becoming obsessed with their looks. Moreover, the very fact that camp was a special environment away from home—something that many camp directors felt was *beneficial* to children's weight loss—was censured for being too artificial, too different to achieve realistic reeducation of the child's habits. Some former fat campers also described having horrendous experiences— one girl who attended Camp Murietta in the 1970s described it as "like being in a concentration camp."[24]

Anecdotal evidence suggested that while the camps were successful in getting children to lose weight at the camp, children rapidly regained the weight once they were home again. Some camps sought to address this problem by extending the reach of the camp beyond the end of the eight-week summer session, through talks and education sessions with parents, follow-up sessions, and discussions about how campers could continue to diet in the face of real-world pressures of parties and school cafeteria food. Today's camps use the Internet—chat rooms, social networking, blogs, and e-mail—to maintain contact with campers after the camp is over.[25]

Camps were also criticized for trying to get children to lose very large amounts of weight very rapidly. It was common for fat camps of the 1960s and 1970s to suggest in their advertisements that campers could achieve an *average* weight loss in the order of twenty to forty-five pounds in eight weeks. By contrast, the orthodox medical position of the time was reticent about suggesting growing children *lose* weight and recommended losses of no more than one or two pounds per week.[26]

And camps were expensive. Adjusted for inflation, they have become even more so since the 1960s. For example, Camps Tahoe and Stanley operating in the late 1960s charged $830, which is about $5,370 in today's dollars. The average eight-week session cost for a fat camp today is in the order of $8,000. Since 2007, there have been some experiments in establishing not-for-profit camps, but the fees are in the order of $6,000 for six weeks— still a substantial investment. Fat camps therefore attracted (and continue to attract) middle- and upper-class families who could afford the high fees. That parents will spend that amount of money illustrates their keen hope that the camp will live up to its transformatory promise.[27]

―――――

Like child diet book writers, fat camp directors also currently face complex popular sentiments about their approach and have responded in similar ways to concerns about child dieting. Fat camps increasingly advertise that they do not offer "diets" but rather offer education about healthy lifestyles. ("At Camp La Jolla, we don't believe in diets—we believe in long-term weight loss success through a healthy lifestyle.") Some fat camps, too, are taking a whole-family approach to "healthy lifestyles," offering options of two- to four-week camps and day camps for the whole family to try to deal with that post-Hilde Bruch idea that the family environment needs to be addressed, not just the one child's habits.[28]

Evidence of how successful fat camps are as weight-loss treatments is difficult to find or evaluate. Camp Seascape was unusual in this respect because the directors invited researchers from the Harvard School of Public Health and the Boston Children's Hospital to collect data on their weight-loss program. The results indicated that the girls had indeed lost fat and gained muscle. Weight losses were between 6.6 to 34.2 pounds and were on average 14.2 pounds. From follow-up studies, it seems about 40 percent of Seascape campers maintained their weight losses. Other camps claimed in their advertising that between 75 and 82 percent of campers kept the weight off; director Tony Sparber of Camp Poconos Trails estimates—perhaps more realistically—"It's a 50–50 chance that they keep it off." More recent formal studies confirm that camps achieve weight losses and psychological improvements over the course of the camp, but the persistence of the losses is highly variable.[29]

If anything, the energy-balance response to childhood obesity and its commercialization—the diet books, the fat camps—has become more and more popular as childhood obesity rates have increased. In 2004, Wellspring Camps opened a new, more intensive venture in the fat camp model: a year-round boarding school for overweight children. The Academy of the Sierras (now Wellspring Academies) operates campuses in California and North Carolina, using diet, exercise, and psychological approaches to weight loss. Tuition is a hefty $6,250 per month, and students attend for a minimum of four months.[30]

A market perspective would suggest that the commercial viability of places like Wellspring Academies or of summer fat camps in general is simply a matter of supply increasing to meet an increasing demand. But this begs the question—why the increasing demand for child weight-loss treatments? That is the subject of the next chapter.

PART 3

Epidemic

CHAPTER 10

Bigger Bodies in a Broken World

Television and the Epidemic of Childhood Obesity

> It wasn't easy to produce a generation of overfed kids—but it
> might well have been inevitable.
>
> *Time* magazine, 2008

In 1985, William Dietz of the Centers for Disease Control
and Steven Gortmaker from Harvard's School of Public Health presented a
paper to the American Pediatric Society on their analysis of national survey
data. They had used skinfold measurements collected since the 1960s to
look at the prevalence of childhood obesity. What they found was that the
proportion of overweight children had nearly doubled over that time. "These
data," they concluded, "indicate that obesity is epidemic in the pediatric
population." Dietz and Gortmaker's statement, and particularly their choice
of the word "epidemic," marked the beginning of a massive increase in public
anxiety about the prevalence of the condition.[1]

Since Gortmaker and Dietz announced their findings, more research has
been done to interrogate the data and to describe the childhood obesity
epidemic in greater detail. The increased prevalence has been found to be
population-wide but more concentrated in some racial groups than others:
increases in obesity rates have been highest for Native American, African
American, and Hispanic children. However, the patterning by socioeconomic group that is seen in adults—where poorer adults are fatter than
wealthier adults—seems not to be the case with childhood obesity in recent
decades. (For example, African American girls from wealthy families are
more likely to be obese than those from poorer families.) The complex patterning by socioeconomic standing and ethnicity shows that, in childhood,
the effects of economics, culture, and biology are not clear-cut.[2]

The big increase in childhood obesity over the space of one generation
was far too short a time span for the culprit to be genetic change. The causes
of the epidemic therefore had to be environmental, and, historically speaking,

173

recent. Although there was some indication that rates of childhood obesity had been slowly increasing since the 1930s, something had changed in the American lifestyle since the 1960s that was quickly making more children fat, and then even fatter.

Childhood obesity researchers, public health activists, and the media have since developed a litany of causal factors. Too much soda drinking; agricultural subsidies promoting cheap corn syrup sweetening; neighborhoods without safe outdoor play spaces or without sidewalks so that children can walk to school; the lure of sedentary activities like television and computer games; government cutbacks in physical education classes in schools; too much homework replacing active playtime; too many unhealthy meals eaten out of the home; indulgent parents giving too many sweet treats and car rides to school or failing to notice their child was beyond puppy fat; junk-food advertisers and manufacturers influencing children to eat unhealthy foods and beverages; poor families buying food that offered many calories for a low cost, as a way of saving money; ethnic groups tolerating high degrees of fatness. Each of these factors has been the subject of medical investigation as to its contribution to the condition. Whether in a popular magazine or newspaper or in a scholarly article, a list like this is de rigueur for any piece on childhood obesity.[3]

Taken together, these factors illustrate a new dimension being added to how childhood obesity is understood: childhood obesity as a symptom of social and cultural failure—failure in globalized corporate capitalism; failure in family interactions; failure in race relations, indeed, the failure of modernity itself. This is all the more troubling since the epidemic comes at the end of a century in which healthy living has become entrenched in American culture as an ideal and is considered a reflection of personal striving and achievement. The epidemic of childhood obesity is understood as both an indicator and a product of failed or failing social conditions.[4]

Complicating this portrayal of the epidemic is a bittersweet feeling that modernity, with all its great achievements, is inherently unnatural and unsuited to how we have evolved. This portrayal rests on the "thrifty genotype" hypothesis, so named by its originator, James Neel, a population geneticist who developed the theory in 1962. Neel proposed the thrifty genotype theory to explain why diabetes was so prevalent in modern societies when, being a debilitating condition affecting people before reproductive maturity, it ought to have been bred out over time. Neel hypothesized that the diabetic had a "thrifty" genotype "in the sense of being exception-ally efficient in the intake and/or utilization of food." That thriftiness would convey a survival benefit on him "during the first 99 per cent or more of man's life on earth, while he existed as a hunter and gatherer, [and when] it was often feast or famine." The diabetic genotype therefore had not been bred out because, once upon a time, it was a survival advantage. The diffi-culty was that the environment had changed and the diabetic genotype's survival advantage didn't apply any more.[5]

Neel's "thrifty gene" idea was extended to obesity and has been popularly seized upon as apparently accounting for the obesity epidemic. Modern humans would be the descendants of people who survived and prospered because they could get fat easily and quickly when the circumstances were favorable. Unfortunately, runs the reasoning, our paleolithic bodies are ill-suited to an environment where there are cheap calories for sale at the 7-Eleven on the corner and a Dunkin' Donuts on the next street over.[6]

This reasoning about why childhood obesity has become epidemic since the 1980s has a ring of inevitability about it. "It wasn't easy to produce a generation of overfed kids," explained *Time* magazine in 2008, "but it might well have been inevitable." Like large-scale agriculture, roads, and anti-biotics, childhood obesity was just another feature of modernity, so the impli-cation runs. You can't have your cake and eat it, too. There is, of course, a problem with this tidy and popular reasoning, as the previous chapters of this book show—although childhood obesity has existed throughout the twentieth century, and has possibly been gradually increasing since the 1930s, it had not reached such massive proportions until, historically speaking, very recently. Even if one accepts the "thrifty gene" idea—which is by no means the case for all geneticists—it still remains that our ancient, paleolithically adapted bodies did fine until about the 1970s.[7]

The history of childhood obesity therefore suggests that we should inquire very closely into the particular choices, decisions, and policies shaping American society in the second half of the twentieth century that have fos-tered increases in childhood obesity, not modernity or development per se. This chapter considers one major aspect of recent American culture that has been implicated in the childhood obesity epidemic: television, and espe-cially televised advertising of unhealthy food to children.

Television advertising of unhealthy food to children illustrates certain wider themes that comprise the idea that the childhood obesity epidemic is a symptom of societal failure—the responsibilities of big business (in this case broadcasters, food producers, and advertisers) to society and to their younger clients in particular; the responsibilities (and practicalities) of parents standing sentry over their child's activities and guiding their child's eating habits; and the reality of modern family life, children's leisure, and food-purchasing habits. Both proponents and opponents of televised junk-food advertising to children have couched their arguments in terms of these themes. But the particulars of their arguments have changed over time, refined by virtue of historical experience to become increasingly sophisticated, litigiously aware, and "PR-savvy."

Since television watching became widespread in America in the 1950s, the technology has been something of a whipping boy for concerns about society, and about its impact on childhood and the family in particular. Worries about television have concerned both the *content* of what is shown—even early on, some people were concerned children's socialization and behavior would be affected by "the scantily clad leg and the off-color gag" on vaudeville programming and the "killing[s] with ice-picks, axes, and poison" in cop shows. The nature of television *watching* itself, taking time away from homework or outdoor play or from more complex and socially rewarding interaction with family members, was also a concern.[8]

One of the early responses of the television industry to public worries and a congressional inquiry was, in 1952, to develop a television code. The code was initiated by the industry body, the National Association of Radio and Television Broadcasters (NARTB), and provided guidance to stations on appropriate programming and advertising. In particular, the 1952 television code set out broadcasters' position on their responsibility to child viewers:

> Television, and all who participate in it are jointly accountable to the American public for respect [sic] for the special needs of children, for community responsibility, for the advancement of education and culture, for the acceptability of the program materials chosen, for decency and decorum in production, and for propriety in advertising . . . Parents in particular should be urged to see to it that out of the richness of television fare, the best programs are brought to the attention of their children.[9]

The television code recommended showing no more than twelve minutes of advertising per hour, except in programs that were "women's services, features, shopping guides, market information, and similar material," which could be happily expected to have more advertisements as part of the nature of the program and the audience. Stations were also cautioned to "exercise the utmost care and discrimination with regard to advertising material, including content, placement and presentation, near or adjacent to programs designed for children." The NARTB's television code board would adjudicate on complaints against code stations. It had the option of censuring stations by disallowing them from displaying the NARTB "Seal of Good Practice" in their publications.[10]

By promising that they would self-regulate, the television broadcasting industry stayed congressional action that might have monitored television more closely. In particular, this experience established a recurring pattern for how government and broadcasters dealt with public complaints against the industry: government would threaten intervention, industry would promise to "do better," and government would grant the industry the chance to demonstrate that they could handle the matter through self-regulation.

———————

The issue of regulating television for reasons to do with children's physical health came to a head in 1977 when a group of children's television activist organizations petitioned the Federal Trade Commission (FTC) to ban candy advertisements during children's programs. The saga of hearings that the petition led to, referred to as the "Kid-Vid" episode, stands as a signal event in the history of attempts to protect child health through government intervention.

The hearings had a lengthy background. Since the late 1960s, a coalition of activist groups including Action for Children's Television (ACT), founded by Peggy Charren; the Center for Science in the Public Interest (CSPI), headed by Michael F. Jacobson; and the Council for Children, Media and Merchandising (CMMM), founded and directed by Robert Choate, had been attempting to have government regulate children's television more closely. The groups wanted regulations to require more educational programming for children and to limit—preferably ban—advertising during children's programs.[11]

Children were, in the late 1960s, just beginning to become an independent commercial force. Increasingly since that time, children began to have considerable sums of money of their own to spend and so became consumers in their own right, as well as influencing parental purchases. (One scholar of child consumers calculated that children's spending has risen from $2.2 million in 1968 to more than $35.6 million in 2000, and that children exert an additional $290 billion in "kidfluence" over adult spending as well.) As a consequence, advertisers increasingly targeted children.[12]

The activist groups opposed this trend: childhood, the groups contended, should be a time protected from the full onslaught of consumerism. They objected to advertising strategies like that outlined by the director of children's programming for one Chicago television station: "if you truly want big sales, you will use the child as your assistant salesman. He sells, he nags, until he breaks down the sales resistance of his mother or father."[13]

And, further, the groups were critical of the nature of the products advertised to children—they had conducted a study and found that 80 percent of advertisements on children's Saturday morning television were for highly sugared cereals, candy, soda, and other nutritionally poor foods. Robert Choate of the Council for Children Media and Merchandising (CCMM) became famous in 1970 when he testified to the Senate Commerce Subcommittee that most breakfast cereals were simply "empty calories"—a provocative description because it had previously been applied only to alcohol. Eating the *box* with milk and raisins, said Choate, was healthier than eating the cereal inside it, and he had data to prove it. (Sixteen months later, cereal manufacturers had reformulated most of their products to be more nutritious.) Intriguingly, given later events, Choate had, in February 1971, proposed a "code for advertising edibles." He proposed that only foods that exceeded a certain nutritional standard could be advertised to children, but this idea was roundly rejected by the food industry, the advertising agencies, and the broadcasting association.[14]

The activist groups had, at various times, petitioned the Federal Communications Commission (FCC) and the FTC to improve the educational content and cut advertising on children's television, but without notable results. Their 1977 petition to the FCC was different, however: they singled out food advertising to children, specifically candy advertising, and linked it not only to ideological issues about protecting childish innocence but also, this time, to medical harms. "The purpose of the [proposed] rule," said ACT, "is to remedy a medical problem."[15]

And the main medical problem they had in mind was *tooth decay.*[16]

Candy advertisements to children had caused "pandemic levels of tooth decay in this country," alleged the groups' petition to the FTC. The American Dental Association also wrote in support. Moreover, the groups argued that research showed that "children are extremely susceptible to . . . advertising appeals, and lack the cognitive ability to decipher or evaluate the risks involved in consuming sugar." Candy commercials were, the ACT petitioned, "deceptive within Section 5 of the Federal Trade Commission Act because they have the capacity to mislead the child into believing that the consumption of these candies produces pleasure not potential tooth decay." Accepting the petition, the FTC issued notice in 1978 that they would hold hearings to take comments on a ban or other restrictions on food advertising to children. An inquiry would be held and a ruling restricting food advertising to children was a possibility.[17]

The response by food producers, broadcasters, and advertising agencies was concerned and massive. Just a single network—ABC—had an estimated $600 million in advertising revenue at stake if a full ban on advertising food to children was instituted. As the activist groups worked together to develop a common stance, so too did the industry groups. Industry's basic position was that government regulation of sugary food advertising to children was unnecessary and industry self-regulation was sufficient.[18]

To develop the details of the strategy, over forty-five representatives from food manufacturing, broadcasting, and advertising companies met at the National Association of Broadcasters (NAB) headquarters in Washington. Representatives from the four broadcast networks, and the American Association of Advertising Agencies, the American Advertising Federation, the Association of National Advertisers, the United States Chamber of Commerce, the Grocery Manufacturers Association, the Cereal Institute, the National Soft Drink Association, and the Foodservice and Lodging Institute were in attendance, along with their lawyers. Their combined efforts in combating the activist petitions were being funded by a "war chest"—alleged by *Broadcasting Magazine* to be $2 million and by the *Washington Star* as being between $15 and $30 million—culled from increased membership dues and donations.[19]

The strategy that the industry representatives developed was threefold. On one front, they would fight a public relations battle in the media against regulating children's advertising. To do this, they hired a public relations firm, Burson-Marsteller, which had a reputation for handling situations where the public was likely to be strongly opposed. (Burson-Marsteller had, for example, represented Nigeria's Ministry of Information in its campaign against allegations of genocide in the late 1960s, and, after the Three Mile Island nuclear reactor accident shortly after the FTC hearings, Burson-Marsteller represented the reactor's construction company.) On the second front, a "big thrust" at the Congressional Commerce and Appropriations Committees would apply political pressure to have the FTC's budget cut. And on the third front, alliances of advertisers, broadcasters, and food producers took the FTC to court with pre-hearing actions seeking to have the hearings dropped because of the stringent evidentiary requirements the FTC had set. In a separate legal action, the industry groups sought to have the chairman of the FTC, Michael Pertshuck, removed from chairing the hearings. Pertshuck was considered biased toward making a ruling on advertising to children—F. Kent Mitchell, a vice president at General Foods, referred to him as the "sparkplug" of the FTC "engine" that needed "taking out." Pertshuck was removed, later reinstated, and then voluntarily stood aside for the hearings. The FTC also agreed to lessen the evidentiary requirements on witnesses. With the court challenges dealt with, the hearings were free to proceed.[20]

Two rounds of public hearings on advertising sugared foods to children took place, one in January and the other in March of 1979. The early days of the hearings were a media storm. The activist groups delivered a bag of decayed teeth to the FTC offices. The Grocery Manufacturers Association brought in a shopping cart of groceries "typically consumed by the American youngster" that could not be advertised if the proposed ban were upheld. Seymour Banks, the vice president of advertising agency Leo Burnett and a font of irascible opinions, spoke about parents' responsibility when their child pestered them for an advertised product:

> What harm is there in that? Even if, as many psychologists claim, a child perceives children in TV advertisements as friends, and not actors selling them something, where's the harm? All a parent has to say is, "Shut up or I'll belt you."[21]

Representative Fred Richmond (D-NY) claimed that the "unholy alliance of Madison Avenue, the television networks, and food manufacturers that is currently besieging the FTC with a high priced, three-piece-suited

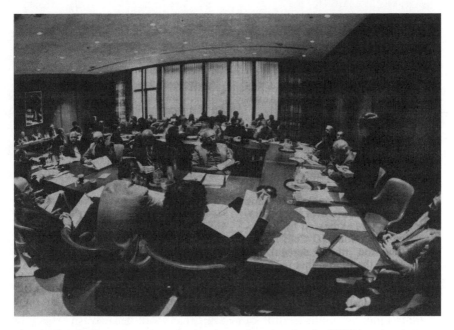

Figure 10.1 Industry strategy meeting in preparation for the FTC hearing into advertising sugary products to children.
Source: "War-Gaming on the Ad-Ban." *Broadcasting,* 13 March 1978, 23.

legion of lawyers" killed any congressional action to improve the nutritional quality of foods advertised to children. A stenographer fainted during "a heated exchange" between the chairman of the hearings and the director of marketing for General Mills. For the first week of proceedings, the "Kid-Vid" hearings, as they became known, were *the* Washington media event.[22]

The arguments presented by both sides in the Kid-Vid saga ranged wide. Did children understand what advertisements were trying to do, asked the FTC? *No,* said the activist groups, citing especially a study by Scott Ward from the Harvard Business School that found only 7 percent of children between five and fifteen years old understood that commercials aimed to "get people to buy the product." *Yes,* said the industry groups, also, ironically, citing Ward's study, which had also found that even very young children could "tell the difference" between commercials and programs. (The two sides were exploiting the subtle variation in Ward's questions—there were two parts to his study, one seeing if children could *define* a commercial and the other seeing if they could define the *intent* of a commercial. Industry emphasized the former, the activist groups the latter.) The activist forces also referred to studies showing that children would ask for and choose foods that they had seen advertised, regardless of the type of food it was— advertising was so persuasive that children would choose vegetables if those were advertised to them on television. The industry forces countered with studies that asked parents about how well they felt their children understood commercials. The interview-based studies had found that parents rated their children as being much more understanding and critical of advertising than observational studies of children indicated.[23]

On the medical front, the activist position was that advertising highly sugared food products to children, in such frequency and without showing the negative health consequences, was deceptive. The result, said activist and public health witnesses, was that industry made money while children suffered health problems. The surgeon general testified as to the dental dangers of foods high in sugar. In a forerunner of later battles, the Massachusetts commissioner for public health pointed out that tooth decay wasn't the only child health problem associated with advertising such products:

> A second but equally serious health hazard associated with these child-directed, advertised foods is that of obesity . . . Children are told approximately 20 times a day that they should consume food products which offer them little but calories.[24]

Industry countered by calling dentists as witnesses who pointed out that tooth decay was caused by many factors, not just sugar. Personal dental hygiene, the food's stickiness, food and drink combinations—all affected whether a person might develop a cavity. And even if highly sugared products *did* cause cavities—which industry by no means conceded—industry witnesses also argued that it "is an American right . . . to be able to buy what you want."[25]

By the second round of Kid-Vid hearings in March 1979, it was apparent to the participants and the media that the momentum had shifted against a complete ban on ads of highly sugared foods to children. Certain arguments made by the industry coalition had had considerable influence in swaying public, and especially political, opinion. One argument was that, in seeking government regulation of children's television content, parents were just trying to pass off their responsibility, or, put more positively, that government would be intruding on a parent's right to control their child's television exposure. Said Kellogg's lawyer, "The last thing we need . . . is a national nanny." Actor Robert Keeshan, who played Captain Kangaroo in the popular children's television program, also testified on behalf of industry groups: "It saddens me to see more government in the living room."[26]

And, argued the industry coalition, parents' rights were not the only rights at stake: industry's constitutionally given right to commercial free speech was also at risk. In a 1976 Supreme Court case, *Virginia State Board of Pharmacy v. Virginia Citizens Consumer Council,* the presiding judge had ruled that in a capitalist economy it was in the public interest that there be a "free flow of commercial information . . . as to who is producing and selling what product, for what reason, and at what price." Therefore, contrary to prior legal opinion that held that only an individual had a right to free speech, commercial speech was also protected under the First Amendment. The American Civil Liberties Union concurred with the industry groups' constitutional argument, and wrote to the FTC saying that the proposed ban would get them into a "first amendment morass." Protecting children's health could not trump companies' First Amendment rights. (A similar commercial free-speech argument was later used to overturn a 2001 Massachusetts law preventing cigarettes from being advertised close to schools and playgrounds.) These two civil liberties arguments successfully reframed the Kid-Vid debate such that *supporting* a ban on sugary food ads to children would be "against the health and well-being of the American child and family"—where "health and well-being" was construed from a rights perspective, rather than a medical one.[27]

On the political front, congressional sentiment was swayed by arguments that regulating children's advertising would cause advertising and product cost increases—an extremely effective argument with the 1970s inflation crisis in full swing and severely damaging the Carter administration. Moreover, the industry coalition had successfully portrayed the FTC as arrogantly usurping Congress's role and "running away with making new laws."[28]

The result was that President Carter was maneuvered into signing Congress's Federal Trade Commission Improvements Act in May 1980. This amended the act, proscribing the FTC's powers such that,

> The Commission shall not have any authority to promulgate any rule in the children's advertising proceeding . . . or in any substantially similar

proceeding on the basis of a determination by the Commission that such advertising constitutes an unfair act or practice in or affecting commerce.

The FTC could still rule on *deceptive* advertising to children, but not *unfair* advertising to children. Unfairness was, however, central to the activist argument. (Advertising sugary cereals to children was unfair since they couldn't understand the intent of the ads nor the implications of eating so much sugary fare.) The amendment decimated what arguments the activist side could present to the FTC, and, with the change of government to President Reagan's deregulatory stance, the FTC discontinued the Kid-Vid inquiry. Tooth decay had been an insufficient medical reason for regulating advertising to children when it was matched against the powerful constitutional and rights-based arguments presented by the industry coalition.[29]

In the 2000s the "new" disease in town—childhood obesity—revitalized calls for restricting junk-food advertising to children and encouraged the FTC to reenter the fray. Comparing the 1970s tooth decay argument for restricting sugary food advertising with the 2000s obesity arguments for restricting junk-food advertising offers both parallels and contrasts. Both episodes saw health-based arguments used to support restricting advertising, but childhood obesity in the 2000s could provide powerful medical reasons for limiting junk-food ads in ways in which tooth decay in the 1970s could not.

For the one part, obesity could justify calls to limit advertisements of more than just sugary foods—the condition could also justify limits on high-fat, high-cholesterol food as well. Obesity therefore provided a rationale for a much wider limitation on advertising to children that appealed to activist groups opposed to the commercialization of childhood in general. (Two of the principal activist groups at the 1970s hearings, ACT and CMMM had, however, disbanded; CSPI had grown and had continued its interest in food marketing.)[30]

Moreover, public sentiment toward vast companies was different in the 2000s compared with the 1970s. The legacies of litigation against "Big Tobacco," Eric Schlosser's book *Fast Food Nation* (2001), and Morgan Spurlock's documentary *SuperSize Me* (2003) had each contributed to a cultural change toward people being more cynical about "Big Food" and more aware of the ways in which companies used advertising to manipulate children's (and adults') food preferences. Journalist Michael Pollan's *The Omnivore's Dilemma* (2006) further augmented interest in food production and processing.[31]

Furthermore, obesity was a far more damaging condition—physically, emotionally and socially—than tooth decay, with research documenting its dangers. Childhood obesity was also obvious—easily seen—making it different from tooth decay and subjecting its sufferers to teasing, and to being discriminated against in college and job prospects.

Unlike in the tooth decay case, childhood obesity was implicated with television in more ways than just the products advertised on it. Studies like Gortmaker and Dietz's 1985 paper implicated both the *nature* of television viewing and the *content* of advertisements as factors in childhood obesity. Sitting watching television was a passive activity that didn't use up much energy; watching television took time away from more active pursuits; children were more likely to snack while watching television and, being distracted, would also not realize how much they were eating; and, lastly, given the content of television advertisements on children's television, children were more likely to want to buy and snack on the high-calorie products being shown. Moreover, although television showed a considerable amount of unhealthy eating, it didn't show the realistic outcomes of such lifestyles: television characters were rarely fat.[32]

With the paper by Gortmaker and Dietz showing that rates of childhood obesity had been rising since at least the 1960s—coinciding with the period in which children were massively targeted by junk-food advertisements on television—this suggested that population-wide measures were needed to address the condition. The surgeon general issued a "call to action" on childhood obesity in 2001. There was support across the political party divide for federal government to "do something." Researchers broadly agreed that reducing the amount of television children watched and limiting junk-food advertising were potential nationwide therapies for childhood obesity. Influential medical organizations like the National Institutes of Health and the American Academy of Pediatrics supported regulating the commercial content of children's television on grounds of its connection with the childhood obesity epidemic.[33]

Responding to escalating anxieties, in 2005 the FTC again took up the issue of advertising food to children. As a first step, with the Department of

Health and Human Services, the FTC hosted a joint government-industry workshop entitled "Perspectives on Marketing, Self-Regulation, and Childhood Obesity."[34]

The Kid-Vid saga and the congressional punishment meted out to the FTC was clearly on everyone's minds—industry, activist, and FTC alike. Industry groups reminded the participants of that damaging and failed episode, while activist groups said that the time was now ripe to revisit the ban idea. The FTC of 2005 under Republican President George W. Bush was *not*, however, interested in reopening the Kid-Vid wounds or trying to strongly regulate advertising to children as had been the case in under President Carter in the 1970s:

> From the FTC's perspective, based on years of experience with advertising, we believe a government ban on children's food advertising is neither wise nor viable.[35]

But, cautioned the FTC chairman, Deborah Platt Majoras,

> It would be, however, equally unwise for industry to maintain the status quo. Not only is downplaying the concerns of consumers bad business, but if industry fails to demonstrate a good faith commitment to this issue [the connection between food marketing and childhood obesity] and take positive steps, others may step in and act in its stead.[36]

The FTC hoped that industry would take action itself and self-regulate.

At the workshop, William Dietz presented the medical arguments and evidence connecting television advertising and childhood obesity; representatives from child health and welfare organizations like the Academy of Pediatrics and from the National Parent Teacher Association spoke about studies showing that children, especially those under eight, could not "understand the inherent bias in advertising [and therefore] interpret commercial claims and appeals as accurate and truthful information." The chairman of the American Association of Advertising Agencies (AAAA) held that the advertising business had "the best example of self-regulation that [he was] aware of in American history," and imposing government control over the top of the industry's own mechanisms was unnecessary.[37]

The self-regulation mechanism that the AAAA chairman was referring to was the Children's Advertising Review Unit (CARU). CARU had been established as a section within the Council of Better Business Bureaus

(CBBB) in 1974 after Coke, General Mills, Mars, and McDonald's—major television advertisers all—wrote to the National Advertising Review Board asking them to institute a review body because "self regulation [was] the most sensible answer to the problems raised by advertising to children" at the FTC Kid-Vid hearings. From 1975 onward, CARU had issued guidelines for advertising directed at children under twelve.[38]

At the time of the 2005 FTC workshop, CARU's guidelines dealt mainly with principles of nondeceptive advertising, but two clauses specifically addressed food ads. Food ads should not "discourage or disparage healthy lifestyle choices, the consumption of fruits or vegetables" and should show the food being used appropriately. (For example, ads should show the advertised food as part of a "nutritionally balanced meal," and snack foods had to be shown as such and not as substitutes for a meal.) The CARU guidelines were therefore intended for ad agencies to use in developing individual advertisements and regulated, to some extent, the advertising techniques used.[39]

How did CARU deal with infringements of the guidelines? For a substantial filing fee (which, at that time, was $2,500 for CARU or CBBB members and $6,000 for nonmembers), CARU would investigate complaints against advertisements not in compliance with its guidelines. CARU also conducted its own monitoring, and the great majority of its cases (95 percent) came from this source rather than external complaints—not surprising, considering the filing fee. CARU would hold confidential proceedings into the matter, and, if it deemed necessary, make recommendations to the advertiser that would be published in a press release.[40]

From 1991, CARU also offered the option of an "expedited hearing" to advertisers who responded quickly to their initial request for information. "Expedited hearings," or "informals" as they were also called, would not only be resolved quickly, but also the detailed report on the outcome would not be published, nor would detailed records be kept. "Informals" were increasingly the more popular route. (In the 1990s, CARU heard 434 "informals" compared with 48 "formals"; from 2000 to 2003, CARU heard 301 informal cases versus 137 formal.) To 2004, CARU had reviewed and reported on about 1,100 advertisements, of which about 14 percent were for food. CARU could ask advertisers to make changes to ads or to pull them entirely. If the advertiser failed to comply, CARU had the option of referring the matter to government agencies like the FTC.[41]

Industry representatives to the FTC workshop held that CARU was an appropriate and sufficient mechanism for regulating advertising to children. But, Senator Harkin (D-Iowa), ranking member of the Labor, Health and Human Services and Education Appropriations Subcommittee differed, for one:

> Now, if CARU is the model, that's a non-starter. CARU, frankly, has become a poster child for how not to conduct self-regulation. Time and again, it has shown itself to be a captive of the industry. It has no real independence, no sanction authority, no teeth. The current situation is like a game with a rule book but no referee. CARU is a tiny group tasked with oversight of a multi-billion-dollar industry, and to me, the deck seems a little bit stacked. And the proof, as we say, is in the eating. Look at the deluge of junk food advertising aimed at kids we see today. CARU has given a green light to all of it.[42]

CARU did not address the *volume* of ads directed at children, the *nature* of the foods advertised, nor the product *mix* across advertisements on children's television. Its guidelines were set by the board of directors of the National Advertising Review Council (NARC)—itself comprised of the Council of Better Business Bureaus, the American Association of Advertising Agencies, the American Advertising Federation, the Association of National Advertisers, the Direct Marketing Association, the Electronic Retailing Association, and the Interactive Advertising Bureau—no parents, no teachers, no members of the public, no medical professionals. The filing fee to make a complaint about an advertisement was substantial, especially for members of the public. And CARU's purpose, as identified by the industry, was threefold: to "increase public trust in advertising," to "maintain a level playing field for settling disputes among competing advertisers," and to "minimize the need for government involvement in the advertising business." CARU served industry interests, argued Senator Harkin and speakers from the health and children's groups, and was not a suitable body to be regulating what children saw. The fox was guarding the henhouse.[43]

The outcome of the 2005 FTC hearings into regulating food advertising to children was to a certain extent a rerun of the old pattern—that is, government threatened they would act if industry couldn't do better. The final report, issued in April 2006, did indeed recommend that industry self-regulation in the form of CARU be continued; the medical recommendation of reducing television watching (which would have meant reducing the audience for child-directed advertising) did not get play in the report. But the report also took note of Senator Harkin's criticism of CARU, concluding that "responsible, industry-generated action and effective self-regulation are critical to addressing the national problem of childhood obesity." The report recommended CARU's guidelines should be expanded, that CARU should take advice from experts on child education and health, and that it should allow parents to lodge complaints with it without charging them the $6,000 filing fee—all of which were adopted. Beyond CARU, the report recommended that producers improve the nutritional profile of children's foods and that advertisers should help by making portion-size packaging and having logos that marked out healthier food choices. Public education about food choices and the importance of exercise was something all parties—government, advertisers, and food producers—could work toward.[44]

The 2005 FTC workshop marked a ramping up of public and government pressure on advertisers and food producers marketing foods to children specifically because of the connection with the childhood obesity epidemic. Over the next few years, the FTC continued to investigate the issue, discovering that in 2006, forty-four major food and beverage companies had spent just over $1.6 billion on advertising to children and that, in 2004, children would have seen an average of 10,700 minutes of advertising or 25,600 ads per year, of which 22 percent were for food. Congress requested that the Institute of Medicine (IOM, part of the National Academy of Sciences) also investigate the connection between food advertising and the epidemic of childhood obesity and report back to it. The IOM released their report, "Food Marketing to Children and Youth: Threat or Opportunity?," in December 2005. They answered their title's question by saying that food marketing was *both* a threat and an opportunity. It was a threat, they said, because "statistically, there is strong evidence that exposure to television advertising is associated with adiposity in children aged 2–11 years and teens aged 12–18 years." And it was an opportunity for food producers and marketers to make and advertise healthier foods to children, restaurants to give nutritional information on their menus and offer healthy options, parent-teacher associations and state governors to work together to improve school food, and for Congress to step in with legislation, using its full range of carrots and sticks—taxes, subsidies, and so forth—to make changes in marketing practices and products.[45]

Childhood obesity had received and would continue to receive far more press and public interest than dental caries ever had. "The backlash is building," said Harkin. With an increasingly high level of public anxiety about the connection between children's health and food advertising, avoiding action would be more risky for companies than had been the case in the 1970s. However, with responsibility for monitoring advertising food to children lying with industry itself, health and activist organizations wondered whether any industry-initiated action would constitute meaningful change or simply be a heat-deflecting publicity maneuver. As the president of the American Advertising Federation pointed out, with the FTC still barred from making a ruling on children's advertising on the basis of unfairness, "there is not a government body in a position to tell the food industry what products to advertise or not." With the FTC hobbled and Congress being concerned but not taking action, activist groups turned to another forum: the courts.[46]

CHAPTER 11

Fat Kids Go to Court

Legal Action as Public Health Response to Childhood Obesity

This is an area of concern about the public health which is going to continue to be targeted by those of us who believe in the motto "sue the bastards."

Public interest litigator John Banzhaf III, 2010

For activist groups like the Center for Science in the Public Interest (CSPI), the disappointment of the Kid-Vid saga in the late 1970s and the pro-self-regulation stance of the Federal Trade Commission (FTC) in the 2000s were signs that they needed to look for new forums beyond federal commissions to promote their agenda. Although there was congressional support for "doing something" nationwide about the epidemic of childhood obesity, it appeared that "reduce" or "regulate" were not words legislators or commissioners were comfortable using in regard to industry. As a result, activist groups instead turned to the state courts: "We are just plain out of branches of government," said CSPI's Margo Wootan. "We've got to go judicial."[1]

The gowned judge, the be-suited lawyers—these are the newest entrants to the range of professionals involved in childhood obesity over the past century. It does, of course, beg the question whether a legal approach is a good idea for addressing a health problem like the epidemic of childhood obesity. Can and should the courts play a useful role in either individual or public health? Legal scholars and commentators have debated this very question, with mixed answers.

Those who are against the courts venturing into this realm point out that there are other public bodies whose job it is to take action on public health matters—regulators like federal or state governments, commissions such as the FTC, and departments like the Health and Education Departments, and so forth. These bodies, so the argument runs, are better able to tackle

191

technical issues, gain public input, address matters beyond what one particular litigant brings, issue broad-reaching regulations or policies, and
monitor the results. And litigation is expensive and long-winded.[2]

The counter position that the courts do in fact have a place in the public
health apparatus holds that those regulatory bodies do not or are not able to
do their job because of political or private pressures and potential backlash.
And, what's more, runs the argument, courts already have a long history of
effectively handling health matters like personal injury claims or class action
suits, and in public health domains of communicable disease, sanitation, car
safety, and tobacco.[3]

For public health workers, there is a sense that while they would like antiobesity policy to be handled and directed through the usual channels of government and health agencies—channels that public health workers know and
commonly work with—they are nonetheless quite happy for litigation to
play a role as well, especially in helping get to grips with the private sector,
whose lobbying efforts might otherwise stymie the government route.[4]

Definitely, the prospect of obesity-related litigation as a "new frontier" of
commercial law has both sides of any potential case excited about the challenges of preparing a case and mounting a defense. This has resulted in a
certain amount of legalistic machismo from lawyers. John "sue the bastards"
Banzhaf, famous as an antitobacco litigator and now the principal leader of
what he calls the "fat litigation" movement, speaks of "hewing" his "legal
weapons" for the fight. Joseph Price, consigliere to General Mills, among
other food producers, countered by quoting *The Godfather:* "If we go to litigation, we're going to go to the mattresses; we're going to dig in, it's going
to be costly and expensive."[5]

Law firm Womble Carlyle Sandridge and Rice teamed up with Burson-
Marsteller (the public relations company that the food, advertising, and
broadcasting groups engaged for the Kid-Vid hearings in 1979) to offer a
thirty-day "Obesity Threat Assessment," "intended to help food companies
understand in detail the threat [of obesity litigation], to outline a strategy,
and to develop an implementation program." Legal pectoral muscles are
being flexed on both sides.[6]

Although America's food industry does indeed "find itself in the
crosshairs" of would-be obesity litigators, as Womble Carlyle put it, legal
posturing aside, very few suits have to date actually reached the courts. In
spite of this, the food industry has started making some of the changes

sought by obesity litigators. But it has been the *threat* of legal action, rather than any decision handed down by judges or juries, that has prompted these changes to the obesogenic environment that children of the 2000s find themselves in.[7]

———————

In 2006, CSPI and the Campaign for a Commercial-Free Childhood (CCFC—on a "mission . . . to reclaim childhood from corporate marketers") teamed up with two Massachusetts parents to announce that they were going to sue Kellogg's and Viacom under Massachusetts's consumer protection laws. Viacom owned Nickelodeon children's cable television channel. Both companies, the activist groups claimed, were "engaged in acts and practices in the Commonwealth of Massachusetts that are both unfair and deceptive with respect to the marketing and sale of foods of poor nutritional quality to children under 8 years old."[8]

The plaintiffs wanted "Nick" to stop advertising high-fat and high-sugar foods during "Nick Jr" programming (for under-eights) and other programming where young children formed a large part of the audience, and for Kellogg's to stop advertising high-fat and high-sugar foods to under-eights. (Journalists covering the suit noted that 27 percent of Kellogg's marketing budget for the United States was directed at the six- to eleven-year-old age group.) The arguments the activist groups mounted could have been taken straight from activist groups' submissions to the FTC hearings in the late 1970s, but this time obesity was top of the list of problems:

> In the short term, these messages [advertisements for high fat and high sugar foods] urge the child to eat a diet that is unbalanced, with nutritionally poor food replacing healthy food . . . Such a diet . . . contributes to poor health characterized by obesity, heart disease, diabetes, cancer, dental caries, and other illnesses.[9]

The complainants alleged that 88 percent of the ads on Nickelodeon were for foods of poor nutritional quality and 60 percent of the foods licensed to carry Nick characters on their packaging were for poor-quality foods. This was unfair on parents, they argued, putting parents in opposition to children's much-loved Nick characters when they were trying to get their children to eat healthily. SpongeBob SquarePants, Nickelodeon's square yellow cartoon figure, had earned $1.5 billion in licensing revenues in 2003 alone, mainly from appearing on cookies, Pop-Tarts, Rice Krispie treats, and candy (although SpongeBob had also spruiked spinach and carrots). Industry watchers estimated that food advertising was around 20 percent of Nickelodeon's total advertising revenue, making the threatened suit a highly strategic one:

> The attack planned by CSPI strikes at the heart of Nickelodeon's financial success: its dominance of the kids advertising market combined with extraordinarily profitable merchandising business. Licensing its characters to other companies, most notably to food manufacturers, is a key element of Nickelodeon's financial strength.[10]

While Kellogg's already had a laudable policy of not advertising to under-sixes, still, the plaintiffs contended, 98 percent of the company's television ads directed at older children were for unhealthy foods. In some cases, Kellogg's advertising actually disparaged healthy food, as in the advertisement for Apple Jacks sugared cereal where "Bad Apple" was defeated by "Sweet Cinna Mon." The suit sought damages that might have come to as much as $1 billion for each company, but the plaintiffs indicated in their press release that it wasn't money that they wanted. They would be happy to settle out of court if the companies undertook to change their food advertising practices.

The potential suit garnered considerable press coverage. ("Suing the pants off SpongeBob.") It was a novel approach to trying to get food companies and broadcasters to stop advertising unhealthy foods to children, and it used heightened anxieties about the childhood obesity epidemic to add pressure. Many journalists interpreted it as a test case of whether "Big Food" would become the next target in health-related lawsuits. If the threatened suit went ahead and was successful, would it prompt a cascade of similar cases against broadcasters, food producers, and advertisers?[11]

Kellogg's alone undertook negotiations with CSPI and CCFC and came to an agreement eighteen months later in 2007. The company pledged that they would devise "Kellogg Nutrient Criteria" that would set out standards for both caloric amounts per serving and the nutrient content of the foods. (Foods could contain no more than two hundred calories per serving, no trans fats, and at most two grams of saturated fat and twelve grams of added sugar. The criteria also set an upper limit on salt content for most products. Eggo waffles, the student's late-night friend, were exempt from this requirement.)

For its advertising slots on television, on the radio, in print, and on the Internet, if children under twelve made up the majority of the audience, Kellogg's pledged that they would only advertise foods that met the "Kellogg Nutrient Criteria." Kellogg's famous licensed characters like Tony the Tiger (Frosted Flakes) and Toucan Sam (Froot Loops) would appear only on foods that met the criteria. Products not meeting the criteria would either be reformulated or not be marketed to children. In exchange, CSPI and CCFC agreed not to sue.[12]

The activist groups were happy with the outcome and praised Kellogg's for "vault[ing] over the rest of the industry." In particular, the groups were pleased about what the actions Kellogg's had taken *signified* (or could be said to signify). Although no legal significance could attach to the agreement since it was an out of court settlement, CCFC suggested that the company's new nutrition policy was,

> a tacit admission that the advertising practices favored by the food industry have had a powerful influence on children's food choices and have had a negative effect on children's health and well-being. For far too long, the food industry has denied that marketing is a factor in children's consumption of unhealthy foods.[13]

Kellogg's, however, preferred to stress that its decision to adopt nutritional criteria for advertising to children was an entirely voluntary initiative on its own part, and "vaulted over" the fact that they had been threatened with a writ. "As we developed the standards, we shared our approach with a number of key stakeholders, including . . . the Center for Science in the Public Interest."[14]

Among the groups that Kellogg's was "sharing its approach with" was the Council for Better Business Bureaus (CBBB), one of the major advertising trade associations that oversaw the Children's Advertising Review Unit (CARU). As the FTC's 2005 workshop on childhood obesity had shown, the council and its members were under public and political pressure to respond to the childhood obesity epidemic in new ways, rather than just pointing to CARU's advertising review role. Organized medicine also favored greater restrictions—the American Academy of Pediatrics released a report in 2006 in which it called for a ban on junk-food advertising to young children, and halving the amount of advertising in general permitted on children's television.[15]

Taking a leaf from Kellogg's negotiations, the CBBB launched the "Children's Food and Beverage Advertising Initiative" in November 2006. Companies who subscribed to the initiative would develop nutrient criteria for foods they could advertise to children, similar to the criteria Kellogg's was then negotiating. The criteria had to be based on government nutritional recommendations or other scientifically based guides like that issued by the Institute of Medicine. Companies had to pledge that at least 50 percent of their outlay on advertising to children under twelve would be for products that satisfied those nutrition criteria. The CBBB would keep records of the criteria that each company developed and would also review whether companies were complying with their pledges. The first ten companies to make pledges under the initiative included Coke, PepsiCo, Hershey, Unilever, McDonald's, General Mills, and Kraft—all major food producers marketing to children. (While broadcasters were not part of the CBBB initiative, several announced similar nutritional criteria for the foods that they would advertise to children. As a case in point, the Walt Disney Company had already, in 2006, adopted nutritional standards for its licensed foods and promotions and on the meals offered at Disney theme parks.)[16]

The Children's Food and Beverage Advertising Initiative was not a public acknowledgement or acceptance by industries that advertising unhealthy foods to children played a role in causing obesity. Press releases announcing the initiative and its growing membership set out the industry position— that *all* foods could have a place in a balanced diet and that parents, especially, had a major role to play:

> While it remains the primary responsibility of parents to guide their children's behavior in these areas, industry members are voluntarily pursuing this initiative as a means of assisting parents in their efforts.[17]

Note that in promoting the initiative, member companies cast themselves as parents' *helpers*. This countered the activist argument being used by CCFC and CSPI in their suit against Kellogg's and Viacom that advertising to children undermined parents' efforts to steer children toward healthy food.

Children's health groups criticized the Children's Food and Beverage Advertising Initiative for still allowing companies to intensively market unhealthy foods to children. The regulations did not address the overall mix of products advertised to children, and the nutrition guidelines were sufficiently generous to still allow quite unhealthy foods to be advertised. Take as an example the long-standing flashpoint of sugar content in children's cereals. Frosted Flakes ("They'rrrrrrre grrrreat!"), at eleven grams of sugar per serving, met Kellogg's nutrition criteria. The criteria allowed for up to twelve grams of added sugar per serving.

The Children's Food and Beverage Advertising Initiative was also criticized on the basis that pledging companies were left to define what *they* meant by "advertising to children." "Family programming," which accounted for the bulk of children's television viewing time but that companies *excluded* from "children's programming," could still therefore feature ads for nutritionally poor products. The fact that the initiative only regulated advertising to children under twelve (and only to 50 percent of the amount spent on *that* and only in particular media), when the majority of food advertisements to children were directed at adolescents, showed that the guidelines were by no means comprehensive. Companies also pledged not to advertise food products in elementary schools, but exempted "displays of food and beverage products, charitable fundraising activities, public service messaging, or items provided to school administrators"—the major component of companies' in-school advertising.[18]

The initiative would, it claimed, "provide companies that advertise foods and beverages to children with a transparent and accountable advertising self-regulation mechanism." But it also provided companies with something to point to as showing that they were responding to the childhood obesity epidemic and so allow them to argue that there was no need for government to impose regulations of its own.[19]

The Children's Food and Beverage Advertising Initiative was useful to companies as both a marketing strategy and a political shield. The first eleven companies to join the initiative announced their commitments during an FTC workshop on childhood obesity held in 2007. (An expansion of the initiative in 2009 to cover 100 percent of advertising to children under twelve, in all media, and which addressed some of the criticism of the initiative, was also announced at an FTC forum.) The workshop itself provided a forum for industry representatives to publicize their actions and to put the focus back on families. "And as for parents," editorialized *Broadcasting and Cable* magazine after announcing the initiative, "wake up and face your responsibility!" *Advertising Age,* the advertising industry's magazine, said the Children's Food and Beverage Advertising Initiative was an excellent idea. The move would do nothing to address childhood obesity, wrote the magazine, but it was a superbly calculated rhetorical strategy:

> Congratulations to food marketers . . . They rose above the sad truth that politicians, parents and the media prefer to blame the easy target of advertising instead of taking on the entrenched social, economic, and educational problems that have led to the obesity issue . . . This goodwill gesture is a smart move. They're calling a tactical retreat that they hope will ultimately win them the ability to continue marketing elsewhere. After all, is it really a huge sacrifice for General Mills to give up marketing Trix to those 12 and under if it can still market Cocoa Puffs to that audience?[20]

The threatened Kellogg's/Nickelodeon lawsuit was part of a broader trend toward using the legal system to achieve changes in the advertising environment that might address the childhood obesity epidemic. In 2003, the Public Health Advocacy Institute—a legal research institute based at Northwestern University—held a conference on the topic of "Legal Approaches to the Obesity Epidemic." The attendees were potential litigants on both sides of the courtroom—representatives from activist and nongovernmental organizations, some private lawyers considering suits against food manufactures, and considerable representation from food companies and their trade organizations. The conference considered *who* might be sued, *how* they might be sued, and *what* the wider ramifications of such a case would be for the obesity epidemic. Since the conference, the potential role of the courts in the obesity epidemic has become the subject of considerable investigation, with full-fledged legal scholars considering the question alongside law students flexing their case-building skills. What area of law might such a case come under? What legal novelties would a case need to deal with? How might an organization defend against a case for causing obesity?[21]

Since the law is, by nature, a historical process, legal scholars have interrogated history for similar cases—their parallels and confounding differences—that may clarify whether the law can play a role in addressing childhood obesity. In this history, tobacco litigation looms large. Indeed, some of the lawyers who were major figures in cases against "Big Tobacco" in the 1990s, such as Richard Daynard (who founded the Tobacco Products Liability Project to gather damning evidence against Big Tobacco) and John Banzhaf (who litigated cases against tobacco advertising and passive smoking), are amongst those promoting the idea that obesity will be the next frontier of public health law. Paradoxically, legal commentators who think obesity litigation is likely to win *and* those who think it likely to fail *both* cite tobacco litigation as evidence for their position.[22]

On the "likely to fail" side, scholars point out that fast food is not like tobacco. It is not illegal for children to eat fast food, while it is illegal for children to smoke cigarettes; parents do not buy their children cigarettes, but they do buy them fast food. Personal injury law as it currently stands would require the plaintiff to demonstrate that one particular food caused his or her obesity—a difficult, if not impossible, task. While it is possible that fast food could be addictive, the current evidence for this is not sufficient for a court challenge. And, perhaps most damagingly to any potential litigant, the public believes that people make free choices as to what they eat and should therefore personally bear the consequences of that choice. Suing somebody for selling you or encouraging you to buy obesity-causing products is just laughable.[23]

On the "likely to win" side, scholars argue that fast food is actually quite a lot like tobacco. Both are vast, international businesses, dominated by a few large companies. Fast food may be addictive, and possibly its manufacturers intentionally made it that way, similar to the way nicotine is addictive and tobacco companies manipulated nicotine levels in cigarettes to make them more addictive. Both Big Tobacco and "Big Food" spend large amounts of money advertising to children (implicitly in the former case, explicitly in the latter), making them vulnerable to perceptions that they exploit children's naïveté. The health consequences involved in each (cancer, obesity) are conditions that are preventable, involve lifestyle choices, cause morbidity and premature death, affect a large proportion of the population, and entail large public and private health costs.[24]

Legal analysts consider that food producers and advertisers are most vulnerable in relation to childhood obesity. Children have been very aggressively marketed to and the defense of personal responsibility is less viable in the case of children (although this is, of course, complicated by the role of parents.) Says the director of litigation for CSPI,

> The discussion of personal responsibility . . . avoids the fact that we're talking about six-year-olds. So, they really don't have much personal responsibility. They're still wetting their pants. They're not fully matured human beings, and they are the subject of this marketing.[25]

Supporters favoring obesity suits take heart that the early suits against Big Tobacco were also thought to be laughable for the same reasons as obesity lawsuits—mainly, that you bear the consequences of personal choice.

A third position holds that the differences between Big Food and Big Tobacco don't matter. Richard Daynard, among others, argues that what "did for" Big Tobacco and forced them into negotiating the Tobacco Master Settlement Agreement in 1998 with the states was *not* that they sold a dangerous product. Rather, the evidence showing that tobacco companies had misbehaved (by making their products more addictive by manipulating the nicotine content and targeting children in advertising) and lied (by denying what they knew about the health effects of their products) were what forced the settlement. Perhaps, wager potential obesity litigants, similar evidence could be found that would be embarrassing to Big Food.[26]

Is there any suggestion that such evidence against "Big Food" exists, or is this simply anticorporation paranoia? Intriguingly, lighting the gleam of battle in the litigator's eye, there are indeed some indications that such evidence might exist. McDonald's, for example, is known to survey its customers and class them as "heavy users" and "super heavy users," depending on how often they eat McDonald's food. If McDonalds had information that eating its food in "super-heavy-user" quantities was unsafe, then it could be held liable for not warning its customers against this. Kellogg's and the Sugar Foundation (the sugar manufacturing industry's trade organization) funded research into obesity metabolism studies in the 1950s. Advertising techniques and methods developed by commercial psychologists for targeting children may also prove to be distastefully (or even deceptively) exploitative of children's developmental attainments and deficiencies. And the legal action taken by industry groups during the Kid-Vid hearings was most suggestive. When the FTC first announced in 1978 that it would hold hearings into food advertising to children, they also set out requirements for witnesses at the public hearing. "Any person who seeks to present information [to the hearing] either orally or in writing," stated the notice,

> shall also present any studies or surveys in the possession, custody or control of the person or the organization he represents . . . which support, contradict or otherwise pertain to the person's presentation.[27]

That evidentiary requirement was a major sticking point for industry groups. They described the requirement as a "hidden subpoena" that would compel them to disclose all they knew about food advertising to children, and a coalition of groups including the Chocolate Manufacturers Association, the Grocery Manufacturers Association, the American Association of Advertising Agencies, Kellogg's, the Association of National Advertisers, and independent advertising agencies took the FTC to court to have the rule-making canceled. The activist groups that were party to the FTC hearings failed to appreciate the potential significance of this move and did not become involved with the case. (Which shows how much activist groups have since learned from tobacco litigation about the importance of the legal discovery process.) The FTC agreed to change the evidentiary requirement, softening it so that only data that witnesses referred to would have to be presented, not *all* the information the person's organization might have on the topic. The case was settled and industry groups kept their secrets about advertising food to children.[28]

Although none of these examples constitutes an evidential "smoking gun" showing that food producers have misbehaved in targeting children, legal analysts interpret signs like these as indications that something incendiary might be smoldering in industry records. Lawyers interested in obesity litigation are therefore very excited about the prospect of a lawsuit against a major food company reaching the discovery stage, during which companies would be compelled to reveal information. Indeed, the parallels with the tobacco litigation would suggest that just getting to that stage without the case being dismissed would be a major development and a stepping-stone for future litigation prospects.

Another position on the prospects of obesity litigation in comparison to tobacco litigation holds that obesity litigation is likely to be *more* successful than tobacco litigation because food is *not* like tobacco. For one, although tobacco companies are not able to make a safer cigarette, it *is* possible to make food healthier by choosing different ingredients or by offering different products. Obesity litigation may therefore be successful in producing changes in the food environment because there are more options for food producers than for cigarette manufacturers. Food producers also often place high value on their reputation for being family-friendly or, particularly, kid-friendly, and this is a critical aspect of their brand that they would want to preserve. Food companies have no wish to be stigmatized as tobacco companies have been. Food producers may therefore be both more able and more willing to improve their offerings than cigarette manufacturers.[29]

Moreover, plaintiffs could argue (and have argued) that fast food is so processed that the average consumer wouldn't even recognize the ingredients as constituting food, let alone know what the biochemical effects on the body are of, for example, dextrose, sodium acid pyrophosphate, TBHQ and dimethylpolysiloxane (ingredients in McDonald's french fries). Consumers therefore can't make a reasonable assessment of the healthfulness of such products. The "personal responsibility" argument that was successful as a defense in tobacco cases may therefore be less persuasive in the case of obesity suits when the food in question is highly processed.[30]

Obesity litigation to date has not, however, been notably successful in the courts. The most prominent case is one following the tobacco personal injury model: an ongoing suit against McDonald's, first brought in 2002 under New York's consumer protection laws by two teenagers (or rather, by their parents on their behalf), Ashley Pelman and Jazlyn Bradley. Pelman and Bradley originally sued on the basis that McDonald's advertised its food as healthy even if eaten daily, that it used marketing techniques to induce children to buy the unhealthy food, that it failed to provide easily accessible nutritional information, and that its food was so processed and addictive that it was more dangerous than a person could reasonably expect hamburgers and milkshakes to be. As a consequence, argued the plaintiffs, they had eaten McDonald's meals so often that they had become obese and suffered from associated health problems.[31]

The girls' lawyer, Samuel Hirsh, struggled to establish the legally novel aspects of the case as it was first pleaded—namely, that McDonald's could be liable for the *cumulative* effects of its products, even if its food was safe for low-level consumption; that McDonald's food was so processed that it was more dangerous than could be reasonably expected; and, critically, that McDonald's—not the girls or their parents—was principally responsible for the girls' illness. McDonald's defense was to attack the weaknesses of Hirsh's case and to appeal to common knowledge:

> It is commonly understood that hamburgers and French fries contain fat and salt and that excessively eating those foods over a prolonged period may have consequences to one's waistline and potentially to one's health.[32]

In the media, Pelman, Bradley, and their parents were excoriated for being graspingly litigious and not taking responsibility for "a lifetime of chowing down Happy Meals."[33]

As the case has moved through a number of stages—pleadings, appeals, amendments, and repleadings—the nature of the plaintiffs' case has changed. More child plaintiffs have sought to join the case, but, most notably, the details of allegations against McDonald's have been amended to focus on the claim that McDonald's deceptively advertised its food as being healthier than it actually was, and had failed to provide nutritional information to allow the children to find out for themselves what they were eating. The suit takes exception to advertising statements such as "meat and potatoes, milk and bread . . . good, basic nutritious food" and that "McDonald's measures up to these [USDA] guidelines" for a healthy diet.[34]

In the most recent development, Judge Pogue of the New York District Court turned down the plaintiffs' request that the suit be certified as a class action.

> Because many foods are high in fat, salt, and cholesterol, low in fiber and certain vitamins, and contain beef and cheese, and because there is no evidence to suggest that all who consume such foods develop the kinds of medical conditions which are at issue in this case, [this] necessarily admits the conclusion that, in the absence of individualized inquiries regarding various other factors, no necessary generalizable causal connection is manifest between the consumption of Defendant's products and the development of certain medical conditions.[35]

Judge Pogue reasoned that a person's obesity, and how different foods might factor into it, was different for each person. So it wasn't possible to consider all the children who wanted to join the Pelman suit as being a "class," having claims and injuries in common with Jazlyn and Ashley. The case stalled in legal limbo . . .

Although the Pelman case has not traveled very far down the legal pathway, and some commentators present it as merely fodder for late night comedians, it has had a notable effect beyond the courtroom. For one, the National Restaurant Association lobbied federal and state politicians to introduce laws banning obesity lawsuits like Pelman's against food producers and restaurants. To date, twenty-three states have passed Orwellian-sounding "Commonsense Consumption Acts" or "Personal Responsibility in Consumption Acts" (dubbed "Cheeseburger Bills" by the media) that prohibit obesity lawsuits. Similar proposals for a federal Cheeseburger Bill were lodged in both the House and Senate but were not passed.[36]

And the other effect of the Pelman case has been that McDonald's and other fast-food restaurants took to offering healthier eating options, changed their advertising messages about the healthfulness of their products, and included nutritional information on packaging. Although struggling in court, outside, the Pelman case had a "win" in shifting the advertising tactics of fast-food restaurants.

———————

The shift in emphasis that the Pelman case has gone through (from trying to attribute childhood obesity to eating a particular food, to focusing on allegations of deceptive advertising) has been an intriguing legal strategy, and one that is shaped by the history of childhood obesity in the United States. Today, childhood obesity is understood as multicausal—an agglomeration of its historical understandings—endocrine, biological, genetic, psychological, familial, behavioral, social, and environmental. It has therefore been impossible for litigators to make a persuasive argument that *this food*, and *only this food*, caused a child's obesity. Judge Pogue's reasoning as to why the Pelman case was unsuitable for a class action simply reflects the historically constructed idea that obesity is complex, individualized, and multifactorial.

Moreover, the historical popularity and persistence of the diet-and-exercise response to obesity gives great power to the defense of personal responsibility. Joseph M. Price, partner in the Faegre Baker Daniels law firm, which represents General Mills, Sara Lee, and Nestle, among other food producers, explained:

> Personal responsibility is, in fact, a legitimate defense in this litigation and I will guarantee you, I have done a lot of jury research over the years, and you all have seen juries react this way. Personal responsibility, in this country, at this time, is significant.[37]

Does the personal responsibility argument apply in the case of childhood obesity, where, as the phrase indicates, the people involved are children? Children clearly have less responsibility for themselves and more need of protection. That protection is offered publicly by society in setting standards for companies to interact with children, and privately by the child herself (to some extent) and by her parents. As the judge pondered in an early hearing on the Pelman case, "where should the line be drawn between an individual's own responsibility to take care of herself, and society's responsibility to ensure that others shield her?" Food producers would like that line to stay where it is or be shifted closer to parents, while child health activists point to the childhood obesity epidemic as evidence that children's nutritional environment is unsafe and companies need to take a larger share of responsibility than they currently do.[38]

The shift in obesity litigation strategy is also a change in approach: from personal injury to consumer fraud. Legislation on consumer protection against deceptive advertising claims varies by state, and certain states' consumer protection legislation is more generous to the potential obesity litigant than others. Some states do not require the plaintiffs to show they have been injured by the deception, merely that the deception took place. Such a requirement would allow plaintiffs to avoid the difficulties of establishing that a particular product caused their obesity, and also blunts the personal responsibility argument—one can't be responsible if one doesn't have accurate information to act on. The large majority of cases claimed as "successes" by obesity litigators have been ones that have pursued this consumer fraud approach. Examples of such cases include a threatened suit against the makers of "Pirate's Booty" puffed rice snacks for incorrectly stating its calorie content and one against Kraft for not disclosing that Oreos contained trans fats. Both cases were settled out of court. The principle involved was "tell the truth"—an ideal that applies to all advertising but one that has been used by obesity litigators to embarrass food producers about the unhealthy nature of their products and push producers to reformulate their products to make them healthier. Critics say that this consumer fraud approach is disingenuous: such cases are not directly to do with obesity but are simply about labeling.[39]

The other line of legal attack, and one that has arguably had greater impact as an intervention against childhood obesity has been threatened suits against school boards and soda bottlers for selling high-calorie drinks in schools. Since the late 1990s, school boards, which are responsible for negotiating food and beverage contracts for products sold in school cafeterias, were able to gain favorable contracts by agreeing to stock only one beverage producer's products in cafeterias or host one company's vending machines in exchange for money, or sporting goods, or other school equipment. Schools became a new battleground for the cola wars, with winning contractors gaining exclusive advertising and display rights for the school's captive youth audience. Cash-tight districts benefited from the money and equipment the winning cola bidder paid—band uniforms, sportswear, library books, computers.[40]

These "pouring rights" contracts—more critically referred to as "Cokes for Kickbacks"—were targeted by obesity litigation lawyers in the mid-2000s as being an area that might prove fruitful. School boards had a duty of care to schoolchildren but, obesity lawyers contended, the boards had failed in their duty by securing contracts for only high-cal beverages. The fact that the boards received payments or other "kickbacks" made the situation worse because lawyers could present this as being a bribe or payoff in exchange for the school intentionally stocking products that would harm the children's health. With tobacco litigation lawyer John Banzhaf threatening that obesity litigators would come after school boards, Los Angeles's and then New York City's school districts announced they would ban soda sales in schools, effective in 2003–2004. Statewide bans followed in California, Maine, and Texas, along with Seattle, Philadelphia, and some smaller school districts.[41]

Although the American Beverage Association (ABA) was against banning sodas in schools, calling the strategy "unfortunate," "an ineffective means of addressing obesity," and "def[ying] science and common sense," they were eventually drawn into negotiating new guidelines for school beverage contracts. In 2006, the three major beverage producers (Coke, Pepsi, and Cadbury Schweppes) and the ABA came to an agreement with the Alliance for a Healthier Generation (a group comprising the American Heart Association and the William J. Clinton foundation). The groups agreed that no sodas—diet or otherwise—would be available in elementary and middle schools, and that along with low-cal milk and juices, only diet sodas would be available in high schools. The ABA pledged to adjust existing pouring rights contracts and to draw up future contracts such that, by the 2008–2009 school year, at least 75 percent of school beverage contracts would meet the guidelines.[42]

There is debate as to how effective the school beverage guidelines measure has been and could be in reducing the incidence of childhood obesity. The ABA itself holds that 98.8 percent of schools' contracts met the guidelines by the end of the 2008–2009 school year, but a study published in the *Archives of Pediatrics and Adolescent Medicine* found that 83.9 percent of elementary students still could buy drinks not allowed by the guidelines at school. In support of antisoda measures, medical evidence suggests that soda *does* contribute to the childhood obesity epidemic and that reducing children's soda consumption reduces their weight, and for these reasons activist groups and public health workers have been keen on introducing taxes on sodas as well as banning soda in schools. Over twenty states now have taxes on soda ranging up to 7 percent in excess of regular local tax; a majority of states now have taxes on sodas sold through vending machines, partly as an antiobesity measure.[43]

The history of childhood obesity that has led to our current understanding of the condition as complex and multicausal is something that has created a point of contention between obesity litigators and those who would defend against such potential suits. A common defense is to say that obesity is caused by a number of things and that targeting one particular product—sodas, say—is going to be ineffective in solving the childhood obesity epidemic. This position has, of course, the appeal of common sense, and the attractive, reasonable idea that "all foods and beverages in moderation can be part of a healthy lifestyle that includes daily physical activity."[44]

Jazlyn Bradley, one of the plaintiffs in the *Pelman v. McDonald's* case, is an example in point about the complexity of childhood obesity. Jazlyn, nineteen years old when the case was filed, was one of ten children, and grew up in a kitchenless apartment in the Bronx. She later lived in a homeless shelter that also didn't have cooking facilities. Poor, black, living in the Bronx, poorly educated, aggressively marketed to, eating McDonald's for three meals a day—many environmental factors, social disparities, and societal failures conspired to cause Bradley's obesity. Using litigation to make McDonald's advertising messages accurately convey how often one should eat their food and to disclose the nutritional content would only go some way toward changing the obesogenic environment that Jazlyn and her fellow plaintiffs grew up in. So, on the one hand, the historical complexity behind our understanding of childhood obesity provides an argument for businesses or organizations who are against imposing limits on any one aspect of obesity causation. And on the other hand, the activist litigator's position, as

CSPI's litigation director explains, is that while incremental or small changes brought about by litigation might not "*solve* the childhood obesity problem," nevertheless, "it's a really good start." Complexity is not a reason to do nothing.[45]

Clearly, the history of childhood obesity presents difficulties for the legal approach. It shapes the choice of which area of law to pursue litigation in, and it offers critical defenses for those who would use them. Moreover, the long-held cultural value of personal responsibility, at the root of the popular diet-and-exercise response to childhood obesity, hovers as a specter over attempts to change more recent environmental contributors to the childhood obesity epidemic. Unedifying it may be, but the litigious approach to the childhood obesity epidemic has the benefit that, rather than require personal action by children themselves in the face of a tempting, manipulative, obesogenic environment, it seeks to change that environment itself. And, in medicine, matching the treatment to the cause is the essence of a rational therapy.

Conclusion

In the United States at the start of the twentieth century, childhood obesity was a condition of little medical significance and relative rarity. In fact, considerable corpulence in a child could make him a local hero, feted by newspapers for his fatness. At the start of the twenty-first century, childhood obesity is epidemically prevalent, and painfully exposes the child and her parents to judgment. Newspapers now report on the condition's risk factors, such as high cholesterol and high blood pressure; its dangerous connection with diabetes and heart disease; and its keenly felt social and emotional harms. Moreover, since the 1960s, the happy understanding of childhood obesity as a temporary condition has given way to a sense that the condition is depressingly difficult to overcome and persists into adulthood. Puberty can change many things, but obesity seems not often one of them.

A recurring issue in childhood obesity's life course has been how to measure and diagnose the condition. Solutions attempted to match the measure to the supposedly harmful features of fatness. Weight-based measures (such as weight in excess of 20 percent of average, or weight-height) were paired with the early twentieth-century idea that obesity's health problems were due to *strain*. Measures therefore captured bulk and heft. With a shift toward thinking that fat itself was harmful because of its metabolic action, measures instead tried to capture body fat content. New technologies and practical considerations (Who would be doing the measuring? Where would they be doing it? With what equipment?) and the changing style of medical research also shaped the choice of diagnostic measures. Obesity researchers borrowed technologies from the military and from physiological research to measure body fat content. But outside of the well-funded physiological lab, they looked for an easy-to-use office-based approximation of body fat content, suitable for mass epidemiological surveys. Since the 1990s, the body mass index (BMI) has become the de facto standard for measuring childhood obesity because, to a certain extent, it fulfills the requirements of correlating with body fat content and is easy to measure and calculate.

Future research into the mechanism of how and why obesity causes health problems may implicate something more refined or specific than total body fat content. In that case, BMI will be discarded and the search will be on again to find a measure that picks out this harmful feature and distinguishes between that "splendid young husky" and the hazardously fat child.

Using a standard based on population measurements—whether of weight or BMI or some other measure—continues to raise the issue of *which* children should form the reference population on whom the standards are based. Should the standards reflect what is *desirable?* If so, which children should be measured to produce these lofty standards? Researchers of the 1920s and 1930s picked middle- to upper-class white children for this job. Or should the standard be based on what is *normal,* taken from a snapshot of the population as a whole? Since the 1970s, U.S. standards have been based on a carefully constructed sample, specially chosen to reflect the nation's mix of ethnicities and socioeconomic levels and regions.

It is not just methodological preferences that have caused the slew of measurement studies since Henry Bowditch's first outing with the tape measure and scales in 1872. Secular change—the fact that children have been getting bigger over the century—has also meant standards have had to be regularly updated. Children of *a particular time* need to provide the standards for *that time.* Standards therefore need to be kept up to date to match the current population.

But when the current population has high levels of obesity, measuring it will not give an indication of what is "normal." The latest BMI standards for American children do not use measurements taken on children after the mid-1990s. Indeed, some countries use standards based on measurements taken no later than the 1970s. Because of the increase in childhood obesity, that century-old idea that standards should reflect the population of the day has broken down. Childhood obesity has meant a return to the past to find acceptable standards for the present.

Theories on what causes childhood obesity have agglomerated and their emphasis has reshuffled over the course of the twentieth century. This process of agglomeration and reemphasis has produced an understanding of the condition as complex and multifactorial. Today, a case of childhood obesity might be explained with a combination of a number of possible contributory factors—endocrinal, biological, genetic, psychological, familial, metabolic, behavioral, social, and environmental. Once the exclusive province of pediatricians, the task of understanding and treating the condition now involves psychologists, educators, diet gurus, committees and commissions, fat camp directors, drug companies, activists, advertisers, food producers, epidemiologists, lawyers, politicians, and first ladies. The expansion in the complexity of the condition and its prevalence has been paralleled with a massive expansion in the types of people who claim a stake or expertise in the matter.

There are two main factors that have driven these additions to how childhood obesity is understood. One is to do with trends or fashions in scientific practice. An enthusiasm for things endocrine in the early decades of the twentieth century saw childhood obesity explained as "gland trouble," treatable with gland-derived drugs. This approach was keenly supported by a vigorous, young drug-manufacturing industry. Vogues in favor of Freudian thinking and the ongoing influence of behaviorism added components of emotions, family, and behavior to the mix from the 1940s onward. The energy-balance idea—calories in balanced by calories out—formed the basis for commercial opportunities in diet-and-exercise treatments especially from the 1960s. Cultural values about childhood as a time for character formation, underscored by the importance of self-responsibility, strongly favored diet and exercise as the dominant idea about cause and treatment. With this heightened emphasis on personal responsibility, it is no surprise that the stigma of fatness in childhood has become more pronounced and more harsh since the 1960s.

The other factor driving the continual renewal and revisiting of the causes and treatments for childhood obesity is failure. As this biography of childhood obesity shows, clinical interventions for weight loss, whether they rely on drugs, diet, or therapy, are disappointingly inconsistent in their success. The sheer difficulty of successfully treating overweight has driven the continued search for new explanations and new avenues of attack. Conversely, disenchantment with obesity treatment (and most sharply with dieting) has also been a contributing factor in fostering fat acceptance and fat activism. Failure has helped give childhood obesity its multifactorial, complex character.

In spite of the rise and fall of gland treatments and the similar fate of amphetamines, there is an ongoing search for a drug treatment for obesity in both childhood and adulthood. The appeal of a pill shows how pharmaceuticals continue to be viewed as powerful and practical responses. Research into the genetics of obesity and of how the body regulates fat stores offer tantalizing but as yet unrealized hopes for a drug treatment. But any potential pill for childhood obesity will also be complicated by the wider issue of whether medicating a child is appropriate. "Appropriateness" involves a complex calculation. Does the drug target the root cause, or does it "merely" treat symptoms? Is the condition harmful enough to justify intervention? Is this the best solution for a child, or are there other measures more suitable to someone who is still growing, still flexible in his habits? The condition, the treatment, and beliefs about childhood all affect how childhood obesity is treated.

Since the 1930s, the medical community has had a sense that childhood obesity was gradually rising in prevalence. When national statistics became available from the 1960s, the numbers showed childhood obesity growing in frequency and degree. The increase appears to have slowed and may have leveled out since about 2000. According to the most recent estimate in 2010, childhood overweight affects 31.7 percent of all American children between two and nineteen years. The term "epidemic," first applied in the mid-1980s, signaled that childhood obesity had expanded from being simply a personal or family problem earlier in the century to also being a public one. Although increased across the board, childhood obesity is most prevalent in certain ethnic groups—particularly among Hispanic and African American children. However, the common assumption that poorer people are fatter (which holds for adults) is not the case in children where the effect of socioeconomic standing varies by ethnic group and sex. In childhood, obesity is not simply a matter of money or its lack, but a complex interplay of economics, culture, and biology.[1]

Journalists like writing about the epidemic of childhood obesity partly because it tells an ironic or unexpected story about progress and our modern way of life. It runs opposite to our standard narrative of progress that Generations Y and Z may be the first generations in recent history to have a shorter life expectancy than their parents. The epidemic has been connected with an excess of things that people cherish and enjoy—car travel, computers, cheap groceries, tasty fast food—but that, ironically, can lead to this health condition. Our environment is one that is conveniently and entertainingly "obesogenic." These unsettling aspects of childhood obesity contribute to the dilemmas in handling the epidemic. It is hard to devise effective interventions when a public health problem is associated with a way of life that is valued and aspired to by many people, and that has many positive aspects.

Running in parallel with this explanation of the epidemic as connected with "too much of a good thing" is also the narrative of the epidemic as connected with the dark side of modernity and failed society. Aggressive advertising of junk food to children, unsafe neighborhoods, fewer home-cooked meals with the family, "screen time" in preference to outdoor play, discrimination and disadvantage expressed in children's health, highly processed and artificial foods, and less physical education in schools—all are factors that researchers have implicated in changing children's environment since the 1960s to become increasingly obesogenic. Framed in this way, the condition is a symptom of modern regrets, such as loss of community, loss of connection with nature, loss of childhood, and lack of racial harmony.

The line of reasoning that connects the childhood obesity epidemic with modern American society—both its positives and negatives—and our bodies' ability to cope in that environment often seems to have an unstoppable momentum to it. Modernity and childhood obesity seem to go hand in hand. But a historian's approach to analyzing this situation is a powerful way of undoing the sense of inevitability in this outcome. Historical analysis can suggest the factors that shaped circumstances, the counterarguments not favored for one reason or another, the moments when decisive choices were made between potentially different courses of action. History picks out the pivot points that can suggest new ways of thinking, new avenues of attack.

What are the options when a health condition affects a large proportion of the population and is also entangled in the structure and nature of the society itself? Is it best to leave it up to individuals or should the public be involved? The debate on these questions reflects how responsibility for child health is apportioned between children, parents, and society.

In making a case for public health interventions, health workers point to not just the private or personal costs of childhood obesity but to the public ones as well. Rising health costs borne by the state and the declining proportion of young people healthy enough for military recruiting show that childhood obesity has a *national* toll. (Some health researchers even point to *global* costs.) The implication of attaching a value in the nation's book-keeping to childhood obesity is that this is not just the child's problem or the parents' problem. Addressing childhood obesity is the country's business, too. But there are also considerable realpolitik issues that influence the direction of public health interventions. Any intervention would have to be *effective* (in reducing obesity either by treating current cases or preventing further increases), *acceptable* (in the sense of being appropriate for children), and *possible* (in the sense of having public and political support, economic feasibility, and surviving the gauntlet of commercial interests).[2]

There are considerable forces favoring getting children to manage their own behavior. For one, the American cultural value for personal responsibility and, for another, the continuing dominance and appeal of the diet-and-exercise cause-and-treatment model both strongly stress individual action. Children are easily reached—they're in schools—and are supposedly more flexible in their habits and not yet set in their ways. However, as a *treatment* for existing obesity, diet-and-exercise approaches are highly irregular in their outcome. Encouraging thoughtful eating and regular exercise may be more successful if the aim is not treatment but *prevention,* although programs tend not to articulate this distinction. Any public health response that aims to get children to be more personally responsible for their diet and exercise will involve a delicate balancing act between making children aware of their eating and exercise habits without this becoming a disordered obsession and without stigmatizing fat children further.[3]

The food and advertising industries—for obvious reasons of self-interest—have also been keen to promote individual action around dietary choices and exercise as the answer. Nickelodeon, for example, explains that its philosophy in regard to childhood obesity is "let the kids lead . . . by empowering them with information." This individualized response would be suited to a situation where childhood obesity was "only" a personal problem, not a public health one. But the high prevalence of childhood obesity and its association with cultural and social factors suggest that structural solutions should play a prominent role in addressing the issue. Indeed, asking kids to "take the lead" against childhood obesity and modify their own behavior without changing the environment is unfair, hypocritical, and an abrogation of adult responsibilities.[4]

The alternative approach of targeting children's eating and exercise *environment* requires society-wide responses, and it requires government, industry, and communities to make them. This approach has the considerable benefit that children would not have to become tender experts, constantly on the defensive against their surroundings. But the issue of food advertising to children and the Kid-Vid saga of the 1970s illustrated just how difficult it can be to achieve change when there are vested interests in not doing so. The turn to the courts by activist groups in the 2000s represents an effort to counter these interests by exerting realpolitik pressure to make companies take actions they might not otherwise have done.

For government, navigating these capricious dynamics and taking a lead in making changes that might effectively address the childhood obesity epidemic has been difficult. Most government programs, such as Mi Cocina and Take the Lead, have taken the individual action line. There are, however, some budding signs that recent government responses are also seeking to tackle the obesogenic environment. In 2010, President Obama announced that he was convening a Task Force on Childhood Obesity, with representatives from various government departments, that would look at ways of "solving the problem of childhood obesity within a generation" through both federal and nongovernmental actions. Although the task force's subsequent report on options was heavily reliant on "encouraging," "promoting" and "empowering" parents, children, and communities, it did contain indications of potential concrete measures that would modify the food and exercise environment.[5]

One suggestion was to institute standards for food advertising to children that are more comprehensive than the Children's Food and Beverage Advertising Initiative. This could be achieved either voluntarily by businesses or imposed by the Federal Communications Commission. Other actions were the Healthy Food Financing Initiative to increase the availability of healthy foods in "food deserts" devoid of grocery stores and Section 4205 of the 2010 Affordable Care Act, which required chain restaurants to display calorie amounts for food items and have more detailed nutritional information easily available. Some of the proposals, such as the effort to improve the healthfulness of meals served under National School Lunch and Breakfast Program, and watering the "food deserts," also stand to address some of the social disparities that have contributed to the socioeconomic patterning of childhood obesity. Closing streets to provide outdoor play areas is a clever way of simultaneously building community and getting children out and active. Michelle Obama, who has lent her articulate glamour to the cause of raising childhood obesity's profile, launched Let's

Move!, the umbrella initiative for implementing the task force's recommendations.[6]

The philosophy of the Let's Move! campaign is that of a "national grassroots movement" to address childhood obesity, but this low-level approach still leaves a number of additional options for action at the federal level. Opportunities exist, for example, to reinstate the FTC's power to rule on unfair advertising to children, to limit political contributions by food producers and advertisers, to develop media literacy education, to make healthier food cheaper than unhealthy food through restructuring subsidies and taxes, and to use market incentives and disincentives for food producers to provide healthier, less processed foods. Recent experience has shown that the legal efforts of quite small grassroots organizations can have wide effects, even without threatened suits coming to court. Large businesses that are sensitive to the family appeal of their brand (and sensitive to the threat of precedent-setting legal action) can be nudged into taking action. Moreover, vigilance and resolve are required when it comes to putting policies into practice. For example, the Healthy, Hunger-Free Kids Act (2010) aimed to improve school meals by (for one) increasing the proportion of vegetables in meals. But when it came to implementing the act, members of Congress representing farm states (Democrats and Republicans alike) and food industry lobbyists ensured that a scant quarter-cup of tomato paste met the definition of "a serving of vegetables." A slice of pizza therefore counted. Let's Move! is commendably broad in its approach, but it will take political courage and fortitude to add more assertive actions and withstand the backlash.[7]

The childhood obesity epidemic—a problem long in the making, gradual in its onset, and broad in its harms—deserves a swift and effective response. The biography of how this formerly rare and insignificant condition became a major threat to children's health is marked with milestones showing the choices made, the options discounted, and the pathways taken. These choices speak to social values as much as to contemporary medical and scientific knowledge. Childhood obesity is not infectious, but it is communicable, spreading via societal choices. May the next milestones in its history be choices that reverse its course.

Notes

Introduction

Epigraphs: "The Fattest Boy." *Chicago Daily Tribune,* 19 January 1896, 40. Hunt Peters, Lulu. *Diet for Children (and Adults) and the Kalorie Kids.* New York: Dodd, Mead, 1924, 176. Bruch, Hilde. "Obese Children Notes 1938." In *Papers of Hilde Bruch.* Houston: Texas Medical Center Archive, 1938. "Miseries of an Overweight Child." *Look Magazine,* 17 November 1967, 36–41, 36. "Affadavit by Ashley Pelman." Supreme Court of the State of New York, County of Bronx: Index no. 24809/02, 2002.

1. "Good natured and amiable . . ." from Emerson, W. R. P. "Overweight in Children." *Boston Medical and Surgical Journal* 185 (1921): 475–476, 475.
2. "Fat children are the victims . . ." from Nixon, N. K. "Obesity in Childhood." *Journal of Pediatrics* 4 (1934): 295–306, 303–304.

   "I was an obese child . . ." from Veeder, B. S. "The Overweight Child." *Journal of the American Medical Association* 83 (1924): 486–489, 489.

   "The fat child is not a happy child" from Hunt Peters, L. "Diet and Health: Answers to Correspondents." *Los Angeles Times,* 14 March 1925, A6.
3. "Most people who are fat in childhood . . ." from Editorial. "Childhood Obesity." *The Lancet,* 257, no. 6659 (1951): 841, 841.
4. The influential early studies on the persistence of childhood obesity into adulthood are Mullins, A. G. "The Prognosis in Juvenile Obesity." *Archives of Disease in Childhood* 33 (1958): 307–314; Abraham, S., and M. Nordsieck. "Relationship of Excess Weight in Children and Adults." *Public Health Reports* 75 (1960): 263–273.

   The 80–85 percent statistic is used in, for example, Huenemann, R. L. "Consideration of Adolescent Obesity as a Public Health Problem." *Public Health Reports* 83 (1968): 491–495; Knittle, J. "Childhood Obesity." *Bulletin of the New York Academy of Medicine* 47 (1971): 579–589; Charney, E., H. Goodman, et al. "Childhood Antecedents of Adult Obesity." *New England Journal of Medicine* 295 (1976): 6–9; Weil, W. "Current Controversies in

Childhood Obesity." *Journal of Pediatrics* 91 (1977): 175–187; Stults, H. "Obesity in Adolescents." *Journal of Pediatric Psychology* 2 (1977): 122–126.

"The main difference . . ." quotation from Brook, C. G. D. "Fat Children." *British Journal of Hospital Medicine* 10 (1973): 30–33, 30.

5. For summary of the comorbidities of childhood obesity and the research basis of this understanding, see, for example, Daniels, S. "The Consequences of Childhood Overweight and Obesity." *The Future of Children* 16 (2006): 47–67.

Studies on discrimination include Richardson, S., N. Goodman, et al. "Cultural Uniformity in Reaction to Physical Disabilities." *American Sociological Review* 26 (1961): 241–247; Maddox, G., K. Beck, and V. Liederman. "Overweight as a Social Deviance and Disability." *Journal of Health and Social Behavior* 9 (1968): 287–298; Richardson, S., and J. Royce. "Race and Physical Handicap in Children's Preference for Other Children." *Child Development* 39 (1968): 467–480; Crandall, C. "Do Parents Discriminate against Their Overweight Daughters?" *Personality and Social Psychology Bulletin* 21 (1995): 724–735; Latner, J. D., and A. Stunkard. "Getting Worse: The Stigmatization of Obese Children." *Obesity Research* 11 (2003): 452–456. An excellent summary is Puhl, R., and J. Latner. "Stigma, Obesity and the Health of the Nation's Children." *Psychological Bulletin* 133 (2007): 557–580.

6. "Fat power" from Fishman, S. G. B. "Life in the Fat Underground." *Radiance* Winter (1998): www.radiancemagazine.com/issues/1998/winter_98/fat_underground.html.

The fat acceptance movement incorporates advocacy organizations, such as NAAFA and the International Size Acceptance Association, as well as unaffiliated activists and advocates who work through books, blogs, and other online and social-networking forums. Its academic arm is called "fat studies"—a cross-disciplinary field that investigates attitudes to fatness, both historically and in recent times, and advocates against fat discrimination. Although all segments of the fat acceptance movement agree on the aim of eliminating fat discrimination, some branches of the movement deny that obesity has any health consequences. Some segments of the movement also reject that there has been a large increase in obesity. The movement's general principles and examples of variations in position within the movement are illustrated in, for example, Campos, P. *The Obesity Myth.* New York: Penguin, 2004; Gard, M., and J. Wright. *The Obesity Epidemic.* New York: Routledge, 2005; Oliver, J. E. *Fat Politics.* New York: Oxford University Press, 2006; O'Hara, L., and J. Gregg. "Human Rights Casualties from the 'War on Obesity.'" *Fat Studies* 1 (2012): 32–46.

7. The term "moral panic" in regard to social and medical attitudes to obesity is particularly associated with law professor and fat activist Paul Campos. See, for example, Campos, P., A. Saguy, et al. "The Epidemiology of Overweight

and Obesity: Public Health Crisis or Moral Panic?" *International Journal of Epidemiology* 35 (2006): 55–60.

HAES is developed in Bacon, Linda. *Health at Every Size.* Dallas: BenBella Books, 2008.

The response to the Campos argument by medical researchers and clinicians is given in other articles in the same edition of the *International Journal of Epidemiology,* for example, Rigby, N. "Commentary: Counterpoint to Campos *et Al.*" *International Journal of Epidemiology* 35 (2006): 79–80; Lobstein, T. "Commentary: Obesity—Public Health Crisis, Moral Panic or a Human Rights Issue?" *International Journal of Epidemiology* 35 (2006): 74–76.

8. "NAAFA Challenges First Lady." *NAAFA Newsletter,* February (2010): 1–2.

Paul Campos, the main advocate of the idea that societal concerns about obesity are simply a "moral panic," has also written on the childhood condition, saying that Michelle Obama's antiobesity campaign is "dangerous nonsense" and will further stigmatize fat children. Campos, P. "Childhood Shmobesity." *New Republic,* 11 February, http://www.newrepublic.com/article /politics/childhood-shmomesity#. 2010. Access date 10 March 2011.

9. The statistic on secular change is from Meredith, H. "Change in the Stature and Body Weight of North American Boys during the Last 80 Years." *Advances in Child Development and Behavior* 2 (1963): 69–114, 81, 89, 95.

See also "Secular Changes in Height and Weights of Children." *Nutrition Reviews* 15 (1957): 205–207; Bakwin, H., and S. McLaughlin. "Secular Increase in Height—Is the End in Sight?" *The Lancet* 284, no. 7371 (1964): 1195–1196; Roche, A. "Secular Trends in Stature, Weight, and Maturation." *Monographs of the Society for Research in Child Development* 44 (1979): 3–27.

10. "The pendulum has swung . . ." quotation from Baird, I. M. "Epidemiological Aspects of Obesity." *British Journal of Hospital Medicine* 10 (1973): 34–36, 34.

Debate on the continuity of secular change is considered in Garn, S. "The Secular Trend in Size and Maturation Timing and Its Implications for Nutritional Assessment." *Journal of Nutrition* 117 (1987): 817–823; Freedman, D., S. Srinivasan, et al. "Secular Increases in Relative Weight and Adiposity among Children over Two Decades." *Pediatrics* 99 (1997): 420–426.

Trends from the 1960s to 1990s discussed in Troiano, R. P., K. M. Flegal, R. J. Kuczmarski, S. M. Campbell, and C. L. Johnson. "Overweight Prevalence and Trends for Children and Adolescents: The National Health and Nutrition Examination Surveys, 1963–1991." *Archives of Pediatrics and Adolescent Medicine* 149 (1995): 1085–1091; Flegal, K. M., and R. P. Troiano. "Changes in the Distribution of Body Mass Index of Adults and Children in the US Population." *International Journal of Obesity* 24 (2000): 807–818; Strauss, R., and H. Pollack. "Epidemic Increase in Childhood Overweight, 1986–1998." *Journal of the American Medical Association* 286 (2001): 2845–2848.

11. "Unduly common" from Stuart, H. "Obesity in Childhood." *Quarterly Review of Pediatrics* 10 (1955): 131–145, 143. "Must be recognized . . ." from Editorial. "The Prognosis in Juvenile Obesity." *Nutrition Reviews* 17 (1959): 99–100, 100. Similar sentiments in Forbes, G. "Overnutrition for the Child: Blessing or Curse?" *Nutrition Reviews* 15 (1957): 193–196; Mullins, "Prognosis in Juvenile Obesity"; Bakwin, H. "Obesity in Children." *Journal of Pediatrics* 54 (1959): 392–400; Asher, P. "Fat Babies and Fat Children." *Archives of Disease in Childhood* 41 (1966): 672–673.

12. Sears's product lines information from Sears, Roebuck and Co. Catalogues (1893–1992/3), Baker Old Class and Historical Collection, Baker Library, Harvard Business School, Boston, Massachusetts.

    Studies from the 1930s to the 1960s estimating the prevalence of childhood obesity include Gray, H., and J. G. Ayres. *Growth in Private School Children.* Chicago: University of Chicago Press, 1931; Johnson, M. L., B. Burke, and J. Mayer. "Relative Importance of Inactivity and Overeating in the Energy Balance of Obese High School Girls." *American Journal of Clinical Nutrition* 4 (1956): 37–44; Huenemann, R. L. "Consideration of Adolescent Obesity."

13. Ogden, C., M. Carroll, et al. "Prevalence of High Body Mass Index in US Children and Adolescents, 2007–2008." *Journal of the American Medical Association* 303 (2010): 241–249.

14. For example, Gordon-Larsen, P., L. S. Adair, and B. Popkin. "The Relationship of Ethnicity, Socioeconomic Factors, and Overweight in US Adolescents." *Obesity Research* 11 (2003): 121–129; Wang, Y., and Q. Zhang. "Are American Children and Adolescents of Low Socioeconomic Status at Increased Risk of Obesity? Changes in the Association between Overweight and Family Income between 1971 and 2002." *American Journal of Clinical Nutrition* 84 (2006): 707–716.

15. For example, explorations of biological bodily differences include Daniels, S., P. Khoury, and J. Morrison. "The Utility of Body Mass Index as a Measure of Body Fatness in Children and Adolescents: Differences by Race and Gender." *Pediatrics* 99 (1997): 804–807; Lee, S., J. Kuk, et al. "Race and Gender Differences in the Relationships between Anthropometrics and Abdominal Fat in Youth." *Obesity* 16 (2008): 1066–1071; Freedman, D. S., J. Wang, et al. "Racial/Ethnic Differences in Body Fatness among Children and Adolescents." *Obesity* 16 (2008): 1105–1111.

    Studies of cultural attitudes and practices affecting obesity rates include Brown, P. "Culture and the Evolution of Obesity." *Human Nature* 2 (1991): 31–57; Furnham, A., and P. Baguma. "Cross-Cultural Differences in the Evaluation of Male and Female Body Shapes." *International Journal of Eating Disorders* 15 (1994): 81–89; Bailey, E. *Food Choice and Obesity in Black America.* Westport, CT: Praeger, 2006; Flynn, K., and M. Fitzgibbon. "Body Images and Obesity Risk among Black Females." *Annals of Behavioral Medicine* 20 (1998): 13–24.

16. Dietz, W. H., S. L. Gortmaker, et al. "Trends in the Prevalence of Childhood and Adolescent Obesity in the United States." *Pediatric Research* 19 (1985): 198A.

17. Christakis, N. A., and J. H. Fowler. "The Spread of Obesity in a Large Social Network over 32 Years." *New England Journal of Medicine* 357 (2007): 370–378.

"The vectors of subsidized agriculture . . ." quotation from Prentice, A. "The Emerging Epidemic of Obesity in Developing Countries." *International Journal of Epidemiology* 35 (2006): 93–99, 93.

Rosenberg, C. E. "Pathologies of Progress: The Idea of Civilization as Risk." *Bulletin of the History of Medicine* 72 (1998): 714–730.

18. See, for example, Magarey, A., L. Daniels, and T. J. Boulton. "Prevalence of Overweight and Obesity in Australian Children and Adolescents." *Medical Journal of Australia* 174 (2001): 561–564; Matsushita, Y., N. Yoshiike, et al. "Trends in Childhood Obesity in Japan over the Last 25 Years from the National Nutrition Survey." *Obesity Research* 12 (2004): 205–214; Stamatakis, E., P. Primatesta, et al. "Overweight and Obesity Trends from 1974 to 2003 in English Children: What Is the Role of Socioeconomic Factors?" *Archives of Disease in Childhood* 90 (2005): 999–1004; Wang, Y., and T. Lobstein. "Worldwide Trends in Childhood Overweight and Obesity." *International Journal of Pediatric Obesity* 1 (2006): 11–25; Kelishadi, R. "Childhood Overweight, Obesity, and the Metabolic Syndrome in Developing Countries." *Endocrinological Reviews* 29 (2007): 62–76; Cheng, Y. J., and T. Cheng. "Epidemic Increase in Overweight and Obesity in Chinese Children from 1985 to 2005." *International Journal of Cardiology* 132, no. 1 (2008): 1–10. An excellent summary is Popkin, B. M. "Using Research on the Obesity Pandemic as a Guide to Unified Vision of Nutrition." *Public Health Nutrition* 8 (2005): 724–729.

"Pandemic" terminology used, for example, in Wang and Lobstein, "Worldwide Trends in Childhood Overweight and Obesity"; Kelishadi, "Childhood Overweight."

The global toll of obesity from a resource standpoint is calculated in Walpole, S., D. Prieto-Merino, et al. "The Weight of Nations: An Estimation of Adult Human Biomass." *Biomed Central Public Health* 12 (2012): 439–445.

19. Omran, A. "Epidemiologic Transition." In *International Encyclopedia of Population*, John A. Ross, ed., 172–183. New York: Free Press, 1982, 172.

20. Strauss and Pollack, "Epidemic Increase in Childhood Overweight"; Wang and Zhang, "Are American Children . . . at Increased Risk of Obesity?"; Wang, Y. "Disparities in Pediatric Obesity in the United States." *Advances in Nutrition* 2 (2011): 23–31.

21. Obama, M. "Remarks by the First Lady on What Health Insurance Reform Means for Women and Families." Washington, DC: White House—Office of the First Lady, 2009.

22. The "nanny state" quotation is from, among others, right-wing "Tea Party" Republican Sarah Palin. See Horowitz, J., and N. M. Henderson. "Some GOP Stalwarts Defend First Lady's Anti-obesity Campaign from Palin's Shots." *Washington Post*, 29 December, http://www.washingtonpost.com/wp-dyn/content/article/2010/12/29/AR2010122901940.html?hpid=topnews. 2010. Access date 25 June 2013; Editorial. "Palin's Food Fight." *Wall Street Journal*, 27 December, http://online.wsj.com/article/SB100014240527487047 74604576036073453559688.html. 2010. Access date 25 June 2013.

23. Brandt, A. M. "Polio, Politics, Publicity, and Duplicity: The Salk Vaccine and the Protection of the Public." *International Journal of Health Services* 8 (1978): 257–270, 265. Similar sentiments in Oshinsky, D. M. *Polio*. Oxford: Oxford University Press, 2005.

24. That the current generation's life expectancy may be less than their parents' is from Olshansky, S. J., D. Passaro, et al. "A Potential Decline in Life Expectancy in the United States in the 21st Century." *New England Journal of Medicine* 352 (2005): 1138–1145. The suggestion is controversial. See, for example, Mann, C. C. "Provocative Study Says Obesity May Reduce U.S. Life Expectancy." *Science* 307, no. 5716 (2005): 1716–1717.

25. Postman, N. *The Disappearance of Childhood*. New York: Vintage Books, 1982.

1. How Big Is Normal?

Epigraph: Evans, W. A. "How to Keep Well." *Chicago Daily Tribune*, 17 January 1932, A7.

1. In the measures used today, Charley's body mass index (BMI) would be 39. This would put him well above the 95th percentile for his age and therefore see him diagnosed as obese. "The Fattest Boy." *Chicago Daily Tribune*, 19 January 1896, 40.

   "Two Remarkable Boys." *New York Times*, 24 April 1892; "Death of the Fat Girl." *New York Times*, 27 October 1883; "The Fat Girl's Body Sold." *New York Times*, 7 November 1883, 1.

2. "Pediatrist" was in usage in the United States until approximately 1930. On the history of pediatrics, see Cone, T. *History of American Pediatrics*. Boston: Little, Brown, 1979; King, C. *Children's Health in America*. New York: Twayne, 1993; Markel, H. "Academic Pediatrics: The View of New York City a Century Ago." *Academic Medicine* 71 (1996): 146–151; Pawluch, D. *The New Pediatrics: A Profession in Transition*. New York: Aldine de Gruyter, 1996.

   Finlayson, J. "Diagnosis." In *Cyclopedia of the Diseases of Children: Medical and Surgical*, J. M. Keating, ed., 73–132. Philadelphia: J.B. Lippincott, 1889, 73–74.

3. On the history of measuring birth weight, see Cone, T. "Pediatric History: De Pondere Infantum Recens Natorum." *Pediatrics* 28 (1961): 490–498.

The textbooks referred to are Dewees, W. *A Treatise on the Physical and Medical Treatment of Children.* Philadelphia: H.C. Carey and I. Lea, 1825; Smith, J. L. *A Treatise on the Diseases of Infancy and Childhood.* Philadelphia: Lea Brothers, 1841. Specialist pediatric textbooks appeared in the United States from the mid-nineteenth century onward.

4. On the history of scales manufacturing in America and their use in domestic settings, see Levine, D. "Managing American Bodies: Diet, Nutrition, and Obesity in America 1840–1920." PhD diss., Harvard University, 2007, chapter 2, "Getting on the Scale."

   "A most important point . . ." quotation from Finlayson, "Diagnosis," 88.

   The stadiometer was invented by Francis Galton, the nineteenth-century English polymath, to efficiently take the heights of large numbers of people visiting the International Hygiene Exhibition in London in 1884. Galton, F. *Memories of My Life.* London: Methuen, 1908; Galton, F. "Some Results of the Anthropometric Laboratory." *Journal of the Anthropometric Institute* 14 (1885): 275–287.

5. An excellent history of measurement studies is Tanner, J. M. *A History of the Study of Human Growth.* Cambridge: Cambridge University Press, 1981.

   See also Kodlin, D., and D. Thompson. "An Appraisal of the Longitudinal Approach to Studies in Growth and Development." *Monographs of the Society for Research in Child Development* 23 (1958); Weigley, E. "Average? Ideal? Desirable? A Brief Overview of Height-Weight Tables in the United States." *Journal of the American Dietetic Association* 84 (1984): 417–423; Brosco, J. "Weight Charts and Well Child Care: When the Pediatrician Became the Expert in Child Health." In *Formative Years: Children's Health in the United States, 1880–2000,* A. M. Stern and H. Markel, eds., 91–120. Ann Arbor: University of Michigan Press, 2002; Knowles, J., and J. Baten. "Looking Backward and Looking Forward: Anthropometric Research and the Development of Social Science History." *Social Science History* 28 (2004): 191–210; Hall, S. *Size Matters.* Boston: Houghton Mifflin, 2006.

6. Bowditch, L. V. *Life and Correspondence of Henry Ingersoll Bowditch.* 2 vols. Boston: Houghton Mifflin, 1902; Fye, W. B. "Growth of American Physiology, 1850–1900." In *Physiology in the American Context, 1850–1940,* G. L. Geison, ed., 47–66. Bethesda, MD: American Physiological Society, 1987; Laszlo, A. "Physiology of the Future: Institutional Styles at Columbia and Harvard." In Geison, *Physiology in the American Context, 1850–1940,* 67–96.

7. Quetelet is notable in the history of statistics for three things: first, he felt that statistical methods could be applied to social scientific data; second, for his concept of the "average man" *(l'homme moyen);* and third, for the technique of fitting distributions to social data. See Stigler, S. *The History of Statistics: The Measurement of Uncertainty before 1900.* Cambridge, MA: Harvard University Press, 1986, especially 161–220.

Bowditch, H. *The Growth of Children.* Boston: Albert J. Wright, State Printer, 1877, 4.

Bowditch, H. "The Relation between Growth and Disease." *Transactions of the American Medical Association* 32 (1881): 371–77, 371.

8. For example, Bowditch, H. "The Growth of Children Studied by Galton's Method of Percentile Grades." In *22nd Annual Report of the State Board of Health of Massachusetts.* Boston: State Board of Health, 1891, 510.

9. "At those periods . . ." from Bowditch, *Growth of Children,* 18.

Clarke's address was published as Clarke, E. *Sex in Education or, a Fair Chance for Girls.* Boston: James R. Osgood, 1875, 38, 78. The book sparked argument and oppositional papers, such as Howe, J. *Sex and Education: A Reply.* Boston: Roberts Brothers, 1874. See Zschoche, S. "Dr. Clarke Revisited: Science, True Womanhood, and Female Collegiate Education." *History of Education Quarterly* 29 (1989): 545–569.

10. Bowditch, H. "Comparative Rate of Growth in the Two Sexes." *Boston Medical and Surgical Journal* 10 (1872): 434–435, 435.

11. Bowditch, *Growth of Children,* 4, 7, 6, 41, 45.

12. Ibid., 12, 20, 21.

13. Ibid., 19.

14. Bowditch, H. *The Growth of Children: A Supplementary Investigation.* Boston: Rand, Avery, 1879, 37.

15. Bowditch, *Growth of Children: A Supplementary Investigation,* 25, 54; Bowditch, *Growth of Children,* 32.

16. See the *Worcester Daily Telegraph,* 5 March 1891, quoted in Cole, D. *Franz Boas: The Early Years, 1858–1906.* Vancouver: Douglas and MacIntyre, 1999, 143.

See also Baker, L. "Franz Boas out of the Ivory Tower." *Anthropological Theory* 4 (2004): 29–51; Benedict, R. "Obituary: Franz Boas." *Science* 97, no. 2507 (1943): 60–62; Lowie, R. "Biographical Memoir of Franz Boas 1858–1942." *National Academy of Sciences—Biographical Memoirs* 24 (1947): 1–22.

Boas's work using his 1890–1892 child measurement data includes Boas, F. "The Growth of Children." *Science* 19, no. 483 (1892): 256–257; Boas, F. "The Growth of Children." *Science* 20, no. 516 (1892): 351–352; Boas, F. "The Growth of Children II." *Science* 19, no. 485 (1892): 281–282; Boas, F. "The Growth of Children." *Science* 5, no. 119 (1897): 570–573; Boas, F, and C. Wissler. "Statistics of Growth." In *Report of the Commissioner of Education for 1904.* 25–132. Washington, DC: United States Bureau of Education, 1905; Boas, F. "Observations on the Growth of Children." *Science* 72, no. 1854 (1930): 44–48.

On Porter's study, see Porter, W. T. "The Physical Basis of Precocity and Dullness." *Transactions of the Academy of Science of St. Louis* 4 (1895): 161–181; Porter, W. T. "The Relation between the Growth of Children and Their Deviation from the Physical Type of Their Sex and Age." *Transactions of the*

Academy of Science of St. Louis 4 (1895): 233–250; Porter, W. T. "The Growth of St. Louis Children." *Transactions of the Academy of Science of St. Louis* 4 (1895): 263–426 and Boas's commentary on the study. Boas, F. "On Dr. William Townsend Porter's Investigation of the Growth of the School Children of St. Louis." *Science* 1, no. 9 (1895): 225–230.

17. Prudden, T. M. "Luther Emmett Holt." *Science* 59, no. 1534 (1924): 452–453; Dunn, P. "Dr Emmett Holt (1855–1924) and the Foundation of North American Pediatrics." *Archives of Disease in Childhood Fetal Neonatal Education* 83 (2000): F221–F223; Duffus, R. L., and L. E. Holt Jr. *L. Emmett Holt: Pioneer of a Children's Century.* New York: D. Appleton-Century, 1940; Park, E., and H. Mason. "Luther Emmett Holt (1855–1924)." In *Pediatric Profiles,* B. Veeder, ed., 33–60. St. Louis, MO: C.V. Mosby, 1957.

18. Further editions were published after Holt's death in 1924. It was retitled *Pediatrics* for the thirteenth edition in 1962. The last edition was the fifteenth, published in 1972.

 Duffus and Holt, *L. Emmett Holt*, 121, ix.

19. Over the many editions of the textbook, Holt revised the number of children that his data was based on so that he could incorporate greater numbers of younger children. In the sixth edition, Holt increased the average weights for younger children by between a half and one pound, and he commented in the seventh edition that older children were also likely to be heavier than the tabulated averages.

20. Duffus and Holt, *L. Emmett Holt*, 117.

 Park, Edwards, and Mason, "Luther Emmett Holt," 53.

 Holt dedicated his little best seller to the lady who had suggested the training school, Mrs. Robert Chapin (Adele Le Bourgeois Chapin), a noted society hostess, extensively involved in nursing and hospital charities. Duffus and Holt, *L. Emmett Holt*, 116.

21. Holt, L. E., Jr. *Holt's Care and Feeding of Children.* New York: D. Appleton-Century, 1943, 19 (italics in original). The height and weight figures in *Care and Feeding* are clearly drawn from the same sources as those for his *Diseases* textbook (namely, Bowditch's, Boas's, and Porter's studies), but are rounded to the nearest quarter-inch or pound.

22. For example, Tweddell, F. *How to Take Care of the Baby: A Mother's Guide and Manual for Nurses.* 2nd ed. Indianapolis, IN: Bobbs-Merrill , 1913; Paddock, C. *Maternitas.* Chicago: Cloyd J. Head, 1905; Kerr, L. *The Baby, Its Care and Development, for the Use of Mothers.* New York: A.T. Huntington, 1908. Holt's *Diseases of Infancy and Childhood,* first published in 1897, carried pictures of scales in its first six editions. After the seventh edition, published in 1917, the books omitted the picture, suggesting that pediatricians were by then perfectly familiar with scales.

 Although many parenting manuals gave tables of both height and weight measurements, most counseled weighing the baby and did not mention taking height (length) measurements. (One exception is Crozer Griffith, J. P. *The Care of the Baby.* Philadelphia: W.B. Saunders, 1900.) Pediatricians therefore regarded measuring height as less important than measuring weight. It is also harder to take accurate length measurements of a baby, making height a less practical indicator.

23. Bowditch, "Growth of Children Studied by Galton's Method," 521.

    On promoting the Bowditch/Boas/Porter data, see, for example, Kerley, C. G. *Short Talks with Young Mothers on the Management of Infants and Young Children.* New York: G.P. Putnam, 1901; Kerr, *The Baby;* Tweddell, *How to Take Care of the Baby;* Smith, R. *The Baby's First Two Years.* Boston: Houghton Mifflin, 1915; Dennett, R. *The Healthy Baby.* New York: MacMillan, 1922.

    Boas appreciated the interpretive shifts involved in using aggregate height-weight data in clinical settings. See his views on the "generalizing approach" in Boas, "Growth of Children"; Boas and Wissler, "Statistics of Growth"; Boas, "Observations."

24. Different towns—Des Moines, Iowa; Shreveport, Louisiana; New York City; Paris; and London—laid claim to having held the first babies' health contest. See Sherbon, F. B. "An Iowa Woman's Great Work for Better Babies." *Chicago Daily Tribune,* 3 August 1913, G2; Richardson, A. S. "New York Joins the Big Movement for Better Babies." *New York Times,* 20 April 1913, SM7; New York Child Welfare Committee, New York Child Welfare. *Handbook of the New York Child Welfare Exhibit.* New York: New York Children Welfare Committee, 1911.

    Contests were widely covered in the news. See, for example, "Baby Contests Growing." *New York Times,* 12 May 1913, 9; "Chicago's Prize Baby." *Chicago Daily Tribune,* 13 August 1920, 7; "Dimpled Cherubs Who Rule Washington Homes." *Washington Post,* 17 January 1915, 8.

    Better Babies contests have been considered by historians including Dorey, A. *Better Baby Contests: The Scientific Quest for Perfect Childhood Health in the Early Twentieth Century.* Jefferson, NC: McFarland, 1999; Meckel, R. *Save the Babies: American Public Health Reform and the Prevention of Infant Mortality, 1850–1929.* Baltimore: Johns Hopkins University Press, 1990; Holt, M. I. *Linoleum, Better Babies, and the Modern Farm Woman, 1890–1930.* Albuquerque: University of New Mexico Press, 1995; Stern, A. M. "Better Babies Contests at the Indiana State Fair: Child Health, Scientific Motherhood, and Eugenics in the Midwest, 1920–1935." In Stern and Markel, *Formative Years,* 121–152.

    The *Woman's Home Companion* served entertainment, advice, and education functions. Child-raising was one topic in particular that the magazine offered help on. In addition to the Better Babies contests, the *Companion* also ran a Prospective Mothers' Circle and a Mothers' Club that supplied readers with pamphlets by mail.

25. "Chicago's Prize Baby." *Chicago Daily Tribune,* 13 August 1920, 7; Holt, M. I. *Linoleum,* 113. Mitchell says that leaders within the African American

community saw Better Babies competitions as a practical defense against high infant mortality and the then-popular eugenic opinion that the black race was dying out. Mitchell, M. *Righteous Propagation*. Chapel Hill: University of North Carolina Press, 2004, especially 95–101. On better babies contests advertised in the "black press," see, for example, "Better Babies Show." *New York Amsterdam News*, 28 March 1923, 9; "Brooklyn Happenings." *Chicago Defender*, 19 August 1922, 9; "At the 'Y's.'" *Chicago Defender*, 8 November 1924, A8; "'Better Baby Contest Held by Homewood Civic Club." *Pittsburgh Courier*, 21 May 1924, 5; Starks, C. "Carrie's Corner." *Pittsburgh Courier*, 30 May 1925, 4.

26. Richardson, "New York Joins the Big Movement"; Sherbon, "Iowa Woman's Great Work."

27. Sherbon, "Iowa Woman's Great Work," G2.

28. On the repeated insistence that the contests are based on "health" assessments, see, for example, Richardson, "New York Joins the Big Movement; "Baby Contests Growing"; Sherbon, "Iowa Woman's Great Work"; "Prize for Best Baby." *Washington Post*, 5 November 1913, 3.

   The term "pathetic grief" from Richardson, "New York Joins the Big Movement," SM7.

29. See, for example, "Daily Procession of Mothers." *Washington Post*, 9 November 1913, 9; "Chicago's Prize Baby";; "Winners in Better Baby Show." *Chicago Daily Tribune*, 29 November 1927, 3.

30. The association's scorecard was based on that used at the 1911 Iowa State Fair. The Iowa organizers took their standards from the January–February 1911 New York Child Welfare exhibit. Holt had been on the health committee for the exhibit and had developed the exhibit materials. The association's score-card awarded points out of one hundred, eighty of which were for physical development. NY Child Welfare Committee. *Handbook of the NY Child Welfare Exhibit*. New York: New York Child Welfare Committee, 1911. The *Woman's Home Companion* scorecard allowed a maximum of one thousand points, broken down as two hundred points for mental development, seven hundred points for a physical exam, and one hundred points specifically for physical measurements.

   Gertrude Lane, director of the *Woman's Home Companion*, quoted in Gray, Norace, and K. M. Gray. "Normal Weight." *Boston Medical and Surgical Journal* 177 (1917): 894–899, 895–896.

   Stern has argued that the Better Babies contests demonstrated the "tyranny of pediatric norms" and that standard tables swept away former measures based on attractiveness. This is too strong a characterization: height-weight recommendations were more fluid, and, moreover, the babies' contest organizers happily altered figures as needed for scoring purposes. Some contests had special award categories for best appearance in the baby parade and popularity contests alongside the health competition. And, far from being neglected, criteria of attractiveness were essential in any winner. The competitions married ideas of "health" to those of "beauty" in judging the winners. Plumpness satisfied both criteria. Stern, A. M. "Beauty Is Not Always Better: Perfect Babies and the Tyranny of Paediatric Norms." *Patterns of Prejudice* 36 (2002): 68–78.

31. Crum, F. "Anthropometric Statistics of Children." *Publications of the American Statistical Association* 15 (1916): 332–336; Crum, F. *Anthropometric Table.* Newark: American Medical Association, Prudential Insurance Company of America, c1916.

Crum was interested in eugenic theories, then popular and prevalent in the United States. He was an assistant statistician to Frederick Hoffman, a significant figure for his racialist analysis of birth and death statistics, in which he concluded that blacks in America would likely die out. See Wilcox, W. "Frederick S. Crum." *Quarterly Publications of the American Statistical Association* 17 (1921): 1020–1021, 1020.

32. Bender, M. "Right Sizes for a Child Are Gamble." *New York Times,* 14 August 1961, 30.

Note that historically within the apparel industry, "clothing" referred to men's wear, while "garments" or "apparel" were gender-neutral terms. I should, therefore, refer to "boys' clothing" and "girls' apparel." This specialization in terminology has significantly eroded since the 1950s, and today the terms are used interchangeably—as I will do.

The early history of the clothing industry in the United States is covered in Cobrin, H. *The Men's Clothing Industry.* New York: Fairchild, 1970; *The New York Story: A History of the New York Clothing Industry.* New York: New York Clothing Manufacturers's Exchange, 1949; Godley, A. "Comparative Labour Productivity in the British and American Clothing Industries, 1850–1950." *Textile History* 28 (1997): 67–80; Solinger, J. *Apparel Manufacturing Analysis.* New York: Textile Book Publishers, 1961; Zakim, M. "A Ready-Made Business: The Birth of the Clothing Industry in America." *Business History Review* 73 (1999): 61–90. Children's clothing specifically is addressed in Buck, A. *Clothes and the Child.* Carlton: Ruth Bean, 1996; Cook, D. *The Commodification of Childhood.* Durham, NC: Duke University Press, 2004.

33. Quotation from Sears Fall/Winter Catalogue 1905–1906, Sears, Roebuck and Co. Catalogues (1893–1992/3), Baker Old Class and Historical Collection, Baker Library, Harvard Business School, Boston, Massachusetts.

Sears's history from Asher, L., and E. Heal. *Send No Money.* Chicago: Argus Books, 1942; Weil, G. *Sears, Roebuck, U.S.A.* New York: Stein and Day, 1977; Emmet, B., and J. Jeuck. *Catalogues and Counters.* Chicago: University of Chicago Press, 1950.

34. On the role of sizing systems in business productivity, see Godley, "Comparative Labour Productivity"; *The Apparel Manufacturing Industry.* New York: Market Planning Service (National Credit Office), 1953; Davis, E. "Why

Ready-Made Clothes Are Poor Fits." *Science News-Letter* 18 (1930): 196–198; Bender, "Right Sizes for a Child Are Gamble"; Emmet and Jeuck, *Catalogues and Counters,* especially 232–235.

35. "Like recipes . . ." quotation in Davis, "Why Ready-Made Clothes Are Poor Fits," 198.

First measurement surveys in United States Bureau of Home Economics. *Manual of Measurements: Study of Body Measurements for Sizing Children's Garments and Patterns.* Washington, DC: United States Department of Agriculture, 1937; O'Brien, R., and M. Girshick. *Children's Body Measurements for Sizing Garments and Patterns.* United States Department of Agriculture, Miscellaneous Publication no. 365. Washington, DC: Government Printing Office, 1939; O'Brien, R., M. Girshick, and E. Hunt. *Body Measurements of American Boys and Girls for Garment and Pattern Construction.* United States Department of Agriculture, Miscellaneous Publication no. 366. Washington, DC: Government Printing Office, 1941; United States Bureau of Home Economics. "Standard Sizes for Children's Clothes." Washington, DC: Bureau of Home Economics, National Consumer-Retailer Council, 1941. See also O'Brien, R. "The Program of Textile Research in the Bureau of Home Economics." *Journal of Home Economics* 22 (1930): 281–287, 283.

Postwar National Bureau of Standards voluntary commercial standards, Commercial Standard CS151-50, "Body Measurements for the Sizing of Apparel for Infants, Babies, Toddlers and Children" (1950); CS 153-48, "Body Measurements for the Sizing of Girls' Apparel" (1949); and CS 155-50, "Body Measurements for the Sizing of Boys' Apparel" (1950); National Institute of Standards and Technology (NIST). "Brief History of Voluntary Standards Published by the U.S. Department of Commerce." National Institute of Standards and Technology, http://ts.nist.gov/Standards/Conformity/briefhis. cfm. 2003. Access date 29 July 2008.

36. A summary of early racially specific studies is Meredith, H. "Stature and Weight of Children of the United States." *American Journal of Diseases of Children* 62 (1941): 909–932.

The Children's Year (1918) study and subsequent standards from Woodbury, R. M. *Statures and Weights of Children under Six Years of Age.* J. Davis and J. Lathorp, eds., Community Welfare Series, no. 3. Washington, DC: Children's Bureau, Government Printing Office, 1921; Woodbury, R. "Special Communications and Reports: Statures and Weights of Children under Six Years of Age." *American Journal of Physical Anthropology* 2 (1919): 195–202; *Children's Year: A Brief Summary of Work Done and Suggestions for Follow-up Work.* Children's Year Follow-up Series, no. 4, Bureau Publication no. 67. Washington, DC: U.S. Department of Labor, Children's Bureau, 1920.

Slews of height-weight studies have been carried out in the United States. Principal among these are those by three large research groups funded by the Laura Spellman Rockefeller Foundation, which had a great interest in child development: namely, the Iowa Child Welfare Research Station study (1918–1974); the Longitudinal Study of Child Health and Development, also known as the Harvard Growth Study (1930–1956); and the Guidance, Berkeley Growth, and Oakland Growth Studies at the California Institute of Child Welfare at the University of California, Berkeley.

On the Laura Spellman Rockefeller Foundation and child development, see, for example, Anderson, J. "Child Development: An Historical Perspective." *Child Development* 27 (1956): 181–196; Schlossman, S. "Philanthropy and the Gospel of Child Development." *History of Education Quarterly* 21 (1981): 275–299; Grant, J. "Constructing the Normal Child: The Rockefeller Philanthropies and the Science of Child Development, 1918–1940." In *Philanthropic Foundations*, E. Lagemann, ed., 131–150. Bloomington: Indiana University Press, 1999.

On Iowa Center, see, for example, Baldwin, B. T. "Studies in Child Welfare: The Physical Growth of Children from Birth to Maturity." *Studies in Child Welfare* 1 (1921): 1–365; Baldwin, B. T., and T. D. Wood. "Weight-Height-Age Tables." *Mother and Child* 4 (1923): supplement 1–11; Jackson, R., and H. Kelly. "Growth Charts for Use in Pediatric Practice." *Journal of Pediatrics* 27 (1945): 215–229; Meredith, H. "A 'Physical Growth Record' for Use in Elementary and High Schools." *American Journal of Public Health* 39 (1949): 878–885; Cravens, H. *Before Head Start: The Iowa Station and America's Children*. Chapel Hill: University of North Carolina Press, 1993.

On the Harvard Growth Study, see the various papers by Walter Dearborn and Frank Shuttleworth in the series Monographs of the Society for Research in Child Development; see also Stuart, H. "The Search for Knowledge of the Child and the Significance of His Growth and Development." *Pediatrics* 24 (1959): 701–709.

The California Institute's work is addressed in Jones, H., and N. Bayley. "The Berkeley Growth Study." *Child Development* 12 (1941): 167–173.

A fourth significant longitudinal growth study is the Fels Longitudinal Study at the Fels Research Institute in Yellow Spring, Ohio, which started in 1929 and is still gathering data. Sontag, L. *The Fels Research Institute for the Study of Human Development*. Yellow Springs, OH: Antioch College Press, 1946; Sontag, L. "The History of Longitudinal Research." *Child Development* 42 (1971): 987–1002; Siervogel, R., A. Roche, S. Guo, D. Mukherjee, and W. Chumlea. "Patterns of Change in Weight/Stature from 2 to 18 Years." *International Journal of Obesity* 15 (1991): 479–485; Roche, A. *Growth, Maturation, and Body Composition: The Fels Longitudinal Study, 1929–1991*. Cambridge: Cambridge University Press, 1992.

NHES and NHANES are discussed in National Center for Health Statistics, "Origin, Program, and Operation of the U.S. National Health Survey." *Vital and Health Statistics* 1 Washington, DC: US Department of Health, Education, and Welfare, 1965; National Center for Health Statistics,

"Plan and Operation of a Health Examination Survey of Youths 12–17 Years of Age." *Vital and Health Statistics* 8. Washington, DC: US Department of Health, Education, and Welfare, 1969; National Center for Health Statistics, "Plan and Operation of the Health and Nutrition Examination Survey, United States, 1971–1973." *Vital and Health Statistics* 10a, 10b. Washington, DC: US Department of Health, Education, and Welfare, 1973; Hamill, P., T. Drizd, et al. "NCHS Growth Charts, 1976." *Monthly Vital Statistics Report* 25 (1976): 1–22; Owen, G. "The New National Center for Health Statistics Growth Charts." *Southern Medical Journal* 71 (1978): 296–297; Dibley, M., J. Goldsby, et al. "Development of Normalized Curves for the International Growth Reference." *American Journal of Clinical Nutrition* 46 (1987): 736–748; Kuczmarski, R. J., C. L. Ogden, et al. "CDC Growth Charts: United States." *Vital and Health Statistics* 314 (2000): 1–28; Kuczmarski, R.J., C.L. Ogden, et al. "2000 CDC Growth Charts for the United States: Methods and Development." *Vital and Health Statistics* 11 (2002).

Development of international growth standards in connection with U.S. survey data is discussed in Dibley et al., "Development of Normalized Curves"; De Onis, M., and J-P. Habicht. "Anthropometric Reference Data for International Use." *American Journal of Clinical Nutrition* 64 (1996): 650–658; De Onis, M., C. Garza, and J-P. Habicht. "Time for a New Growth Reference." *Pediatrics* 100 (1997): e8; De Onis, M., C. Garza, et al. "Comparison of the WHO Child Growth Standards and the CDC 2000 Growth Charts." *Journal of Nutrition* 137 (2007): 144–148.

37. *Infant Care* was produced by the bureau from 1914. The Children's Year data were included in the later editions. Apple, R. *Mothers and Medicine: A Social History of Infant Feeding, 1890–1950.* Madison: University of Wisconsin Press, 1987; Children's Bureau. *The Story of Infant Care.* Washington, DC: U.S. Department of Health, Education, and Welfare, 1965, 1.

2. Measuring Up

Epigraph: Illingworth, R. S. "Obesity." *Journal of Pediatrics* 53 (1958): 117–130, 117.

1. Veeder, B. "The Overweight Child." *Journal of the American Medical Association* 83 (1924): 486–489, 486.

2. The rise of concern about adult obesity in America and especially dietary treatment is discussed in Stearns, P. *Fat History.* New York: New York University Press, 1997; Schwartz, H. *Never Satisfied: A Cultural History of Diets, Fantasies, and Fat.* New York: Free Press, 1986; Gilman, Sr. *Fat: A Cultural History of Obesity.* Cambridge: Polity, 2008; Levenstein, H. *Paradox of Plenty: A Social History of Eating in Modern America.* Oxford: Oxford University Press, 1993.

Banting, W. *A Letter on Corpulence, Addressed to the Public.* 2nd ed. London: Harrison and Sons, 1863, 7–8, 14, 22–23.

3. The role of nutrition in childhood mortality is discussed in Hardy, A. "Rickets and the Rest: Child-Care, Diet and the Infectious Children's Diseases, 1850–1914." *Social History of Medicine* 5 (1992): 389–412.

    Death rates from Shulman, S. "A History of Pediatric Infectious Diseases." *Pediatric Research* 55 (2004): 163–176.

    The theory on the decline in infectious disease mortality due to social and environmental change is most associated with McKeown, T. *The Role of Medicine*. Princeton, NJ: Princeton University Press, 1979.

4. Emerson, W. R. P. "Overweight in Children." *Boston Medical and Surgical Journal* 185 (1921): 475–476, 476. Similar sentiments may be found in Evans, F., and J. Strang. "A Departure from the Usual Methods in Treating Obesity." *American Journal of Medical Science* 177 (1929): 339–348; Nixon, N. K. "Obesity in Childhood." *Journal of Pediatrics* 4 (1934): 295–306.

5. Reviews of advertising using children include Alexander, V. "The Image of Children in Magazine Advertisements from 1905 to 1990." *Communication Research* 21 (1994): 742–765; Muncaster, A., E. Sawyer, and K. Kapson. *The Baby Made Me Buy It*. New York: Crown, 1991; Margerum, E. "The Child in American Advertising, 1890–1960." In *Images of the Child*, H. Eiss, ed., 335–354. Bowling Green, OH: Bowling Green State University Press, 1994; Viser, V. "Mode of Address, Emotion, and Stylistics: Images of Children in American Magazine Advertising, 1940–1950." *Communication Research* 24 (1997): 83–101.

    Product-specific histories include Bradley, L. "Millais's *Bubbles* and the Problem of Artistic Advertising." In *Pre-Raphaelite Art in Its European Context*, S. Casteras and A. Craig Faxon, eds. Madison, NJ: Fairleigh Dickinson University Press, 1995; Chen, A. *Campbell Kids*. New York: Abrahams, 2004; Wyman, C. *Jello*. San Diego, CA: Harcourt, 2001.

    On the history of children in film (although not the body shape of child actors), see Goldstein, R., and E. Zornow. *The Screen Image of Youth*. Metuchen, NJ: Scarecrow Press, 1980; Sinyard, N. *Children in the Movies*. London: Batsford, 1992.

    An insightful exploration of the fat boy character in ensemble films is Mosher, J. "Survival of the Fattest: Contending with the Fat Boy in Children's Ensemble Films." In *Where the Boys Are*, M. Pomerance and F. Gateward, eds., 61–82. Detroit: Wayne State University Press, 2005.

6. Starr, L. *Hygiene of the Nursery*. Philadelphia: Blakiston, 1889, 24.

    Chen, *Campbell Kids*.

7. We can speculate as to why attractiveness in children has become slimmer over the twentieth century. The comparative rarity of fatness in children in the early twentieth century may have made it more appealing; its increasing prevalence may have encouraged the appeal of the slimness that is now more unusual. The changing nature of filmic storytelling to more psychologically complicated child roles and darker themes may have driven a tendency to cast children with

more angular features. Scholars of advertising have also noted connections between economic prosperity, parenting style, and the advertising appeal of children. See, for example, Margerum, "Child in American Advertising"; Alexander, "Image of Children in Magazine Advertisements."

8. The Association of Life Insurance Medical Directors and the Actuarial Society of America. "Medico-Actuarial Mortality Investigation." *Medico-Actuarial Mortality Investigation* 2 (1913): 5–9, 44–47. See also Dublin, L. "Body Build and Longevity." In *Delamar Lectures, 1925–1926*, 113–127. Baltimore, MD: Williams and Wilkins, 1927; Marks, H. "Body Weight: Facts from Life Insurance Records." In *Body Measurements and Human Nutrition*, J. Brožek, ed., 107–121. Detroit: Wayne University Press, 1956; Weigley, E. "Average? Ideal? Desirable? A Brief Overview of Height-Weight Tables in the United States." *Journal of the American Dietetic Association* 84 (1984): 417–423; Bray, G. "Life Insurance and Overweight." *Obesity Research* 3 (1995): 97–99.

9. For example, Preble, W. "Obesity and Malnutrition." *Boston Medical and Surgical Journal* 922 (1915): 740–744; Dublin, "Body Build and Longevity."

10. "So far as we know . . ." quotation from Veeder, "Overweight Child," 488; "the tax put upon the heart . . ." from Emerson, "Overweight in Children", 475–476; "games requiring more skill . . ." from Veeder, "Overweight Child," 487.

11. Emerson, "Overweight in Children," 475.

12. For example, Bronstein, I., L. J. Halpern, and A. W Brown. "Obesity in Children." *Journal of Pediatrics* 21 (1942): 485–496; Stuart, H. "Obesity in Childhood." *Quarterly Review of Pediatrics* 10 (1955): 131–145; Illingworth, "Obesity." *Journal of Pediatrics* 53 (1958): 117–130.

Baldwin, B. T., and T. Wood. "Weight-Height-Age Tables." *Mother and Child* 4, (1923): supplement 1–11, 3.

13. Illingworth, "Obesity," 117.; Bakwin, H. "Obesity in Children." *Journal of Pediatrics* 54 (1959): 392–400; Evans and Strang, "Departure from the Usual Methods"; Bronstein, Halpern, and Brown, "Obesity in Children"; Stuart, "Obesity in Childhood."

Bronstein, Halpern, and Brown, "Obesity in Children," 486.

Pediatrics textbooks advised using deviations from average weight to diagnose obesity but also cautioned using clinical judgment. See, for example, Holt, L. E., and J. Howland. *Holt's Diseases of Infancy and Childhood*. 10th ed. L. E. Holt Jr. and R. McIntosh, eds. New York: Appleton, 1933, 21; Bruch, H. "Overnutrition: Obesity." In *Pediatrics*, L. E. Holt Jr., R. McIntosh and H. Barnett, eds., 255–258. New York: Appleton-Century-Crofts, 1962; Paulsen, E. "Obesity in Children and Adolescents." In *Pediatrics*, H. Barnett and A. Einhorn, eds., 214–221. New York: Appleton-Century-Crofts, 1972, 214–216.

14. Nixon, "Obesity in Childhood," 295.

15. Barlow, S., W. Dietz, et al. "Medical Evaluation of Overweight Children and Adolescents" *Pediatrics* 110 (2002): 222–228.

16. An example of the Children's Bureau's cautions is Children's Bureau. *Infant Care,* Washington, DC: Government Printing Office, 1945.

    The medical profession's wish for sole rights over school health determinations is addressed in "Note on Height-Weight-Age Tables for Children." *American Journal of Physical Anthropology* 18 (1933): 155–157; Starr, P. *The Social Transformation of American Medicine.* New York: Basic Books, 1982, 187–189.

    "Zealous, if misguided" quotation from Dearborn, W., and J. Rothney. *Predicting the Child's Development.* Cambridge, MA: Sci-Art Publishers, 1941, 44.

17. Compare, for example, Faber, H. "Variability in Weight for Height in Children of School Age." *American Journal of Diseases of Children* 30 (1925): 328–335; Gray, H., and J. G. Ayres. *Growth in Private School Children.* Chicago: University of Chicago Press, 1931.

18. Meredith, H. "A 'Physical Growth Record' for Use in Elementary and High Schools." *American Journal of Public Health* 39 (1949): 878–885, 878; Stuart, H., and H. Meredith. "Use of Body Measurements in the School Health Program." *American Journal of Public Health and the Nation's Health* 36 (1946): 1365–1386.

19. Meredith, "'Physical Growth Record,'" 882.

20. Ibid.

21. "En considérant les valeurs comme des nombres abstrait." Quetelet, A. *Sur L'homme et le développement de ses facultés, ou essai de physique sociale.* Paris: Bachelier, 1835, 3. See also Lurgin, C. "Quetelet's Scientific Work." *Science* 60, no. 1555 (1924): 351–352; Porter, T. "The Mathematics of Society: Variation and Error in Quetelet's Statistics." *British Journal for the History of Science* 18 (1985): 51–69; Stigler, S. *The History of Statistics.* Cambridge, MA: Harvard University Press, 1986.

22. "D'après des recherches nombreuses que j'ai faites sur la corrélation entre les tailles et les poids des homes adults, j'ai cru pouvoir conclure que les poids sont simplement *comme les carrés des hauteurs*." Quetelet, *Sur L'homme et le développement de ses facultíes,* 97.

23. Keys, A., F. Fidanza, et al. "Indices of Relative Weight and Obesity." *Journal of Chronic Diseases* 25 (1972): 329–343.

24. Livi, R. "L'indice ponderale o il rapporto tra la statura e il peso." *Atti Soc Romana di Antrop* 5 (1897): 125–152, reproduced in French as Livi, R. "L'indice pondéral ou rapport entre la taille et le poids." *Archives Italiennes de Biologie* 32 (1899): 229–378.

25. Wetzel, N. "Physical Fitness in Terms of Physique, Development and Basal Metabolism." *Journal of the American Medical Association* 116 (1941): 1187–1195. See also Wetzel, N. "Assessing the Physical Condition of Children." *Journal of Pediatrics* 22 (1943): 82–110, 208–225, 329–361; Wetzel, N. "Growth." In *Medical Physics,* O. Glasser, ed., 513–569. Chicago: Year Book, 1944.

26. Wetzel, "Physical Fitness," 1189–1190, 1191.

27. Tanner, J. M. "The Assessment of Growth and Development in Children." *Archives of Disease in Childhood* 27, (1952): 10–33, 25. See also Baer, M. J., I. Torgoff, and D. Harris. "Differential Impact of Weight and Height on Wetzel Developmental Age." *Child Development* 33 (1962): 737–750; Bruch, H. "The Grid for Evaluating Physical Fitness (Wetzel)." *Journal of the American Medical Association* 118 (1942): 1289–1293.

28. Examples using the Wetzel grid include Wheatley, G. "Trends in School Health Services." *Review of Educational Research* 13 (1943): 490–498; Garn, S. "Individual and Group Deviations from 'Channelwise' Grid Progression in Girls." *Child Development* 23 (1952): 193–206; Baer, Torgoff, and Harris, "Differential Impact." Studies using the Wetzel grid to determine the prevalence of obesity are Bruch, "Grid"; Dupertuis, C. W., and N. Michael. "Comparison of Growth in Height and Weight between Ectomorphic and Mesomorphic Boys." *Child Development* 24 (1953): 203–214; Johnson, M. L., B. Burke, and J. Mayer. "Relative Importance of Inactivity and Overeating in the Energy Balance of Obese High School Girls." *American Journal of Clinical Nutrition* 4 (1956): 37–44; Rauh, J., D. Schumsky, and M. Witt. "Heights, Weights, and Obesity in Urban School Children." *Child Development* 38 (1967): 515–530.

29. For example, McCloy, C. *Appraising Physical Status.* G. Stoddard, ed. Vol. 12. Studies in Child Welfare. Iowa City: University of Iowa, 1936; Wolff, "A Study of Height"; Franzen, R. "Validity of Comparisons of Current Methods for Estimating Physical Status." *Child Development* 8 (1937): 221–222.

30. Pearl, R. "An Index of Body Build." *American Journal of Physical Anthropology* 26 (1940): 315–348, 320; Meredith, H., and S. Culp. "Body Form in Childhood." *Child Development* 22 (1951): 3–14, 5; Davenport, C. B. "Height-Weight Index of Build." *American Journal of Physical Anthropology* 3 (1920): 467–475.

31. Hamill, P., T. Drizd, et al. "NCHS Growth Charts, 1976." *Monthly Vital Statistics Report* 25 (1976): 1–22; Hamill, P., T. Drizd, et al. "NCHS Growth Curves for Children: Birth–18 Years." In National Center for Health Statistics. *Data from the National Health Survey.* Washington, DC. United States Department of Health, Education, and Welfare, 1977; Owen, G. "The New National Center for Health Statistics Growth Charts." *Southern Medical Journal* 71 (1978): 296–297; Hamill, P., T. Drizd, C. L. Johnson, R. B. Reed, A. F. Roche, and W. M. Moore. "Physical Growth: National Center for Health Statistics Percentiles." *American Journal of Clinical Nutrition* 32 (1979): 607–629.

The National Health Survey Act of 1956 authorized making regular health surveys of the population to base regulatory and policy decisions on. For the first National Health Examination Survey (NHES I, 1959–1962), the National Center for Health Statistics collected data on certain chronic diseases of adults between eighteen and seventy-nine years of age. NHES II (1963–1965) and NHES III (1966–1970) looked at the health, growth, and development of children and adolescents. Renamed the National Health and Nutrition Examination Surveys (to incorporate questions on diet), NHANES I (1971–1975) looked at people aged between one and seventy. The 1976 tables were based on data from NHES II to NHANES I. In the second cycle, NHANES II (1976–1980), the age range was expanded to include children from six months, and the third NHANES III (1988–1994) expanded to include an even greater age range, down to two months old. After 1999, surveys continued without a break between cycles. About 7,500 people were surveyed in each of the first three NHES cycles, and 25,000 in NHANES I. Between 25,000 and 40,000 people were surveyed in the later NHANES rounds. National Centre for Health Statistics, "Origin, Program, and Operation of the U.S. National Health Survey." *Vital and Health Statistics* 1. Washington, DC:US Department of Health, Education, and Welfare, 1965; National Centre for Health Statistics, "Plan and Operation of the Second National Health and Nutrition Examination Survey, 1976–1980." *Vital and Health Statistics* 15. Washington, DC: US Department of Health, Education, and Welfare, 1981; Kuczmarski, R.J., C.L. Ogden, S.S. Guo, et al. "2000 CDC Growth Charts for the United States: Methods and Development." *Vital and Health Statistics* 11 (2002).

The exception to this whole-of-population reference group was the part of the table for infants up to one year of age. NHES had not gathered data on children this young. To fill the gap, the NCHS used data from the Fels Longitudinal Study, conducted since 1929 at Yellow Springs, Ohio. The Fels study was made on children in the area close to the Fels Institute and was not, therefore, representative of the United States as a whole. Sontag, L. *The Fels Research Institute for the Study of Human Development.* Yellow Springs, OH: Antioch College Press, 1946; Roche, A. *Growth, Maturation, and Body Composition: The Fels Longitudinal Study, 1929–1991.* Cambridge: Cambridge University Press, 1992.

See also commentary in Dibley, M., J. Goldsby, et al. "Development of Normalized Curves for the International Growth Reference." *American Journal of Clinical Nutrition* 46 (1987): 736–748.

32. Roche, A., and J. McKigney. "Reports of Meetings: Physical Growth of Ethnic Groups Comprising the United States Population." *American Journal of Clinical Nutrition* 28 (1975): 1071–1074; Owen, "New National Center for Health Statistics."

33. Hamill et al., "Physical Growth," 628.

34. An excellent review of ways of measuring obesity prevalence is Troiano, R., and K. Flegal. "Overweight Prevalence among Youth in the United States: Why So Many Different Numbers?" *International Journal of Obesity* 23, supplement (1999): S22–S27.

The recommendation regarding ethnic groups is from Roche and McKigney, "Reports of Meetings," 1072.

3. Sugar, Spice, Frogs, Snails

Epigraph: Seltzer, C., and J. Mayer. "A Simple Criterion of Obesity." *Postgraduate Medicine* 38 (1965): A101–A07, A106.

1. For example, in the physiology textbooks by William Zoethout, the first twelve editions to 1955 repeat this tripartite function of fat. Zoethout, W. *A Textbook of Physiology.* 2nd ed. St. Louis: C.V. Mosby, 1925; Zoethout, W., and W. W. Tuttle. *A Textbook of Physiology.* 12th ed. St. Louis: C.V. Mosby, 1955.

2. Cahill illustrates the exponential increase in papers on the physiology of adipose tissue since the early 1950s. Cahill, G. "Metabolic Role of Adipose Tissue." *Transactions of the American Clinical Climatological Association* 73 (1962): 22–29. A good review is Redinger, R. "Fat Storage and the Biology of Energy Expenditure." *Translational Research* 142 (2009): 52–60.

   An early study of the effects of fat location is Vague, J. "The Degree of Masculine Differentiation of Obesities." *American Journal of Clinical Nutrition* 4 (1956): 20–34. Vague showed that "gynoid" (lower-body) fat tended not to be associated with cardiovascular and metabolic conditions, whereas "android" (upper-body) fat was. Similar findings reviewed in Snijder, M. B., R. M. van Dam, et al. "What Aspects of Body Fat Are Particularly Hazardous and How Do We Measure Them?" *International Journal of Epidemiology* 35 (2006): 83–92.

   The Minnesota starvation experiment, conducted by Ancel Keys and his team at the University of Minnesota from 1944 to 1945, showed that a starved body would not metabolize all its fat reserves. Keys, A., J. Brožek, et al. *The Biology of Human Starvation.* Minneapolis: University of Minnesota Press, 1950; Taylor, H., and A. Keys. "Adaptation to Caloric Restriction." *Science* 112, no. 2904 (1950): 215–218; Lasker, G. "The Effects of Partial Starvation on Somatotype." *American Journal of Physical Anthropology* 5 (1947): 323–342. On the controversial use of conscientious objectors as experimental subjects, see Tucker, T. *The Great Starvation Experiment.* Minneapolis: University of Minnesota Press, 2006.

   The increasing attention being given by physiologists to fat and its involvement in metabolic processes can be traced in evolving editions of textbooks, such as, for example, Arthur C. Guyton's *Textbook of Medical Physiology* or William D. Zoethout's (later William Tuttle's) *Textbook of Physiology.* As a case in point, the 1956 edition of Guyton's textbook contains twenty-seven entries under the heading "fat"; the 2000 edition has sixty-five. Guyton, A. *Textbook of Medical Physiology.* Philadelphia: W.B. Saunders, 1956; Guyton, A., and J. Hall. *Textbook of Medical Physiology.* 10th ed. Philadelphia: W.B. Saunders, 2000.

3. "Inference of fatness" quotation from Seltzer and Mayer, "Simple Criterion of Obesity," A106.

4. Widdowson was a leading figure in nutrition studies who worked on wartime rationing in the United Kingdom and instituted vitamin and mineral fortification of flour. She is also known for her study of German orphans and the effects of loving attention. She experimented extensively on herself, believing that the investigator must be willing to undergo what was asked of subjects. Cadaver analysis was, presumably, an exception. Ashwell, M. "Elsie May Widdowson." *Biographical Memoirs of Fellows of the Royal Society* 48 (2002): 483–506; Ashwell, M. *McCance and Widdowson: A Scientific Partnership of 60 Years.* London: British Nutrition, 1993.

   Overviews of direct analysis methods in Widdowson, E. M. "Chemical Analysis of the Body." In *Human Body Composition,* J. Brožek, ed., 31–48. Oxford: Pergamon, 1965; Sheng, H-P., and R. Huggins. "A Review of Body Composition Studies with Emphasis on Total Body Water and Fat." *American Journal of Clinical Nutrition* 32 (1979): 630–647; Pierson, R. N. "A Brief History of Body Composition: From F. D. Moore to the New Reference Man." *Acta Diabetologica* 40, supplement (2003): 114–116.

   "Uniform dark brown suspension" from Widdowson, "Chemical Analysis of the Body," 33.

   "Heroic" and "tedious" quotation from Pitts, G. C. "Studies of Gross Body Composition by Direct Dissection." *Annals of the New York Academy of Sciences* 100 (1963): 11–22.

5. Knight, G. S., A. H. Beddoe, et al. "Body Composition of Two Human Cadavers by Neutron Activation and Chemical Analysis." *American Journal of Physiology: Endocrinology and Metabolism* 250 (1986): E179–E85, E181.

6. A number of studies of fetuses and stillborn babies were carried out by German physiologists at the turn of the century. Overviews include Moulton, C. R. "Age and Chemical Development in Mammals." *Journal of Biological Chemistry* 62 (1923): 79–97; Widdowson, E. M., and J. W. T. Dickerson. "Chemical Composition of the Body." In *Mineral Metabolism,* C. L. Comar and F. Bronner, eds., 2–247. New York: Academic Press, 1964.

   "They are of a more manageable size" from Widdowson and Dickerson, "Chemical Composition of the Body," 38.

7. See, for example, Sappol, M. *A Traffic of Dead Bodies.* Princeton, NJ: Princeton University Press, 2002; Roach, M. *Stiff.* New York: Norton, 2003; Watson, K. *Forensic Medicine in Western Society.* Oxford: Routledge, 2011, chapter 6.

   "Chemical derangement" quotation from Forbes, G. "Methods for Determining Composition of the Human Body." *Pediatrics* 29 (1962): 477–494, 478.

8. Behnke received his medical training at Stanford and also worked as a research fellow in physiology in the School of Public Health at Harvard. After his retirement from the navy in 1959, Behnke continued his research on body

composition at the University of California in Berkeley. He died in 1992. Bray, G. "Measurement of Body Composition: An Improving Art." *Obesity Research* 3 (1995): 291–293. A summary of the issues Behnke was trying to address is in Behnke, A. "Physiologic Studies Pertaining to Deep Sea Diving and Aviation, Especially in Relation to the Fat Content and Composition of the Body." *Harvey Lectures* 37 (1941–1942): 198–226.

9. Other gases, such as helium, are less absorbed by the body, and so helium-oxygen mixtures were (and are) also used by deep-sea divers. Breathing pure oxygen for long periods is not a solution to the problem of the body absorbing other gases—divers breathing pure oxygen can suffer from "oxygen poisoning," which starts as a feeling of euphoria, the "rapture of the deep," and progresses to vision impairment, nausea, and loss of consciousness.

   The football players study is Welham, W. C., and A. Behnke. "The Specific Gravity of Health Men." *Journal of the American Medical Association* 118 (1942): 498–501. Behnke also included a correction for "residual air"—the air remaining in a person's lungs even after exhaling which would contribute slightly to buoyancy. Later refinements of densitometry included corrections for gas trapped in a person's gastrointestinal tract.

10. Behnke, A., B. G. Feen, and W. C. Welham. "The Specific Gravity of Healthy Men." *Journal of the American Medical Association* 118 (1942): 495–498.

11. Siri, W. E. "The Gross Composition of the Body." In *Advances in Biological and Medical Physics*, C. A. Tobias and J. Lawrence, eds., 239–280. New York: Academic Press, 1956; Brožek, J., F. Grande, et al. "Densiometric Analysis of Body Composition." *Annals of the New York Academy of Sciences* 100 (1963): 113–140.

12. Not only would there be the matter of dunking the cadaver in the densitometry tank and stopping it from filling up with water, but also making corrections for lung volume and gastrointestinal tract gases would be extremely difficult. One would have to suck the air out of the cadaver's lungs and keep them evacuated. Moreover, gastrointestinal tract bacteria quickly make a dead body bloat with trapped gas.

13. Brožek, J., and A. Keys. "The Evaluation of Leanness-Fatness in Man." *British Journal of Nutrition* 5 (1951): 194–206.

14. Rauh, J., and D. Schumsky. "Lean and Non-lean Body Mass Estimates in Urban School Children." In *Human Growth*, D. B. Cheek, ed., 242–252. Philadelphia: Lea and Febiger, 1968, 251.

15. For example, Mayer, J. "Some Aspects of the Problem of Regulation of Food Intake and Obesity." *New England Journal of Medicine* 274 (1966): 610–616; Wilmore, J., and J. McNamara. "Prevalence of Coronary Heart Disease Risk Factors in Boys, 8 to 12 Years of Age." *Journal of Pediatrics* 84 (1974): 527–533; Lohman, T. G. "Applicability of Body Composition Techniques and Constants for Children and Youths." *Exercise Sport Science Review* 14 (1986): 325–357.

Haschke, F., S. Fomon, and E. Ziegler. "Body Composition of a Nine-Year-Old Reference Boy." *Pediatric Research* 15 (1981): 847–849.

16. On the history of radiation detectors and especially of the Los Alamos Laboratory's role in their development, see Petersen, D. "Los Alamos Radiation Detectors for Biology and Medicine." *Los Alamos Science* 23 (1995): 274–279; Voelz, G., D. Petersen, and D. Daugherty. "Tracer Studies at Los Alamos." *Los Alamos Science* 23 (1995): 256–273.

17. Anderson, E., R. Schuch, et al. "The Los Alamos Human Counter." *Nucleonics* 14 (1956): 26–29, 26.

18. The team was comprised of Wright Langham (the team leader), with F. Newton Hayes (an organic chemist who developed the liquid used as the scintillator), Ernest Anderson, Robert Schuch, and Jim Perrings. Anderson, Perrings, and Schuch worked on the detector instrumentation; they had previously worked on carbon decay.

    Experimenters had tried using scintillation as a way of detecting radiation since 1903, but they had had to manually count the light flashes—a time-consuming and error-prone task. With the invention of the photomultiplier tube in the late 1940s—a device that could detect the flashes of light and turn them into an electrical signal—scintillation counters became a feasible method for routinely detecting radiation. Petersen, "Los Alamos Radiation Detectors."

    On the prototype detector, see Reines, F., R. I. Schuch, et al. "Determination of Total Body Radiation Using Liquid Scintillation Counters." *Nature* 172, no. 4377 (1953): 521–523.

    On HUMCO-1 and the measurement program, see Anderson, E. C., and W. H..Langham. "Average Potassium Concentration of the Human Body as a Function of Age." *Science* 130, no. 3377 (1959): 713–714; Anderson, Schuch, et al, "Los Alamos Human Counter."

19. Anderson and Langham, "Average Potassium Concentration of the Human Body," 713.

20. The Los Alamos and Rochester teams (who had built their own scintillation counter in 1959) argued over who had first suggested that the technique could be useful in studying and defining obesity. See Woodward, K. T., T. T. Trujillo et al. "Correlation of Total Body Potassium with Body-Water." *Nature* 178, no. 4524 (1956): 97–98; Anderson and Langham. "Average Potassium Concentration of the Human Body"; Forbes, G., J. Gallup, and J. Hursh. "Estimation of Total Body Fat from Potassium-40 Content." *Science* 133, no. 3446 (1961): 101–102; Anderson, E. C., and W. H. Langham. "Estimation of Total Body Fat from Potassium-40 Content." *Science* 133, no. 3468 (1961): 1917; Forbes, G., and J. Hursh. "Estimation of Total Body Fat from Potassium-40 Content: Reply." *Science* 133, no. 3468 (1961): 1918.

21. Forbes, G. "Lean Body Mass and Fat in Obese Children." *Pediatrics* 34 (1964): 308–314, 313. See also Forbes, Gallup, and Hursh, "Estimation of Total Body

Fat from Potassium-40 Content"; Forbes, G. "Body Composition in Adolescence." In *Human Growth*, F. Falkner and J. M. Tanner, eds., 239–271. New York: Plenum Press, 1978.

22. Moulton, "Age and Chemical Development in Mammals," 95–96.

23. Researchers using Moulton's argument to justify using adult equations for children include Novak, L. "Total Body Water and Solids in Six- to Seven-Year-Old Children: Differences between the Sexes." *Pediatrics* 38 (1966): 483–489; Rauh and Schumsky, "Lean and Non-lean Body Mass Estimates"; Forbes, G., and G. H. Amirhakimi. "Skinfold Thickness and Body Fat in Children." *Human Biology* 42 (1970): 401–418.

Examples of researchers *not* accepting that adult equations should be used with children include Pařízková, J. "Total Body Fat and Skinfold Thickness in Children." *Metabolism* 10 (1961): 794–807; Young, C., S. Sipin, and D. Roe. "Body Composition of Pre-adolescent and Adolescent Girls I. Density and Skinfold Measurements." *Journal of the American Dietetic Association* 53 (1968): 25–31.

24. Haschke, Fomon, and Ziegler, "Body Composition of a Nine-Year-old Reference Boy"; Lohman, T. G. "Skinfolds and Body Density and Their Relation to Body Fatness." *Human Biology* 53 (1981): 181–225; Lohman, T., R. Boileau, and M. Slaughter. "Body Composition in Children and Youth." In *Advances in Pediatric Sport Sciences*, Bar-Or, O., ed., 29–57. Champaign, IL: Human Kinetics, 1984; Lohman, "Applicability of Body Composition Techniques."

Estimation of age 15 from Lohman, Boileau, and Slaughter, "Body Composition in Children," 37; estimation of age 16 for girls, 18 for boys from Lohman, "Applicability of Body Composition Techniques," 334.

25. Lohman, "Applicability of Body Composition Techniques," 325, 353. See also Forbes, "Body Composition in Adolescence"; Haschke, Fomon, and Ziegler, "Body Composition of a Nine-Year-Old Reference Boy"; Boileau, R. A., T. G. Lohman, et al. "Hydration of the Fat-Free Body in Children during Maturation." *Human Biology* 56 (1984): 651–666; Lohman, Boileau, and Slaughter, "Body Composition in Children and Youth"; Slaughter, M. H., T. G. Lohman, and R. A. Boileau. "Skinfold Equations for Estimation of Body Fatness in Children and Youth." *Human Biology* 60 (1988): 709–723.

26. Neutron activation measurement is related to potassium counting. It involves irradiating the person and then using a total body scintillator to measure the radiation that his or her body gives off. See Cohn, S. H., C. S. Dombrowski, H. R. Pate, and J. S. Robertson. "A Whole-Body Counter with an Invariant Response to Radionuclide Distribution and Body Size." *Physics in Medicine and Biology* 14 (1969): 645–658; Vaswani, A., I. Zanzi, et al. "Changes in Body Chemical Composition with Age Measured by Total Body Neutron Activation." *Metabolism* 25 (1976): 85–96.

Bioelectrical impedance relies on the fact that bone and body fat do not conduct electricity well, whereas water-containing body tissues (both inside and outside cells) do. Cell membranes also conduct some electricity and absorb some current as a capacitor does. Electrical leads are connected to a person's hands and ankles, and a small current is run through them. The body acts as an electrical circuit in which there are two parallel pathways: one (the extracellular pathway) with a resistor, and the other (the intracellular and cell membrane pathway) acting as a resistor and capacitor in series. Depending on the frequency of the applied current, the current will travel along these two pathways in different proportions. The resistance of the body can be used to give an estimate of the water content, from which fat content is then calculated. See Presto, E., J. Wang, et al. "Measurement of Total Body Conductivity: A New Method for Estimation of Body Composition." *American Journal of Clinical Nutrition* 37 (1983): 735–739.

DEXA (sometimes DXA) was originally developed to assess bone density. X-rays of different frequencies are absorbed differently by different tissue types. By using two different X-ray frequencies and taking measurements of how these two wavelengths are absorbed by different parts of a person's body, it is possible to calculate the amount of bone, fat, and lean tissues. See Peppler, W. W., and R. B. Mazess. "Total Body Bone Mineral and Lean Body Mass by Dual-Photon Absorptiometry." *Calcified Tissue International* 33 (1981): 353–359; Mazess, R. B., W. W. Peppler, and M. Gibbons. "Total Body Composition by Dual Photon (^{153} Gd) Absorptiometry." *American Journal of Clinical Nutrition* 40 (1984): 834–839.

4. Insides Made Easy

Epigraph: Keys, A., F. Fidanza, et al. "Indices of Relative Weight and Obesity." *Journal of Chronic Diseases* 25 (1972): 329–343, 329, 341.

1. Rauh, J., and D. Schumsky. "Lean and Non-lean Body Mass Estimates in Urban School Children." In *Human Growth,* D. Cheek, ed., 242–252. Philadelphia: Lea and Febiger, 1968, 242.

2. For example, Meredith, H., and H. Stuart. "Use of Body Measurements in the School Health Program." *American Journal of Public Health* 37 (1947): 1435–1438; Pařízková, J. "Total Body Fat and Skinfold Thickness in Children." *Metabolism* 10 (1961): 794–807, 794; Lowe, C., D. Coursin, et al. "Measurement of Skinfold Thickness in Childhood." *Pediatrics* 42 (1968): 538–543; Lohman, T. G. "Skinfolds and Body Density and Their Relation to Body Fatness." *Human Biology* 53 (1981): 181–225; Weststrate, J., and P. Deurenberg. "Body Composition in Children: Proposal for a Method for Calculating Body Fat Percentage from Total Body Density or Skinfold-Thickness Measurements." *American Journal of Clinical Nutrition* 50 (1989): 1104–1115.

An excellent overview of the issues of this approach is Brožek, J., and A. Keys. "The Evaluation of Leanness-Fatness in Man." *British Journal of Nutrition* 5 (1951): 194–206.

3. For example, Keys, A. "Obesity Measurement and the Composition of the Body." In *Overeating, Overweight and Obesity: Proceedings of the Nutrition Symposium Held at the Harvard School of Public Health. Boston, Massachusetts, October 29, 1952.* New York: National Vitamin Foundation, 1953; Goran, M. "Measurement Issues Related to Studies of Childhood Obesity." *Pediatrics* 101 (1998): 505–518.

4. Keys, A., F. Fidanza, et al. "Indices of Relative Weight and Obesity." *Journal of Chronic Diseases* 25 (1972): 329–343; Benn, R. T. "Some Mathematical Properties of Weight-for-Height Indices Used as Measures of Adiposity." *British Journal of Preventative Social Medicine* 25 (1971): 42–50, 42.

5. Billewicz, W. Z., W. F. F. Kemsley, and A. M. Thomson. "Indices of Adiposity." *British Journal of Preventative Social Medicine* 16 (1962): 183–188, 187.

Khosla, T., and C. R. Lowe. "Indices of Obesity Derived from Body Weight and Height." *British Journal of Preventative Social Medicine* 21 (1967): 122–128, 122, 124.

"All the weight-height indices" is a simplification. Precisely, Quetelet's index was the most highly correlated of all indices of the form w/h^n where the exponent n is a whole number between 1 and 3. Indices with a non-whole-number exponent were found to correlate slightly more highly with body fat than Quetelet's index but have not since been used in practice because they are more confusing to calculate, and the value of the exponent tends to be sex- and age-specific. See, for example, Benn, "Some Mathematical Properties of Weight-for-Height Indices."

6. Keys et al., "Indices of Relative Weight and Obesity," 341.

7. National Institutes of Health Consensus Development Conference Statement. "Health Implications of Obesity." *Annals of Internal Medicine* 103 (1985): 1073–1077; Burton, B. T., W. R. Foster, et al. "Health Implications of Obesity." *International Journal of Obesity* 9 (1985): 155–169, 157; Van Italie, T. "Health Implications of Overweight and Obesity in the United States." *Annals of Internal Medicine* 103 (1985): 983–988.

8. An excellent summary of the use of BMI in government health reports is Kuczmarski, R. J., and K. Flegal. "Criteria for Definition of Overweight in Transition." *American Journal of Clinical Nutrition* 72 (2000): 1074–1081. On the varying cutoffs and diagnostic categories, see, for example, National Center for Health Statistics. "Health United States, 1985." Washington, DC: Public Health Service, 1985; Committee on Diet and Health. "Diet and Health: Recommendations for Reducing Chronic Disease Risk." Washington, DC: National Academy Press, 1989; United States Department of Health and Human Services. "Healthy People 2000: National Health Promotion and

Disease Prevention Objectives." Washington, DC: United States Government Printing Office, 1990.

The 1997 WHO conference is reported in World Health Organization. "Obesity: Preventing and Managing the Global Epidemic." Geneva: World Health Organization, 1997.

9. For example Roche, A., R. Siervogel, et al. "Grading Body Fatness from Limited Anthropometric Data." *American Journal of Clinical Nutrition* 34 (1981): 2831–2838 (compares BMI with hydrodensitometry, skinfolds); Deurenberg, P., J. Weststrate, and J. Seidell. "Body Mass Index as a Measure of Body Fatness." *British Journal of Nutrition* 65 (1991): 105–114 (compares BMI with hydrodensitometry); Daniels, S., P. Khoury, and J. Morrison. "The Utility of Body Mass Index as a Measure of Body Fatness in Children and Adolescents: Differences by Race and Gender." *Pediatrics* 99 (1997): 804–807 (compares BMI with DEXA); Malina, R., and P. Katzmarzyk. "Validity of the Body Mass Index as an Indicator of the Risk and Presence of Overweight in Adolescents." *American Journal of Clinical Nutrition* 70, supplement (1999): 131–136 (compares BMI with hydrodensitometry and dilution techniques).

An example of complications in using the BMI is the study by Freedman et al., which suggests that insights from indirect body-composition analysis techniques imply that we should use racially specific BMI cutoff points to diagnose childhood obesity. Freedman, D. S., J. Wang, et al. "Racial/Ethnic Differences in Body Fatness among Children and Adolescents." *Obesity* 16 (2008): 1105–1111.

10. See Siervogel, R., A. Roche, S. Guo, D. Mukherjee, and W. Chumlea. "Patterns of Change in Weight/Stature from 2 to 18 Years." *International Journal of Obesity* 15 (1991): 479–485; Hammer, L., H. Kraemer, et al. "Standardized Percentile Curves of Body-Mass Index for Children and Adolescents." *American Journal of Diseases of Children* 145 (1991): 259–263.

11. Researchers who consider the fact that BMI varies with height in children to be a bad thing include, for example, Bellizzi, M., and W. Dietz. "Workshop on Childhood Obesity: Summary of the Discussion." *American Journal of Clinical Nutrition* 70, supplement (1999): 173–175. The converse opinion, that the variation with height is not necessarily bad, is expressed in Maynard, L. M., W. Wisemandle, et al. "Childhood Body Composition in Relation to Body Mass Index." *Pediatrics* 107 (2001): 344–350.

12. Yanovski, J. A., S. Z. Yanovski, et al. "Differences in Body Composition of Black and White Girls." *American Journal of Clinical Nutrition* 64 (1996): 833–839; Daniels, Khoury, and Morrison, "Utility of Body Mass Index"; Duncan, J. S., Duncan E. K., and G. Schofield. "Accuracy of Body Mass Index (BMI) Thresholds for Predicting Excess Body Fat in Girls from Five Ethnicities." *Asia Pacific Journal of Clinical Nutrition* 18 (2009): 404–411.

World Health Organization. "Appropriate Body-Mass Index for Asian Populations and Its Implications for Policy and Intervention Strategies." *The Lancet* 363, no. 9412 (2004): 157–163; National Institute for Health Care Excellence. "Assessing Body Mass Index and Waist Circumference Thresholds for Intervening to Prevent Ill Health and Premature Death among Adults from Black, Asian and Other Minority Ethnic Groups in the UK." *NICE Public Health Guidance.* PH46, London: National Institute for Health Care Excellence, 2013.

NICE's recommended BMI cutoffs for Asian adults are 2 to 3 BMI points lower than those for white and black adults.

13. Kuczmarski, R., C. Ogden, et al. "CDC Growth Charts: United States." *Vital and Health Statistics* 314 (2000): 1–28, 6; Kuczmarski, R.J., C.L. Ogden, S.S. Guo, and et al. "2000 CDC Growth Charts for the United States: Methods and Development." *Vital and Health Statistics* 11, (2002).

On criticism of the BMI as a measure of obesity, see, for example, Nevill, A., A. Stewart, et al. "Relationship between Adiposity and Body Size Reveals Limitations of BMI." *American Journal of Physical Anthropology* 129 (2006): 151–156; Garn, S., W. Leonard, and V. Hawthorne. "Three Limitations of the Body Mass Index." *American Journal of Clinical Nutrition* 44 (1986): 996–997; Poskin, E. M. E. "Defining Childhood Obesity: Fiddling Whilst Rome Burns." *Acta Paediatrica* 90 (2001): 1361–1367.

Studies giving BMI standards from NHANES data include Hammer, Kraemer, et al. "Standardized Percentile Curves of Body-Mass"; Rosner, B., R. Prineas, et al. "Percentiles for Body Mass Index in U.S. Children 5 to 17 Years of Age." *The Journal of Pediatrics* 132 (1998): 211–222; Must, A., G. Dallal, and W. Dietz. "Reference Data for Obesity: 85th and 95th Percentiles of Body Mass Index (Wt/Ht²) and Triceps Skinfold Thickness." *American Journal of Clinical Nutrition* 53 (1991): 839–846.

14. For example, see the review by Horlick, M. "Editorial: Body Mass Index in Childhood: Measuring a Moving Target." *Journal of Clinical Endocrinology and Metabolism* 86 (2001): 4059–4060. One solution suggested by an International Obesity Taskforce (IOTF) workshop in 1997 was to quantify the risk that obesity in childhood would persist into adulthood. The taskforce did not pursue the option, however, despite the considerable volume of scholarship amassed on the issue since it was first systematically investigated in the late 1950s. See, for example, Mullins, A. G. "The Prognosis in Juvenile Obesity." *Archives of Disease in Childhood* 33 (1958): 307–314; Abraham, S., and M. Nordsieck. "Relationship of Excess Weight in Children and Adults." *Public Health Reports* 75 (1960): 263–273; Charney, E., H. Goodman, et al. "Childhood Antecedents of Adult Obesity." *New England Journal of Medicine* 295 (1976): 6–9; Guo, S., and W. Chumlea. "Tracking of Body Mass Index in Children in Relation to Overweight in Adulthood." *American Journal of Clinical Nutrition* 70, supplement (1999): 145–148.

15. Himes, J. H., and W. Dietz. "Guidelines for Overweight in Adolescent Preventative Services." *American Journal of Clinical Nutrition* 59 (1994): 307–316.

16. The percentile tables of BMI that the expert committee recommended be used were from Must, Dallal, and Dietz, "Reference Data for Obesity."

17. Himes and Dietz, "Guidelines for Overweight in Adolescent Preventative Services," 308–309.

18. "Not intended to define or diagnose obesity . . ." quotation from ibid., 307.

    That the cutoffs are used both to define and diagnose obesity as well as serve as a screening tool is the case both in the United States and internationally (although the cutoffs and reference data used internationally are different.) See, for example, Flegal, K. "Defining Obesity in Children and Adolescents: Epidemiologic Approaches." *Critical Reviews of Food Science and Nutrition* 33, no. 4 (1993): 307–312; Guillaume, M. "Defining Obesity in Childhood: Current Practice." *American Journal of Clinical Nutrition* 70, supplement (1999): 126–130; Cole, T. J., M. C. Bellizzi, K. M. Flegal, and W. H. Dietz. "Establishing a Standard Definition for Child Overweight and Obesity Worldwide: International Survey." *British Medical Journal* 320, (2000): 1–6.

19. Kuczmarski, Ogden, et al., "CDC Growth Charts, 6.

20. Koplan, J., C. Liverman, and V. Kraak, eds. *Preventing Childhood Obesity.* Institute of Medicine. Washington, DC: National Academies Press, 2005.

21. See for example, Susser, M. "Epidemiology in the United States after World War II." *Epidemiology Review* 7 (1985): 147–177; Marks, H. *The Progress of Experiment.* Cambridge: Cambridge University Press, 1997; Rothstein, W. *Public Health and the Risk Factor.* Rochester, NY: Rochester University Press, 2003.

5. Something Wrong Inside

Epigraph: Lisser, H. "The Frequency of Endogenous Endocrine Obesity and Its Treatment by Glandular Therapy." *California and Western Medicine* 22 (1924): 509–514, 510.

1. A sample of the various theories on causes and treatments, along with reprints of influential papers, can be found in the series of articles by obesity researcher George Bray. See, for example, Bray, G. "Amphetamine: The Janus of Treatment for Obesity." *Obesity Research* 2 (1994): 286–292; Bray, G. "Measurement of Body Composition: An Improving Art." *Obesity Research* 3 (1995): 291–293; Bray, G. "Archeology of Mind: Obesity and Psychoanalysis." *Obesity Research* 5 (1997): 153–156.

2. For varying approaches to the issue of past therapeutics, compare Ackerknecht, E. *Therapeutics from the Primitives to the 20th Century.* New York: Hafner Press, 1973; Shorter, E. *Bedside Manners.* New York: Simon and Schuster, 1985;

Rosenberg, C. E. "The Therapeutic Revolution." In *Explaining Epidemics*, C. E. Rosenberg, ed., 9–31. Cambridge: Cambridge University Press, 1992.

3. On drug manufacturing and regulation in the United States, see, for example, Liebenau, J. "Ethical Business: The Formation of the Pharmaceutical Industry in Britain, Germany, and the United States before 1914." *Business History* 30 (1988): 116–129; Swann, J. "FDA and the Practice of Pharmacy." *Pharmacy in History* 36 (1994): 55–70; Rasmussen, N. "Steroids in Arms." *Medical History* 46 (2002): 299–324; Tone, A., and E. Watkins, eds. *Medicating Modern America*. New York: New York University Press, 2007.

4. On the treatment of myxoedema, see "The Curability of Myxoedema." *Therapeutic Gazette* 14 (1890): 718–719; Murray, G. "Note on the Treatment of Myxoedema by Hypodermic Injections of an Extract of the Thyroid Gland of a Sheep." *British Medical Journal* 2 (1891): 796–797; MacKenzie, H. "A Case of Myxoedema Treated with Great Benefit by Feeding with Fresh Thyroid Glands." *British Medical Journal* 2 (1892): 940–941; Ginn, S., and J. Vilensky. "Experimental Confirmation by Sir Victor Horsley of the Relationship between Thyroid Gland Dysfunction and Myxoedema." *Thyroid* 16 (2006): 743–747.

On Brown-Séquard and his rejuvenation, see Brown-Séquard, C. E. "The Effects Produced on Man by Subcutaneous Injections of a Liquid Obtained from the Testicles of Animals." *The Lancet* 134, no. 3438 (1889): 105–107, 106; see also Brown-Séquard, C. E. "On a New Therapeutic Method Consisting in the Use of Organic Liquids Extracted from Glands and Other Organs (II)." *British Medical Journal* 1 (1893): 1212–1214. On the response to Brown-Séquard's claims, see, for example, Hammond, W. "On Certain Organic Extracts." *New York Medical Journal* 57 (1893): 93–96; Editorial. "A Forlorn Hope." *Journal of the American Medical Association* 8 (1889): 344; Editorial. "Animal Extracts as Therapeutic Agents." *British Medical Journal* 1 (1893): 1279.

On the early history of endocrinology more broadly, see Borell, M. "Brown-Séquard's Organotherapy and Its Appearance in America at the End of the Nineteenth Century." *Bulletin of the History of Medicine* 50 (1976): 309–320; Borell, M. "Organotherapy, British Physiology, and the Discovery of the Internal Secretions." *Journal of the History of Biology* 9 (1976): 235–268; Hall, D. "The Critic and the Advocate." *Journal of the History of Biology* 9 (1976): 269–285; Borell, M. "Setting the Standards for a New Science." *Medical History* 22 (1978): 282–290; Hamilton, D. *The Monkey Gland Affair*. London: Chatto and Windus, 1986; Sengoopta, C. *The Most Secret Quintessence of Life:Sex, Glands, and Hormones, 1850–1950*. Chicago: University of Chicago Press, 2006.

5. Starling, E. "The Chemical Correlation of the Functions of the Body." *The Lancet* 166, no. 4275 (1905): 339–341, 339, 340.

6. See, for example, Advertisement: "Fresh and Fragrant the Laughing Mouth of Youth—It Can Always Be Yours" (Pebeco Tooth Paste). *Chicago Daily Tribune,* 7 November 1926, 15; Advertisement: "1468 Gland Tests Made by Physician" (Glandogen). *Los Angeles Times,* 15 November 1923, I15; Advertisement: "Money-Back Gland Remedy Restores Vigorous Health!" (Glendage). *Los Angeles Times,* 19 January 1928, 16; Advertisement: "Tropical Fish Thrive on New Glandular Food" (Glandex). *New York Times,* 5 March 1933, SM17.

7. Kraus, F. "The Present Status of Animal Therapeutics." *Journal of the American Medical Association* 26 (1896): 528–532, 528; Waller, H. "Some Observations on Thyroid Medication." *The Prescriber* 7 (1913): 98–101, 98; Stephenson, T, and H. R. Harrower. "A Review of Hormone Therapy." *The Prescriber* 7 (1913): 89–108, 89.

   On postulated actions of organotherapeutics, see Brown-Séquard, "On a New Therapeutic Method"; Strauss, S. "Endocrine Gland Extracts I: Their Manufacture and Use." *New York Medical Journal* 63 (1921): 395–397; Clark, A. J. "The Experimental Basis of Endocrine Therapy." *British Medical Journal* 52 (1923): 51–53; Dardel, J. "The Present State of Organotherapeutics." *The Practitioner,* June (1912): 852–861.

8. "Spare eaters . . ." quotation from Shaw, H. B. *Organotherapy.* Chicago: W.T. Keener, 1905, 60.

   For Von Noorden's classification, see Von Noorden, K. *Die Fettsucht (Obesity).* Wien: Alfred Hölder, 1900, 24. Von Noorden's classification was brought to the attention of English readers in Von Noorden, K. *Obesity, Metabolism and Practical Medicine.* Chicago: V.T. Keener, 1907. On the use of Von Noorden's classification, see Lisser, "Frequency of Endogenous Endocrine Obesity"; Rony, H. "Juvenile Obesity." *Endocrinology* 16 (1932): 601–610; Nixon, N. K. "Obesity in Childhood." *Journal of Pediatrics* 4 (1934): 295–306; Gordon, M. "Endocrine Obesity in Children." *Journal of Pediatrics* 10 (1937): 204–220.

   "Poor eater . . ." quotation from Bruch, H. "Mothers [Clinical Notes]," c1940. Papers of Hilde Bruch, Texas Medical Center Archive, Houston.

9. Lisser, "Frequency of Endogenous Endocrine Obesity," 510.

10. "Endocrine therapy is indicated . . ." quotation from Gordon, "Endocrine Obesity in Children," 218.

    "It is remarkable . . ." Emerson, W. P. "Overweight in Children." *Boston Medical and Surgical Journal* 185 (1921): 475–476, 476.

11. Veeder, B. "The Overweight Child." *Journal of the American Medical Association* 83 (1924): 486–489, 489.

12. Barker, L. F. "The Obesities—Their Origins and Some of the Methods of Reducing Them." *California and Western Medicine* 37 (1932): 73–81, 76; Veeder, "Overweight Child," 487.

13. For example, Gordon, "Endocrine Obesity in Children."

14. "Gland-ridden world" phrase from Thorne, V. B. "The Craze for Rejuvenation."
    New York Times, 4 June 1922, 18, 26.

    For examples of instructions on how to make one's own gland preparations,
    see Cunningham, R. H. "The Physiological Effects of Preparations of the
    Ductless Glands." *Medical News* 77 (1900): 83–86; Dardel, "Present State of
    Organotherapeutics"; Strauss, "Endocrine Gland Extracts I."

    "To the slaughter houses . . ." quotation from Strauss, "Endocrine Gland
    Extracts I," 395.

    "Sickly, disagreeable odor" quotation from Cunningham, "Physiological
    Effects," 84.

    "Most rigid antiseptic precautions . . ." quotation from Hammond, "On
    Certain Organic Extracts," 94. For criticism of the injection vogue, see Hun,
    H. "The Uses and Abuses of Animal Extracts as Medicines." *New York Medical
    Journal*, January (1895): 33–37, 33.

15. After his military service, William Hammond practiced in New York. He was
    profoundly influenced by Brown-Séquard's use of testicular extract and was
    among the first American physicians to promote the technique. He founded a
    number of gland- and organ-based drug manufacturing companies in the
    1890s. See Blustein, B. *Preserve Your Love for Science: The Life of William A.
    Hammond*. Cambridge: Cambridge University Press, 1991.

    Harry Harrower had, until 1988, been written out of histories of the
    Association for the Study of Internal Secretions (now the Endocrine Society).
    See Pottenger, R. M. "The Association for the Study of Internal Secretions."
    Endocrinology 30 (1942): 846–852; Lisser, H. "The Endocrine Society: The
    First Forty Years (1917–1957)." *Endocrinology* 80 (1967): 5–28; Wilhelmi, A.
    "The Endocrine Society." *Endocrinology* 123 (1988): 2–42; Schwartz, T.
    "Henry Harrower and the Turbulent Beginnings of Endocrinology." *Annals of
    Internal Medicine* 131 (1999): 702–706.

    Examples of Harrower's publications include Harrower, H. *Practical
    Hormone Therapy*. London: Bailliere, Tindall and Cox, 1914; Harrower, H. *A
    Manual of Pluriglandular Therapy*. Glendale, CA: Harrower Laboratory, 1924;
    Harrower, H. *An Endocrine Handbook*. Glendale, CA: Harrower Laboratory,
    1939.

    Prominent historians of early pharmaceutical and patent medicine manu-
    facturing usually make a definite distinction and see no similarities between
    "rational" therapies and proprietary medicines. See, for example, Liebenau, J.
    Medical Science and Medical Industry. London: MacMillan, 1987; Young, J. H.
    The Toadstool Millionaires. Princeton, NJ: Princeton University Press, 1961;
    Young, J. H. *The Medical Messiahs: A Social History of Health Quackery in
    Twentieth-Century America*. Princeton, NJ: Princeton University Press, 1992.

16. Quantities from Strauss, "Endocrine Gland Extracts I," 396.

17. Setting up subsidiary companies was a strategy that all the "Big Five" meat-
    packing companies (Armour, Swift, Wilson, Morris, Cudahy) adopted to

shore up their declining profits in the 1890s. Swift, for example, established feed, fertilizer, and finance operations; Wilson, a sporting-goods company, used leather, bristle, and gut supplied by the parent company. On meat-packing in the United States and its significance in economic and industrial history, see Arnould, R. "Changing Patterns of Concentration in American Meat Packing, 1880–1963." *Business History Review* 45 (1971): 18–34; Walsh, M. *The Rise of the Midwestern Meat Packing Industry.* Lexington: University Press of Kentucky, 1982; Skaggs, J. *Prime Cut: Livestock Raising and Meatpacking in the United States, 1607–1983* College Station: Texas A&M University Press, 1986.

Armour's family of companies has been divided up. Armour thyroid is currently made by Forest Laboratories.

For the vast range of products that meat-packing companies derived from animals, see "Packers Waste None of Their Products." *Washington Post,* 29 November 1923, 6.

18. "Among conservative physicians . . ." quotation from Jacobsen, W. W., and A. Cramer. "Clinical Results of Anterior Pituitary Therapy in Children." *Journal of the American Medical Association* 109 (1937): 101–108, 101.

"I suggest the administration . . ." quotation from Clark, "Experimental Basis of Endocrine Therapy," 53.

19. Earlier studies had suggested that obese people *did* have low basal metabolic rates, but corrections to take into account the obese person's greater surface area than a slim person of the same height altered the outcome. For a review of basal metabolic rate calculation, see Newburgh, L. H. "Obesity." *Archives of Internal Medicine* 70 (1942): 1033–1096. Studies on obese children showing normal or raised BMR include Kerley, C. G. "Basal Metabolism Studies in Obesity in Children." *Journal of Pediatrics* 2 (1933): 729–732; Talbot, F., and J. Worcester. "The Basal Metabolism of Obese Children." *Journal of Pediatrics* 16 (1940): 146–150.

20. Talbot, F., E. Wilson, and J. Worcester. "Basal Metabolism of Girls." *American Journal of Diseases of Children* 53 (1937): 273–347, 340.

21. Newburgh, L. H. "The Cause of Obesity." *Journal of the American Medical Association* 97 (1931): 1659–1663, 1660–1661.

22. Bruch, H. "Obesity in Relation to Puberty." *Journal of Pediatrics* 19 (1941): 365–375, 374. For other criticism of the diagnosis of Fröhlich's syndrome, see Nixon, "Obesity in Childhood"; Bruch, H. "The Frohlich Syndrome." *American Journal of Diseases of Children* 58 (1939): 1282–1289; Bronstein, I. P., L. J. Halpern, and A. W. Brown. "Obesity in Children." *Journal of Pediatrics* 21 (1942): 485–496.

23. Rosenberg, C. E. "Framing Disease: Illness, Society, and History." In *Framing Disease: Studies in Cultural History,* C. Rosenberg and J. Golden, eds., xiii–xxvi. New Brunswick, NJ: Rutgers University Press, 1992; Rosenberg, "Therapeutic Revolution."

6. The Enduring Promise

Epigraphs: Bett, W. R, L. Howells, and A. D. McDonald. *Amphetamine in Clinical Medicine*. London: Livingstone, 1955, 30.

1. Details on the development, patenting, and commercial use of amphetamines can be found in Rasmussen, N. *On Speed*. New York: New York University Press, 2008. See also Jackson, C. "Before the Drug Culture Barbiturate/Amphetamine Abuse in American Society." *Clio Medica* 11 (1976): 47–58; Anglin, M. D., C. Burke, et al. "History of the Methamphetamine Problem." *Journal of Psychoactive Drugs* 32 (2000): 137–141; Iverson, L. "Medical Uses of Amphetamines." In *Speed, Ecstasy, Ritalin*, ed. L. Iverson, 29–70. Oxford: Oxford University Press, 2006.

   The effect of amphetamine is discussed in, for example, Wilbur, D., A. MacLean, and E. Allen. "Clinical Observation on the Effect of Benzedrine Sulfate." *Journal of the American Medical Association* 109 (1937): 549–554

   In 1937, the American Medical Association's Council on Pharmacy and Chemistry ruled that the new drug could be used to good effect in treating narcolepsy, but that for depression and fatigue it should only be used under a doctor's close supervision, meaning only on institutionalized patients. Council on Pharmacy and Chemistry (AMA). "Present Status of Benzedrine Sulfate." *Journal of the American Medical Association* 109 (1937): 2064–2069.

2. Nathanson, M. H. "The Central Action of Beta-Aminopropylbenzene (Benzedrine)." *Journal of the American Medical Association* 108 (1937): 528–531, 529.

   Lesses, M., and A. Myerson. "Benzedrine Sulfate as an Aid in the Treatment of Obesity." *New England Journal of Medicine* 218 (1938): 119–124.

   News of the drug in the popular press includes Clendening, L. "Hardships of Reducing." *Washington Post*, 2 April 1938, X11; Cutter, I. "Obesity Treatment Aided by Benzedrine Sulfate." *Chicago Daily Tribune*, 22 February 1938, 10; "Drug for Hangovers." *New York Times*, 5 June 1938, 54; "Drug Held Cure for Alcoholism." *New York Times*, 28 December 1938, 17.

3. Details on the Food and Drug Administration's approvals of these compounds can be found in Colman, E. "Anorectics on Trial." *Annals of Internal Medicine* 143 (2005): 380–385.

4. Studies investigating the use of amphetamine in children include Bruch, H., and I. Waters. "Benzedrine Sulfate (Amphetamine) in the Treatment of Obese Children and Adolescents." *Journal of Pediatrics* 20 (1942): 54–64; Kunstadter, R. "Experience with Benzedrine Sulfate in the Management of Obesity in Children." *Journal of Pediatrics* 17 (1940): 490–501; Mossberg, H-O., and A. R. Frisk. "Evaluation of the Effect of D-Amphetamine Sulfate in the Treatment of Obesity in Children." *Acta Paediatrica* 39 (1950): 243–250; Lorber, J., and J. Rendle-Short. "Obesity in Childhood: A Controlled Trial of Phenmetrazine, Amphetamine Resinate, and Diet." *Quarterly Review of*

Pediatrics 16 (1961): 93–96; Jones, H. E. "A Trial of Diethylpropion in the Treatment of Childhood Obesity." *Practitioner* 118 (1962): 229–231; Lorber, J. "Obesity in Childhood: A Controlled Trial of Anorectic Drugs." *Archives of Disease in Childhood* 41 (1966): 309–312; Lorber, J. "Obesity in Childhood." *Clinical Pediatrics* 6 (1967): 325–326.

The study that found a weight loss of one pound a week was Rendle-Short, J. "Obesity in Childhood: A Clinical Trial of Phenmetrazine." *British Medical Journal* 1 (1960): 703–704.

The Danish research study was Andersen, H., and F. Quaade. "The Effect of D-Amphetamine on Obese Children." *Danish Medical Bulletin* 1 (1954): 118–123, 122.

"Children eagerly confirmed . . ." quotation from Bruch and Waters, "Benzedrine Sulfate," 57.

5. Bett, Howells, and McDonald, *Amphetamine in Clinical Medicine*, 30.
6. Studies in which children were given amphetamines for obesity include Bakwin, H. "Obesity in Children." *Journal of Pediatrics* 54 (1959): 392–400; Mullins, A. G. "The Prognosis in Juvenile Obesity." *Archives of Disease in Childhood* 33 (1958): 307–314; Gordon, H., and L. F. Hill. "Obesity in Pediatric Practice." *Pediatrics* 20 (1957): 540–546; Steiner, M. "The Management of Obesity in Childhood." *Medical Clinics of North America*, January (1950): 223–234.

The recommended adult dosages are given in Council on Pharmacy and Chemistry (AMA). *New and Non-Official Remedies*. Philadelphia: Lippincott, 1950, 270.

Adult dosages used in practice described in, among others, Nathanson, "Central Action of Beta-Aminopropylbenzene"; Roberts, E. "The Treatment of Obesity with an Anorexigenic Drug." *Annals of Internal Medicine* 34 (1951): 1324–1330; Freed, S. C., and M. Mizel. "The Use of Amphetamine Combinations for Appetite Suppression." *Annals of Internal Medicine* 36 (1952): 1492–1497.

7. An example of the "hunger center" theory is Nathanson, "Central Action of Beta-Aminopropylbenzene," 529.

Dog study result reported in Harris, S., A. C. Ivy, and L. Searle. "The Mechanism of Amphetamine-Induced Loss of Weight." *Journal of the American Medical Association* 134 (1947): 1468–1475.

8. Lesses and Myerson. "Benzedrine Sulfate," 119.
9. The fact that amphetamines helped a person not to feel fatigue led to its use by the U.S., German, and Japanese military during World War II for soldiers and pilots. Historians trace the later blossoming of amphetamine abuse in the United States to this use. See Anglin et al., "History of the Methamphetamine Problem"; Jackson, "Before the Drug Culture."

"Sense of power . . ." quotation from Cutter, "Obesity Treatment," 10.
10. Lorber, "Obesity in Childhood: A Controlled Trial," 312.

11. Andelman, M., C. Jones, and S. Nathan. "Treatment of Obesity in Under-privileged Adolescents." *Clinical Pediatrics* 6 (1967): 327–330, 327, 330.

12. "No reports . . ." quotation from Wilbur, MacLean, and Allen, "Clinical Observation," 553.

    Studies showing the limited effectiveness of amphetamines include Adlersberg, D., and M. Mayer. "Results of Prolonged Medical Treatment of Obesity." *Journal of Clinical Endocrinology* 8 (1948): 624–625; Lorber and Rendle-Short, "Obesity in Childhood: A Controlled Trial"; Editorial. "Obesity in Childhood." *The Lancet* 288, no. 7458 (1966): 327; Lorber, "Obesity in Childhood."

    The history of diet drugs is considered in Colman, "Anorectics on Trial."

13. On the FDA's regulation of amphetamine-based diet drugs, see Colman, "Anorectics on Trial"; Iverson, "Medical Uses of Amphetamines."

    Editorial. "Drugs and Obesity." *Journal of the American Medical Association* 204 (1968): 118–119, 118.

14. For example, Grollman, A. "Drug Therapy of Obesity in Children." In *Childhood Obesity*, P. Collipp, ed., 83–96. Acton, MA: Publishing Sciences, 1975, 267.

    "They don't work" quotation from Eden, A. N. *Growing Up Thin*. New York: David McKay, 1975, 12.

    The AAP's recommendations may be found in Yaffe, S., C. Bierman, et al. "Use of D-Amphetamine and Related Central Nervous System Stimulants in Children." *Pediatrics* 51 (1973): 302–305, 303, 304.

    Yaffe et al. "Use of D-Amphetamine," 304.

15. Edelstein, B. *The Woman Doctor's Diet for Teen-Age Girls*. Englewood Cliffs, NJ: Prentice-Hall, 1980, 76.

16. The FDA had approved propanolamine in the mid-1970s for use as a nasal decongestant and, later, for weight loss. Director, Center for Drug Evaluation and Research. "FDA Letter to Manufacturers of Drug Products Containing Phenylpropanolamine (PPA)." 3 November 2000.

17. One most fortunate outcome in this change of opinion was that children, unlike adults, did not share in the renewed vogue in the 1990s for diet pills, notably "Fen-Phen" (fenfluramine-phentermine), a long-acting amphetamine derivative later found to cause heart-valve damage. Fen-Phen was withdrawn from sale in 1997, and a massive lawsuit was litigated against Wyeth, the manufacturer. See Colman, "Anorectics on Trial"; Rasmussen, *On Speed*, 241–242.

18. There are intriguing parallels here with a more recent controversy relating to children and drug treatment. Children with attention deficit hyperactivity disorder (ADHD, also ADD) are sometimes prescribed an amphetamine-related drug, Ritalin, to help manage their willful and difficult behavior. Some popular and medical commentators have controversially suggested that the drug is not treating a physical problem but is making up for deficiencies in parenting.

The following illustrate the different perspectives on the Ritalin issue: Accardo, P., and J. Accardo. "Say No to Drugs?" *Journal of Pediatrics* 147 (2005): 286–287; Rafalovich, A. *Framing ADHD Children.* Lanham, MD: Lexington Books, 2004, especially chapter 4; Rosemond, J. *The Diseasing of America's Children.* Nashville, TN: Thomas Nelson, 2008.

19. Historical moments in the homeostasis concept are addressed in Cannon, W. B. *The Wisdom of the Body.* New York: Norton, 1932; Cannon, W. B., and A. L. Washburn. "An Explanation of Hunger." *American Journal of Physiology* 29 (1912): 441–454; Lashley, K. S. "Experimental Analysis of Instinctual Behavior." *Psychological Review* 45 (1938): 445–471; Mayer, J. "Regulation of Energy Intake and Body Weight." *Annals of the New York Academy of Sciences* 63 (1955): 15–43.

A third "thermostatic theory" relating to body temperature was suggested by physiologist John Brobeck, but this mechanism failed to satisfy certain requirements of a homeostatic regulating signal. Brobeck, J. R. "Physiology of Appetite." In *Overeating, Overweight and Obesity: Proceedings of the Nutrition Symposium Held at the Harvard School of Public Health, Boston, Massachusetts, October 29, 1952.* New York: National Vitamin Foundation, 1953.

20. Ingalls, A., M. Dickie, and G. D. Snell. "Obese, a New Mutation in the House Mouse." *Journal of Heredity* 41 (1950): 317–318; "Obituary: Margaret M. Dickie, 1922–1969." *Journal of Heredity* 60 (1969): 162.

21. Zhang, Y., R. Proenca, et al. "Positional Cloning of the Mouse *Obese* Gene and Its Human Homologue." *Nature* 372, no. 1 (1994): 425–432, quotation 431. An excellent short history of the *ob/ob* mouse and Friedman's work can be found in Castracane, V. D., and M. Henson. "The Obese *(Ob/Ob)* Mouse and the Discovery of Leptin." In *Leptin,* V. D. Castracane, ed., 1–9. New York: Springer, 2006.

22. Halaas, J., K. Gajiwala, et al. "Weight-Reducing Effects of the Plasma Protein Encoded by the *Obese* Gene." *Science* 269, no. 5223 (1995): 543–546, 543.

23. Stone, R. "Rockefeller Strikes Fat Deal with Amgen." *Science* 268, no. 5211 (1995): 631, 631.

24. On the failure of the *ob* gene to account for most cases of human obesity and the rarity of *ob* mutations in humans, see Maffei, M., M. Stoffel, et al. "Absence of Mutations in the Human Ob Gene in Obese/Diabetic Subjects." *Diabetes* 45 (1996): 679–682; Montague, C., S. Farooqui, et al. "Congenital Leptin Deficiency Is Associated with Severe Early-Onset Obesity in Humans." *Nature* 387, no. 26 (1997): 903–908; Friedman, J., and J. Halaas. "Leptin and the Regulation of Body Weight in Mammals." *Nature* 395, no. 22 (1998): 763–770, 768.

A summary of obesity genetics in humans is Rankinen, T., A. Zuberi, et al. "The Human Obesity Gene Map: The 2005 Update." *Obesity* 14 (2006): 529–644.

25. Pelleymounter, M. A., M. J. Cullen, et al. "Effects of the *Obese* Gene Product on Body Weight Regulation in *Ob/Ob* Mice." *Science* 269, no. 5223 (1995): 540–543; Halaas et al., "Weight-Reducing Effects."

26. Quotation from Considine, R., M. Sinha, et al. "Serum Immunoreactive-Leptin Concentrations in Normal-Weight and Obese Humans." *New England Journal of Medicine* 334 (1996): 292–295, 292.

  An example of the gloomy outlook for leptin's prospects as an antiobesity drug is Rohner-Jeanrenaud, F. "Obesity, Leptin, and the Brain." *New England Journal of Medicine* 334, (1996): 324–325.

27. Chicurel, M. "Whatever Happened to Leptin?" *Nature* 404, no. 6 (2000): 538–540; Friedman and Halaas, "Leptin and the Regulation."

28. Friedman and Halaas, "Leptin and the Regulation," 769.

29. On the brief reprisal of hope in leptin, see Miller, M., D. Duhl, et al. "Cloning of the Mouse *Agouti* Gene Predicts a Secreted Protein Ubiquitously Expressed in Mice Carrying the *Lethal Yellow* Mutation." *Genes and Development* 7 (1993): 454–467; Miltenberger, R., R. Mynatt, et al. "The Role of the *Agouti* Gene in the Yellow Obese Syndrome." *The Journal of Nutrition* 127 (1997): 1902S–1907S.

  For an overview of obesity genetics and reviews of the importance of the *ob* mouse and leptin research, see Schwartz, M., S. Woods, et al. "Central Nervous System Control of Food Intake." *Nature* 404, no. 6 (2000): 661–671; Barsh, G. "From Agouti to *Pomc*." *Nature Medicine* 5 (1999): 984–985; Rankinen et al., "Human Obesity Gene Map."

30. For commentary, see Prodi, E., and S. Obici. "The Brain as a Molecular Target for Diabetic Therapy." *Endocrinology* 147 (2006): 2664–2669. An example of a study into restoring leptin sensitivity is Ozcan, L., Ergin A. S., et al. "Endoplasmic Reticulum Stress Plays a Central Role in Development of Leptin Resistance." *Cell Metabolism* 9 (2009): 35–51.

31. For example, Morton, G. J., D. E. Cummings, et al. "Central Nervous System Control of Food Intake and Body Weight." *Nature* 443, no. 21 (2006): 289–295.

32. Frederich, R. C., A. Hamann, et al. "Leptin Levels Reflect Body Lipid Content in Mice: Evidence for Diet-Induced Resistance to Leptin Action." *Nature Medicine* 1 (1995): 1311–1314; Lin, S., T. C. Thomas, et al. "Development of High Fat Diet-Induced Obesity and Leptin Resistance in C57b1/6j Mice." *International Journal of Obesity and Related Metabolic Disorders* 24 (2000): 639–646.

33. Amylin Pharmaceuticals, and Takeda Pharmaceutical Company. "Amylin and Takeda Discontinue Development of Pramlintide/Metreleptin Combination Treatment." Amylin Pharmaceuticals, Takeda Pharmaceutical Company, 5 August 2011 http://www.takeda.com/press/article_42791.html. 2011. Access date 21 February 2012.

7. Feeling Fat

Epigraph: Moore, Judith. *Fat Girl.* New York: Hudson Street Press, 2005, 77.

1. Nixon, N. K. "Obesity in Childhood." *Journal of Pediatrics* 4 (1934): 295–306, 302.

   Preston, J., and H. Decker. "APA Interviews of Hilde Bruch (Transcript)," 1974–1975, 58. Papers of Hilde Bruch, Texas Medical Center Archive, Houston.

2. Bruch's family life in Germany is covered extensively in the biography written by the wife of her nephew (and adopted son): Bruch, J. H. *Unlocking the Golden Cage.* Carlsbad: Gürze Books, 1996. Émigré physicians' experiences are addressed in Genizi, H. "New York Is Big—America Is Bigger: The Resettlement of Refugees from Nazism, 1936–1945." *Jewish Social Studies* 46 (1984): 61–72; Breitman, R., and A. Kraut. *American Refugee Policy and European Jewry, 1933–1945.* Bloomington: Indiana University Press, 1987.

3. Preston and Decker, "APA Interviews," 58–59, 157, and also Bruch, H. "Unpublished Paper: Obesity in Children," 1939. Papers of Hilde Bruch, Texas Medical Center Archive, Houston; Bruch, H. "Obesity in Childhood: II. Basal Metabolism and Serum Cholesterol of Obese Children." *American Journal of Diseases of Children* 58 (1939): 1001–1022.

4. Preston and Decker, "APA Interviews," 59–60.

5. Witenberg, E. "Janet Mackenzie Rioch (1905–1974), the Transference Phenomenon in Psychoanalytic Theory." In *Pioneers of Interpersonal Psychoanalysis,* D. Stern, C. Mann, S. Kantor, and G. Schlesinger, eds., 43–60. Hillsdale, NJ: Analytic Press, 1995; Preston and Decker, "APA Interviews," 60–61.

   Rioch worked with Helen Flanders Dunbar, who was the leading figure in psychosomatic medicine in America. See Powell, R. "Helen Flanders Dunbar (1902–1959) and a Holistic Approach to Psychosomatic Problems." *Psychiatric Quarterly* 49 (1977): 133–152.

   On Freudianism in America in this period, see Hale, N. *The Rise and Crisis of Psychoanalysis in America: Freud and the Americans, 1917–1985.* Oxford: Oxford University Press, 1995; Paris, J. *The Fall of an Icon: Psychoanalysis and Academic Psychiatry.* Toronto: University of Toronto Press, 2005; Gifford, S. "The Psychoanalytic Movement in the United States, 1906–1991." In *History of Psychiatry and Medical Psychology,* E. Wallace and J. Gach, eds., 629–656. New York: Springer, 2008.

6. Bruch, H., and G. Touraine. "Obesity in Childhood: V. The Family Frame of Obese Children." *Psychosomatic Medicine* 2 (1940): 141–206. Bruch borrowed the term "frame" from physics (as in "frame of reference") to suggest that data were only meaningful if the frame of reference were specified. Preston and Decker, "APA Interviews," 62.

7. Bruch and Touraine, "Obesity in Childhood: V.," 205.

8. For example, Bruch, H. "Obese Children Notes 1940" and "Obese Children Notes 1940 (II)," 1940. Papers of Hilde Bruch, Texas Medical Center Archive, Houston.

9. Bruch, H. "Psychiatric Aspects of Obesity in Children." *American Journal of Psychiatry* 99 (1943): 752–757.

10. "Spaghetti and macaroni . . ." quotation from Bruch, H. "Obesity in Childhood: III. Physiologic and Psychological Aspects of the Food Intake of Obese Children." *American Journal of Diseases of Children* 59 (1940): 739–781, 751. Gilman has argued that Bruch represented the female, Jewish child as the epitome of the fat child. This is not correct. Italian children appear as commonly in Bruch's work as do Jewish children (there were large numbers of children from groups in the area close to the Babies Hospital where Bruch worked); Bruch refers to boys as well as girls in her case examples. Bruch's family frame theory was not gendered, nor did it involve any ethnic component. Gilman, S. "Obesity, the Jews and Psychoanalysis." *History of Psychiatry* 17 (2006): 55–66.

    Bruch introduced the term "thin fat person" in 1947 in Bruch, H. "Psychological Aspects of Obesity." *Psychiatry* 10 (1947): 373–381. She found the concept highly useful and continued to use it thereafter. See, for example, Bruch, H. "Psychological Aspects of Obesity." *Bulletin of the New York Academy of Medicine* 24 (1948): 73–86, 85; Bruch, H. "Thin Fat People." *Medical Opinion* 2 (1973): 50–56; Bruch, H. *Eating Disorders: Obesity, Anorexia Nervosa and the Person Within.* New York: Basic Books, 1973, 194–210.

    "Probably the most important therapeutic tool . . ." quotation from Bruch, H. "Obesity and Overnutrition." In *Current Pediatric Therapy*, S. Gellis and B. Kagan, eds., 2–3. Philadelphia: W.B. Saunders, 1964, 3. Similar sentiments may be found in Bruch, H. "Dietary Treatment of Obesity in Childhood." *Journal of the American Dietetic Association* 20 (1944): 361–364; Bruch, H., and D. McCune. "Psychotherapeutic Aspects of Pediatric Practice." *Pediatrics* 2 (1948): 405–409; Bruch, H. "Psychological Aspects of Obesity," *Psychiatry.*

11. Bruch, H. "Fat Children Grown Up." *American Journal of Diseases of Children* 90 (1955): 501.

12. Bruch, "Psychological Aspects of Obesity," *Psychiatry,* 378, 376. Similar sentiments in Bruch, "Dietary Treatment of Obesity in Childhood"; Bruch, "Psychological Aspects of Obesity," *Bulletin.*

13. On criticism of Bruch's "family frame" theory, see, for example, Hamburger, W. W. "Emotional Aspects of Obesity." *Medical Clinics of North America* 35 (1951): 483–499; Tolstrup, K. "On Psychogenic Obesity in Children." *Acta Paediatrica* 42 (1953): 289–304; Quaade, F. *Obese Children.* Kobenhavn: Dansk Videnskabs Forlag A/S, 1955; Burchinal, L. G. "Test of the Psychogenic Theory of Obesity for a Sample of Rural Girls." *American Journal of Clinical Nutrition* 7 (1959): 288–294.

Bruch's new theory is addressed in, for example, Bruch, H. "Developmental Obesity and Schizophrenia." *Psychiatry* 24 (1958): 65–70; Bruch, H. "Transformation of Oral Impulses." *Psychiatric Quarterly* 35 (1961): 458–481; Bruch, H. "Falsification of Bodily Needs and Body Concept in Schizophrenia." *Archives of General Psychiatry* 6 (1962): 18–24; Bruch, H. "Disturbed Communication in Eating Disorders." *American Journal of Orthopsychiatry* 33 (1963): 99–104.

On schizophrenia, see for example, Howells, J., ed. *The Concept of Schizophrenia: Historical Perspectives.* Washington, DC: American Psychiatric Press, 1991.

14. Bruch, "Falsification of Bodily Needs and Body Concept in Schizophrenia."

Bruch's theory here was similar to that of anthropologist and social scientist Gregory Bateson's "double-bind," which Bruch also referred to in her work. Bateson also thought that the mother's inconsistent communication was to blame for causing schizophrenia. He, however, considered childhood to be the critical period and verbal communication to be the major means by which the mother confused the child; Bruch thought infant experiences were at root.

Bruch's conceptualization was also strongly influenced by fellow psychoanalyst Harry Stack Sullivan's views on infancy and interpersonal relationships. See Chapman, A. H. *Harry Stack Sullivan.* New York: G.P. Putnam, 1976; Fiscalini, J. "Harry Stack Sullivan (1892–1949)." In *Pioneers of Interpersonal Psychoanalysis,* D. B. Stern, C. H. Mann, S. Kantor, and G. Schlesinger, eds., 1–26. Hillsdale, NJ: Analytic Press, 1995.

15. Preston and Decker, "APA Interviews," 95.

16. Bruch's later explorations of eating disorders include Bruch, H. "Conceptual Confusion in Eating Disorders." *Journal of Nervous and Mental Disease* 133 (1961): 46–54; Bruch, "Disturbed Communication in Eating Disorders"; Bruch, H. *The Importance of Overweight.* New York: W.W. Norton and Company, 1957; Bruch, H. "Obesity and Anorexia Nervosa." *Psychosomatics* 19 (1978): 208–212; Bruch, *Eating Disorders.*

17. Watson, J. B. "Psychology as the Behaviorist Views It." *Psychological Review* 20 (1913): 158–177, 158.

18. Cushman, P. *Constructing the Self, Constructing America.* Reading, MA: Addison-Wesley, 1995; Schnog, N. "On Inventing the Psychological." In *Inventing the Psychological,* J. Pfister and N. Schnog, eds., 3–16. New Haven, CT: Yale University Press, 1997; Proctor, R. W., and D. J. Weeks. *The Goal of B. F. Skinner and Behavior Analysis.* New York: Springer-Verlag, 1990.

The practical application of behaviorism is addressed extensively in Rutherford, A. *Beyond the Box: B. F. Skinner's Technology of Behavior from Laboratory to Life, 1950s–1970s.* Toronto: University of Toronto Press, 2009; Eysenck, H. J. "Behavioral Psychotherapy." In *Clinical Psychology: Historical and Research Foundations,* C. E. Walker, ed., 417–442. New York: Plenum Press, 1991.

19. Meyer, V., and A. H. Crisp. "Aversion Therapy in Two Cases of Obesity." *Behavioral Research Therapy* 2 (1964): 143–147, 145, 144, italics added.

20. Thorpe, J. G., E. Schmidt, et al. "Aversion-Relief Therapy: A New Method." *Behavioral Research and Therapy* 2 (1964): 71–82, 73.

21. "Not symptomatic . . ." quotation from Brownell, K., and A. Stunkard. "Behavioral Treatment of Obesity in Children." *American Journal of Diseases of Children* 132 (1978): 403–412, 404.

   The early study on nurses was Ferster, C. B., J. I. Nurnberger, and E. E. Levitt. "The Control of Eating." In *Behavioral Treatments of Obesity*, J. P. Foreyt, ed., 309–326. Oxford: Pergamon Press, 1977. (Reprinted from *Journal of Mathetics* 1 [1962]: 87–109.)

   Stuart, R., and B. Davis. *Slim Chance in a Fat World*. Champaign, IL: Research Press, 1972.

   Research studies using behavioral therapy to treat obesity in children include Aragona, J., J. Cassady, and R. Drabman. "Treating Overweight Children through Parental Training and Contingency Contracting." *Journal of Applied Behavior Analysis* 8 (1975): 269–278; Rivinus, T. M., T. Drummond, and L. Combrinck-Graham. "A Group Behavior Treatment Program for Overweight Children." *Pediatric and Adolescent Endocrinology* 1 (1976): 55–61; Wheeler, M., and K. Hess. "Treatment of Juvenile Obesity by Successive Approximation Control of Eating." *Journal of Behavioral Therapy and Experimental Psychology* 7 (1976): 235–241; Epstein, L., L. Parker, et al. "Descriptive Analysis of Eating Regulation in Obese and Nonobese Children." *Journal of Applied Behavioral Analysis* 9 (1976): 407–415; Kingsley, R., and J. Shapiro. "A Comparison of Three Behavioral Programs for the Control of Obesity in Children." *Behavior Therapy* 8 (1977): 30–36.

   For summaries of approaches in children, see Jordan, H., and L. Levitz. "Behavior Modification in the Treatment of Childhood Obesity." In *Childhood Obesity*, M. Winick, ed., 141–150. New York: John Wiley, 1975; Brownell and Stunkard, "Behavioral Treatment of Obesity in Children"; Stunkard, A. J. "Behavioral Treatment of Obesity: The Current Status." *International Journal of Obesity* 2 (1978): 237–248; Spence, S. H. "Behavioral Treatments of Childhood Obesity." *Journal of Child Psychology and Psychiatry* 27 (1986): 447–455.

22. "Call attention . . ." quotation from Wheeler and Hess, "Treatment of Juvenile Obesity," 236.

23. Jordan and Levitz, "Behavior Modification," 147.

24. "Encouraging . . ." and "produced a favorable climate . . ." quotations from Brownell and Stunkard, "Behavioral Treatment of Obesity in Children," 403, 404.

25. Stunkard, "Behavioral Treatment," 237.

26. Spence, "Behavioral Treatments"; Golan, M., V. Kaufman, and D. R. Shahar. "Childhood Obesity Treatment." *British Journal of Nutrition* 95 (2006): 1008–

1015; Epstein, L. H., M. D. Myers, et al. "Treatment of Pediatric Obesity." *Pediatrics* 101 (1998): 554–570; Drohan, S. H. "Managing Early Childhood Obesity in the Primary Care Setting." *Pediatric Nursing* 28 (2002): 599–610.

27. Rosenberg, C. E. "The Therapeutic Revolution." In *Explaining Epidemics,* C. E. Rosenberg, ed., 9–31. Cambridge: Cambridge University Press, 1992.

28. Garn, S., and D. Clark. "Trends in Fatness and the Origins of Obesity." *Pediatrics* 57 (1976): 443–456; Garn, S., S. Bailey, et al. "Effect of Remaining Family Members on Fatness Prediction." *The American Journal of Clinical Nutrition* 34 (1981): 148–153; Garn, S., P. Cole, and S. Bailey. "Effect of Parental Fatness Levels on the Fatness of Biological and Adoptive Children." *Ecology of Food and Nutrition* 6 (1977): 91–93.

   Smaller-scale studies before this had also shown strong parent-child and sibling body similarities. See Childs, B. "Familial Aspects of Obesity." *Pediatrics* 20 (1957): 547–549; Atkinson, R., and E. Ringuette. "A Survey of Biographical and Psychological Features in Extraordinary Fatness." *Psychosomatic Medicine* 29 (1967): 121–133.

   Notable twin studies suggesting a genetic component to obesity include Börjeson, M. "The Aetiology of Obesity in Children." *Acta Paediatrica Scandanavica* 65 (1976): 279–287; Stunkard, A., T. T. Foch, and Z. Hrubec. "A Twin Study of Human Obesity." *Journal of the American Medical Association* 4 (1986): 51–54; Silvertoinen, K., B. Bokholm, J. Kaprio, and T. Sorensen. "The Genetic and Environmental Influences on Childhood Obesity." *International Journal of Obesity* 34 (2010): 29–40.

29. Garn and Clark, "Trends in Fatness."

   Studies showing similarities between parents and adopted children include Garn, Stanley, S. Bailey, and P. Cole. "Similarities between Parents and Their Adopted Children." *American Journal of Physical Anthropology* 45 (1976): 539–543; Garn, Cole, and Bailey, "Effect of Parental Fatness."

   "It is clear that fatness and obesity . . ." quotation from Garn, S., M. LaVelle, and J. Pilkington. "Obesity and Living Together." In *Obesity and the Family,* D. Kallen and M. Sussman, eds., 33–47. New York: Haworth Press, 1984, 33.

   "While fatness follows family lines . . ." quotation from Garn, LaVelle, and Pilkington, "Obesity and Living Together," 45. See also Chlouverakis, C. S. "Controversies in Medicine (II): Nature and Nurture in Human Obesity." *Obesity/Bariatric Medicine* 3 (1974): 28–31.

30. Montague, C., S. Farooqi, et al. "Congenital Leptin Deficiency Is Associated with Severe Early-Onset Obesity in Humans." *Nature* 387, no. 26 (1997): 903–908.

31. For example, Farooqi, I. S., and S. O'Rahilly. "Recent Advances in the Genetics of Severe Childhood Obesity." *Archives of Disease in Childhood* 83 (2000): 31–34; Feng, N., D. Adler-Wailes, et al. "Sequence Variants of the

POMC Gene and Their Associations with Body Composition in Children." *Obesity Research* 11 (2003): 619–624; Rankinen, T., A. Zuberi, et al. "The Human Obesity Gene Map: The 2005 Update." *Obesity* 14 (2006): 529–644; Wheeler, E., N. Huang, et al. "Genome-Wide SNP and CNV Analysis Identified Common and Low-Frequency Variants Associated with Severe Early-Onset Obesity." *Nature Genetics* 45 (2013): 513–517.

32. Mason, E. "Obesity in Pet Dogs." *Veterinary Record* 86 (1970): 612–616; Christakis, N., and J. H. Fowler. "The Spread of Obesity in a Large Social Network over 32 Years." *New England Journal of Medicine* 357 (2007): 370–378.

33. On trends in rates of breast-feeding, see Martinez, G., and J. Nalezienski. "The Recent Trend in Breastfeeding." *Pediatrics* 64 (1979): 686–692. On breast-feeding and obesity, see Addy, D. P. "Infant Feeding." *British Medical Journal* 1 (1976): 1268–1271; Himes, J. H. "Infant Feeding Practices and Obesity." *Journal of the American Dietetic Association* 75 (1979): 122–125; Elliott, K. G., C. L. Kjolhede, E. Gournis, and K. M. Rasmussen. "Duration of Breastfeeding Associated with Obesity during Adolescence." *Obesity Research* 5 (1997): 538–541; von Kries, R., B. Koletzko, et al. "Breast Feeding and Obesity." *British Medical Journal* 319 (1999): 147–150; Armstrong, J., J. J. Reilly, et al. "Breastfeeding and Lowering the Risk of Childhood Obesity." *The Lancet* 359, no. 8 (2002): 2003–2004.

On the potential mechanism whereby breast-feeding protects against childhood obesity, see, for example, Kramer, M. "Do Breast-Feeding and Delayed Introduction of Solid Foods Protect against Subsequent Obesity?" *Journal of Pediatrics* 98 (1981): 883–887; Gilman, M., S. Rifas-Shiman, et al. "Risk of Overweight among Adolescents Who Were Breastfed as Infants." *Journal of the American Medical Association* 285 (2001): 2461–2467.

34. Jain, A., S. Sherman, et al. "Why Don't Low-Income Mothers Worry about Their Preschoolers Being Overweight?" *Pediatrics* 107 (2001): 1138–1146; Baughcum, A., L. Chamberlin, et al. "Maternal Perceptions of Overweight Preschool Children." *Pediatrics* 106 (2000): 1380–1386.

35. An overview of studies into prenatal factors and childhood obesity is Rogers, I. "The Influence of Birthweight and Intrauterine Environment on Adiposity and Fat Distribution in Later Life." *International Journal of Obesity and Related Metabolic Disorders* 27 (2003): 755–777. See also Oken, E., and M. W. Gillman. "Fetal Origins of Obesity." *Obesity Research* 11 (2003): 496–506; Oken, E., E. M. Taveras, K. Kleinman, J. W. Rich-Edwards, and M. W. Gillman. "Gestational Weight Gain and Child Adiposity at Age 3 Years." *American Journal of Obstetrics and Gynecology* 196 (2007): e1–e8.

36. Knittle, J., and J. Hirsch. "Infantile Metabolism as a Determinant of Adult Adipose Tissue Metabolism and Cellularity." *Clinical Research* 15 (1967): 323; Knittle, J. "Childhood Obesity." *Bulletin of the New York Academy of Medicine* 47 (1971): 579–589.

37. This concept has variously been called "danger periods," "sensitive periods," and, most recently, "critical periods." See, for example, Stuart, H. "Obesity in Childhood." *Quarterly Review of Pediatrics* 10 (1955): 131–145; Brook, C. G. D. "Evidence for a Sensitive Period in Adipose-Cell Replication in Man." *The Lancet* 300, no. 7778 (1972): 624–627; Cheek, D. "Insulin, Early Cell Growth and Excess Adipose Tissue." *Obesity and Bariatric Medicine* 2 (1973): 190–193; Brook, C. G. D. "Critical Periods in Childhood Obesity." In *Obesity Symposium*, W. L. Burland and P. Samuel, eds., 85–104. New York: Churchill Livingstone, 1973; Dobbing, J. "Fat Cells in Childhood Obesity." *The Lancet* 305, no. 7900 (1975): 224; Knittle, J. "Can Obesity Be Prevented?" In *Childhood Obesity*, P. Collipp, ed., 1–14. Acton, MA: Publishing Sciences, 1975; Dietz, W., and S. Gortmaker. "Preventing Obesity in Children and Adolescents." *Annual Review of Public Health* 22 (2001): 337–353; Daniels, S., D. Arnett, et al. "Overweight in Children and Adolescents." *Circulation* 111 (2005): 1999–2012.

38. Garn and Clark, "Trends in Fatness," 450.

39. The early study examining fathers' contribution to children's fatness is Garn and Clark, "Trends in Fatness."

    More recent studies include Le Stunff, C., D. Fallin, and P. Bougnères. "Paternal Transmission of the Very Common Class I *INS* VNTR Alleles Predisposes to Childhood Obesity." *Nature Genetics* 26 (2001): 96–99; Sheau-Fang, N., R. C. Y. Lin, D. R. Laybutt, et al. "Chronic High-Fat Diet in Fathers Programs B-Cell Dysfunction in Female Rat Offspring." *Nature* 467 (2010): 963–966.

40. Gable, S., and S. Lutz. "Household, Parent, and Child Contributions to Childhood Obesity." *Family Relations* 49 (2000): 293–300; Faith, M., K. Scanlon, et al. "Parent-Child Feeding Strategies and Their Relationships to Child Eating and Weight Status." *Obesity Research* 12 (2004): 1711–1722.

41. Edelstein, B. *The Woman Doctor's Diet for Teen-Age Girls.* Englewood Cliffs, NJ: Prentice-Hall, 1980, 24.

42. The term is commonly used in both popular diet books and studies of eating behaviors. For example, Edelstein, *Woman Doctor's Diet for Teen-Age Girls*, 24; Wiatt, C., and B. Schroeder. *The Diet for Teenagers Only.* New York: Regan Books, 2005, 169–177; Fletcher, A. *Weight Loss Confidential.* New York: Houghton Mifflin, 2006, 24–25.

43. As a subgenre, the self-written account of "life as a fat person" has a long history. See, for example, Cheyne, G. *An Essay of Health and Long Life.* London: George Strahan and J. Leake, 1724; Shapin, S. "Trusting George Cheyne: Scientific Expertise, Common Sense, and Moral Authority in Early Eighteenth-Century Dietetic Medicine." *Bulletin of the History of Medicine* 77 (2003): 263–297; Banting, W. *A Letter on Corpulence, Addressed to the Public.* 2nd ed. London: Harrison and Sons, 1863.

44. Moore, *Fat Girl*, 77.

45. For example, Wilensky, A. *The Weight of It*. New York: Henry Holt, 2004; Berman, M. S., and L. Shames. *Living Large: A Big Man's Ideas on Weight, Success, and Acceptance*. New York: Rodale, 2006; Shanker, W. *The Fat Girl's Guide to Life*. New York: Bloomsbury, 2004; Moore, *Fat Girl*; Scott, J. *Off the Scales: A Battle to Beat Teenage Obesity*. Stansted, UK: Kenton, 2009; Wheatley, S. *'Til the Fat Girl Sings*. Avon, WI: Adams Media, 2006; Hope, J. *Big, Bold and Beautiful*. Toronto: MacMillan, 1996; Klein, S. *Moose: A Memoir of Fat Camp*. New York: William Morrow, 2008.

8. Kalorie Kids

Epigraph: West, R. *The Teen-Age Diet Book*. New York: Bantam, 1959, 3.

1. Historians examining adult obesity have concentrated on dietary responses above all other treatments. This reflects the fact that dietary concerns are of long standing and also shows how dominant they have become in the current approach to fatness. See Schwartz, H. *Never Satisfied: A Cultural History of Diets, Fantasies, and Fat*. New York: Free Press, 1986; Levenstein, H. *Paradox of Plenty: A Social History of Eating in Modern America*. Oxford: Oxford University Press, 1993; Stearns, P. *Fat History*. New York: New York University Press, 1997; Gilman, S. *Diets and Dieting*. New York: Routledge, 2008; Gilman, S. *Fat: A Cultural History of Obesity*. Cambridge: Polity, 2008.

2. Corlin, J., and M. Miller. *The Scarsdale Nutritionist's Weight Loss Program for Teenagers*. New York: Fireside, 1983, 95. For an overview of Atwater's work, see Hargrove, J. "The History of the Calorie in Nutrition." *Journal of Nutrition* 136 (2006): 2957–2961.

3. Corlin and Miller, *Scarsdale Nutritionist's Weight Loss Program*, 95.

4. Veeder, B. "The Overweight Child." *Journal of the American Medical Association* 83 (1924): 486–489, 487.

5. Editorial. "Childhood Obesity." *The Lancet* 257, no. 6659 (1951): 841, 841.

6. This dieting prescription or slight variations on it, often in combination with other treatment options, can be found in much research and popular advice on treating childhood obesity. See, for example, "Metabolism of the Very Obese Child." *Journal of the American Medical Association* 75 (1920): 1291; "Dieting Improves Health of Over-Fat Children." *The Science News-Letter* 28 (1935): 340–341; Bruch, H. "Obesity in Childhood: III. Physiologic and Psychological Aspects of the Food Intake of Obese Children." *American Journal of Diseases of Children* 59 (1940): 739–781; Stuart, H. "Obesity in Childhood." *Quarterly Review of Pediatrics* 10 (1955): 131–145; Huenemann, R. "Consideration of Adolescent Obesity as a Public Health Problem." *Public Health Reports* 83 (1968): 491–495; Stults, H. "Obesity in Adolescents." *Journal of Pediatric Psychology* 2 (1977): 122–126; Cusack, R. "Dietary Management of Obese Children and Adolescents." *Pediatric Annals* 13 (1984): 455–464; Dietz, W., and S. Gortmaker. "Preventing Obesity in Children and Adolescents." *Annual*

Review of Public Health 22 (2001): 337–353; Daniels, S., D. Arnett, et al. "Overweight in Children and Adolescents." *Circulation* 111 (2005): 1999–2012; Hassink, S. *A Clinical Guide to Pediatric Weight Management and Obesity.* Philadelphia: Wolters Kluwer, 2007.

7. Bess Marvin's interest in dieting is mentioned in, for example, Keene, C. *The Secret of Shadow Ranch.* New York: Grosset and Dunlap, 1931; Keene, C. *The Secret of Red Gate Farm.* New York: Grosset and Dunlap, 1931. See Dyer, C., and N. Romalov, eds. *Rediscovering Nancy Drew.* Iowa City: University of Iowa Press, 1995.

   Studies of the prevalence and reasons for child dieting are Deisher, R. W., and C. A. Mills. "The Adolescent Looks at His Health and Medical Care." *American Journal of Public Health* 53 (1963): 1928–1936; Dwyer, J., J. Feldman, and J. Mayer. "Adolescent Dieters: Who Are They?" *American Journal of Clinical Nutrition* 20 (1967): 1045–1056; Huenemann, R., M. Hampton, et al. "Adolescent Food Practices Associated with Obesity." *Proceedings of American Societies for Experimental Biology* 25 (1966): 4–10; Nylander, I. "The Feeling of Being Fat and Dieting in a School Population." *Acta Socio-Medica Scandanavica* 3 (1971): 17–26. One study that concentrated on weight-loss behaviors in boys is Tipton, C., and T.-K. Tcheng. "Iowa Wrestling Study: Weight Loss in High School Students." *Journal of the American Medical Association* 214 (1970): 1269–1274.

8. On self-help culture, see Anker, R. *Self-Help and Popular Religion in Early American Culture.* Westport, CT: Greenwood, 1999; Starker, S. *Oracle at the Supermarket.* New Brunswick, NJ: Transaction, 1989.

   Notable early studies of the connection between child smoking and weight concerns include Tucker, L. "Cigarette Smoking Intentions and Obesity among High School Males." *Psychological Reports* 52 (1983): 530; Charlton, A. "Smoking and Weight Control in Teenagers." *Public Health* 98 (1984): 277–281; Feldman, W. C., and S. Corbett. "Relationship between Higher Prevalence of Smoking and Weight Concern amongst Adolescent Girls." *Canadian Journal of Public Health* 76 (1985): 205–206. These studies found that children were more likely to smoke and smoke heavily if they were also concerned about their weight and believed smoking helped control appetite. More recent studies confirming the dieting-smoking-weight-loss connections include Huseth, A. L., K. M. Thompson, et al. "Smoking and Weight Control in Adolescent Females." *Eating Behavior* 1 (2000): 123–135; Cawley, J., S. Markowitz, and J. Tauras. "Lighting Up and Slimming Down: The Effect of Body Weight and Cigarette Prices on Adolescent Smoking Initiation." National Bureau of Economic Research Working Paper Series 9561, Cambridge, MA 2003.

9. The most significant study in this regard is Richardson, S., N. Goodman, A. Hastorf, and S. Dornbusch. "Cultural Uniformity in Reaction to Physical Disabilities." *American Sociological Review* 26 (1961): 241–247. Richardson et al. showed children pictures of children with different visible handicaps—one

in a wheelchair, one with only one hand, an obese child, and so forth—and asked the children to say which they "liked best," then "next best," and so on down to establish a rank order. The authors found that children consistently ranked the obese child lowest. Latner and Stunkard repeated the study in 2003 and found that the degree of stigmatization of obese children had become even more extreme. Latner, J. D., and A. Stunkard. "Getting Worse: The Stigmatization of Obese Children." *Obesity Research* 11 (2003): 452–456.

10. Hunt Peters, L. *Diet and Health with Key to the Calories.* Chicago: Reilly and Lee, 1918.

11. Ibid., 20.

12. On readers' likely familiarity with calories, see Hargrove, "History of the Calorie in Nutrition."

    "Kal'-o-ri" quotation from Hunt Peters, *Diet and Health,* 23.

    Hunt Peters's personal weight-loss methods described in Hunt Peters, *Diet and Health,* 109–110.

13. Korda, M. *Making the List: A Cultural History of the American Bestseller, 1900–1999.* New York: Barnes and Noble, 2001, 46–50.

    On newspaper syndicates, see Watson, E. *A History of Newspaper Syndicates in the United States, 1865–1935.* Chicago: Elmo Scott Watson, 1936.

14. Hunt Peters, L. "Answers to Correspondents." *Los Angeles Times,* 28 January 1925, B7.

15. Hunt Peters, L. "Answers to Correspondents." *Los Angeles Times,* 5 August 1922, I110.

16. Hunt Peters, L. "The Fat Child I." *Los Angeles Times,* 5 February 1924, A6.

17. Hunt Peters, "The Fat Child I." The specifics of the reduction plan (the "reduction rules") are given in Hunt Peters, L. "The Fat Child II." *Los Angeles Times,* 6 February 1924, A7.

18. Hunt Peters, L. *Diet for Children (and Adults) and the Kalorie Kids.* New York: Dodd, Mead, 1924, 174–175.

19. Ibid., ix.

20. Ibid., 176.

21. Ibid., 177–178.

22. For example, the 1943 edition of *Holt's Care and Feeding of Children* (first published 1894) was the first edition to include guidance on how to slim a fat child. Holt, L. E., Jr. *Holt's Care and Feeding of Children.* New York: D. Appleton-Century, 1943.

    Hunt Peters died while traveling to a meeting at the Royal Sanitary Institute in London. Although she did diet frequently and may have damaged her health by doing so, there is, however, no definitive evidence for this. Largo, M. "Lulu Hunt Peters." In *Genius and Heroin,* 222–223. New York: Harper, 2008.

23. Kain, I. J. *Rx for Slimming.* Philadelphia: David McKay, 1940; Kain, I. J. *Stay Slim for Life.* New York: Doubleday, 1958.

Kain, I. J. "Exercise without Tension Gives Supple Figure, Says Skater." *Washington Post,* 24 May 1941, 9.

24. Osgood, N. "Ida Jean Kain Practices What She Preaches." *St. Petersberg Times,* 20 March 1956, 21; Kain, I. J. "Hollywood Director Cuts down Weight by Diet and Swimming." *Washington Post,* 23 September 1936, 13; Kain, I. J. "Contentment Is the Best Beautifier, Believes Mary Pickford." *Washington Post,* 5 November 1936, 19.

25. "Some insurance against tuberculosis" quotation from Kain, I. J. "Children and Youths Need Some Extra Weight to Fight Disease." *Washington Post,* 16 December 1937, 19.

    "Curves and a round face" quotation from Kain, I. J. "Teen Age Hates to Be Fat—And Why Not!" *Washington Post,* 4 September 1942, B2.

    Famous child dieters from Kain, I. J. "Too Much Weight Is a Handicap Even to Young Children." *Washington Post,* 28 July 1939, 17.

26. Kain, I. J. "Subteen Laziness Lures Fat." *Washington Post,* 6 March 1960, F21; Kain, I. J. "Small Fry Problem: Obesity." *Washington Post,* 7 July 1959, B5.

27. Kain, I. J. "Shirley Temple Gives Advice to Teen Agers." *Washington Post,* 5 February 1945, 10.

28. "There is a general impression . . ." quotation from Editorial. "Childhood Obesity." *The Lancet* 257, no. 6659 (1951): 841.

29. On the risk factor concept, see Beck, U. *Risk Society.* London: Sage, 1992; Rosenberg, C. E. "Banishing Risk." *Perspectives in Biology and Medicine* 39 (1995): 28–42; Aronowitz, R. "The Social Construction of Coronary Heart Disease Risk Factors." In *Making Sense of Illness,* 111–144. Cambridge: Cambridge University Press, 1998; Rothstein, W. *Public Health and the Risk Factor.* Rochester, NY: Rochester University Press, 2003.

30. See, for example, Dawber, T. R., F. E. Moore, and G. V. Mann. "Coronary Heart Disease in the Framingham Study." *American Journal of Public Health and the Nation's Health* 27 (1957): 4–24; *Build and Blood Pressure Study.* 2 vols. Chicago: Society of Actuaries, 1959; Dawber, T. *The Framingham Study.* Cambridge, MA: Harvard University Press, 1980.

31. The two influential studies were Mullins, A. G. "The Prognosis in Juvenile Obesity." *Archives of Disease in Childhood* 33 (1958): 307–314; Abraham, S., and M. Nordsieck. "Relationship of Excess Weight in Children and Adults." *Public Health Reports* 75 (1960): 263–273.

    On the spread of this thinking about the risks of childhood obesity, see, for example, Bruch, H. "Fat Children Grown Up." *American Journal of Diseases of Children* 90 (1955): 501; Illingworth, R. S. "Obesity." *Journal of Pediatrics* 53 (1958): 117–130; Huenemann, "Consideration of Adolescent Obesity"; Knittle, J. "Childhood Obesity." *Bulletin of the New York Academy of Medicine* 47 (1971): 579–589; Charney, E., H. Goodman, et al. "Childhood Antecedents of Adult Obesity." *New England Journal of Medicine* 295 (1976): 6–9.

More recent studies confirming the persistence of childhood obesity are Guo, S., A. Roche, et al. "The Predictive Values of Childhood Body Mass Index Values for Overweight at Age 35y." *American Journal of Clinical Nutrition* 59 (1994): 810–819; Guo, S., and W. Chumlea. "Tracking of Body Mass Index in Children in Relation to Overweight in Adulthood." *American Journal of Clinical Nutrition* 70, supplement (1999): 145–148.

32. Atkins, R. *Dr. Atkins' Diet Revolution.* New York: McKay, 1972. West is listed as an author in the copyright application but in the published book is only mentioned in the acknowledgments. Copyright Office. *Catalog of Copyright Entries.* July–December. Washington, DC: Library of Congress, 1972, 2398.

33. For example, Greenfield, D., D. Quinlan, et al. "Eating Behavior in an Adolescent Population." *International Journal of Eating Disorders* 6 (1987): 99–111; Casper, R., and D. Offer. "Weight and Dieting Concerns in Adolescents, Fashion or Symptom?" *Pediatrics* 86 (1990): 384–390; Hill, A., S. Oliver, and P. Rogers. "Eating in the Adult World: The Rise of Dieting in Childhood and Adolescence." *British Journal of Clinical Psychology* 31 (1992): 95–105; Schur, E., M. Sanders, and H. Steiner. "Body Dissatisfaction and Dieting in Young Children." *International Journal of Eating Disorders* 27 (2000): 74–82; Field, A., C. Camargo, et al. "Peer, Parent, and Media Influences on the Development of Weight Concerns and Frequent Dieting among Preadolescent and Adolescent Girls and Boys." *Pediatrics* 107 (2001): 54–60; van den Berg, P., D. Neumark-Sztainer, et al. "Is Dieting Advice from Magazines Helpful or Harmful?" *Pediatrics* 119 (2007): e30–e37.

34. "Way-of-life" book quotation from West, *Teen-Age Diet Book,* 3. Other books that insist they are not dieting books include Eden, A. *Growing Up Thin.* New York: David McKay, 1975; Levine, J., and L. Bine. *Helping Your Child Lose Weight the Healthy Way.* New York: Citadel, 1996; Boutaudou, S. *Weighing In.* New York: Amulet, 2006.

    "You'll lose many pounds and inches in a hurry" quotation from Stillman, I., and S. Sinclair Baker. *The Doctor's Quick Teenage Diet.* New York: Paperback Library, 1971, 11.

    Woolfolk, D. *The Teenage Surefire Diet Cookbook.* New York: Franklin Watts, 1979, 6.

35. "As a young person" quotation from McGraw, J. *The Ultimate Weight Solution for Teens.* New York: Free Press, 2003, xvii.

    Writers using their own history of weight loss in their pitch include Lindauer, L. *The Fast-and-Easy Teenage Diet.* New York: Award, 1973; Mason, G. *Help Your Child Lose Weight and Keep It Off.* New York: Grossett and Dunlap, 1975; Lukes, B. *How to Be a Reasonably Thin Teenage Girl without Starving, Losing Your Friends or Running Away from Home.* New York: Atheneum, 1986; Meyer, C. *I Was a Teenage Loser (You Can Be One, Too).* Milwaukee, WI: SHR Press, 2007.

Doctors or health professionals who had lost weight and wrote a diet book for children include Edelstein, B. *The Woman Doctor's Diet for Teen-Age Girls*. Englewood Cliffs, NJ: Prentice-Hall, 1980; Silberstein, W., and L. Galton. *Helping Your Child Grow Slim*. New York: Simon and Schuster, 1982; Cohen, M., and L. Abramson. *Thin Kids*. New York: Beaufort, 1985; Pescatore, F. *Feed Your Kids Well*. New York: John Wiley, 1998.

Mothers who wrote diet books, and who note the fact that they are mothers as part of their claims to authority, include Woolfolk, *Teenage Surefire Diet Cookbook;* Wiatt, C., and B. Schroeder. *The Diet for Teenagers Only*. New York: Regan Books, 2005; Fletcher, A. *Weight Loss Confidential*. New York: Houghton Mifflin, 2006.

36. Stillman and Baker, *Doctor's Quick Teenage Diet*.
37. Lukes, *How to Be a Reasonably Thin Teenage Girl*, 4.
38. Matthews, D., A. Zullo, and B. Nash. *The You Can Do It! Kids' Diet*. New York: Holt, Rinehart and Winston, 1985, 19.
39. "Punkers" from Ibid., 64.
40. Corlin and Miller, *Scarsdale Nutritionist's Weight Loss Program*, 11.
41. West, *Teen-Age Diet Book*, 38.
42. Matthews et al., *You Can Do It! Kids' Diet*, 64.
43. West, *Teen-Age Diet Book*, 3; Stillman and Baker, *Doctor's Quick Teenage Diet*, 7.
44. Boutaudou, *Weighing In*, 101.
45. Surveys of children's reasons for dieting that have found this include Dwyer, Feldman, and Mayer, "Adolescent Dieters"; Nylander, "Feeling of Being Fat"; Greenfield, Quinlan, et al. "Eating Behavior"; Maloney, M. J., J. McGuire, S. R. Daniels, and B. Specker. "Dieting Behavior and Eating Attitudes in Children " *Pediatrics* 84 (1989): 482–489; Casper and Offer, "Weight and Dieting Concerns"; Schur, Sandes, and Steiner, "Body Dissatisfaction and Dieting"; Field, Camargo, et al., "Peer, Parent, and Media Influences"; van den Berg, Neumark-Sztainer, et al., "Dieting Advice from Magazines." A good exploration of why children diet is Hill, Oliver, and Rogers, "Eating in the Adult World."
46. Matthews et al., *You Can Do It! Kids' Diet*, 19–20.
47. Ibid., 225. A similar approach is taken by Lukes, *How to Be a Reasonably Thin Teenage Girl*.
48. Tipton and Tcheng. "Iowa Wrestling Study"; Lakin, J., S. Steen, and R. Oppliger. "Eating Behaviors, Weight Loss Methods, and Nutrition Practices among High School Wrestlers." *Journal of Community Health Nursing* 7 (1990): 223–234.
49. Bartell, S. S. *Dr. Susan's Girls-Only Weight Loss Guide*. New York: Parent Positive Press, 2006.

On feminism and girl dieting, see Brumberg, J. *The Body Project: An Intimate History of American Girls*. New York: Vintage, 1997.

50. Nichter, M. *Fat Talk: What Girls and Their Parents Say about Dieting.* Cambridge, MA: Harvard University Press, 2000.

51. Meyer, *I Was a Teenage Loser,* 1.

    Scott, J. *Off the Scales: A Battle to Beat Teenage Obesity.* Stansted, UK: Kenton, 2009.

52. Mason, *Help Your Child Lose Weight,* 13.

    On the history of parenting styles, see James, A., and A. Prout, eds. *Constructing and Reconstructing Childhood.* London: Falmer Press, 1997; Stearns, P. *Anxious Parents: A History of Modern Childrearing in America.* New York: New York University Press, 2003.

53. Mason, *Help Your Child Lose Weight,* 14.

54. "Love . . . listening . . . and limits . . ." quotation from David, L. *Slimming for Teenagers.* New York: Pocket Books, 1966, 74.

    "Stick to your guns" quotation from Eden, *Growing Up Thin,* 9, 10. Similar sentiments in Wolff, J., and D. Lipe. *Help for the Overweight Child.* New York: Stein and Day, 1978.

55. Bartell, *Dr. Susan's Girls-Only Weight Loss Guide,* 110.

56. Ibid., 110.

57. McGraw, *Ultimate Weight Solution for Teens,* 154.

58. Bartell, *Dr. Susan's Girls-Only Weight Loss Guide,* 111.

59. The first books in each series are Rowling, J. K. *Harry Potter and the Sorcerer's Stone.* U.S. paperback ed. New York: Scholastic, 1999; Riordan, R. *The Lightning Thief.* New York: Miramax, 2006.

60. Classic children's literature is characterized by the *absence* of adult characters, which allows the child characters to take the lead in adventures of their own. In this recent trend in children's literature, adults are present, but are ineffective.

61. Austin, S. B. "Fat, Loathing and Public Health." *Culture, Medicine and Psychiatry* 23 (1999): 245–268; Wilson, T. "The Controversy over Dieting." In *Eating Disorders and Obesity,* C. Fairburn and K. Brownell, eds., 93–97. New York: Guilford, 2002; Pitman, T., and M. Kaufman. *All Shapes and Sizes.* New York: Harper Perennial, 1994.

    On the fat acceptance movement's position on dieting, see, for example, Fishman, S. G. B. "Life in the Fat Underground." *Radiance,* Winter 1998, www.radiancemagazine.com/issues/1998/winter_98/fat_underground.html; Campos, P. *The Obesity Myth.* New York: Penguin, 2004; Oliver, J. E. *Fat Politics.* New York: Oxford University Press, 2006; O'Hara, L., and J. Gregg. "Human Rights Casualties from the 'War on Obesity.'" *Fat Studies* 1 (2012): 32–46.

    HAES philosophy and its rejection of dieting derives from Bacon, L. *Health at Every Size.* Dallas: BenBella Books, 2008.

62. National Institutes of Health. *Gastrointestinal Surgery for Severe Obesity.* NIH Consensus Statement. Washington, DC: National Institutes of Health, 1991;

United States Food and Drug Administration (FDA). "Medical Devices: Gastric Banding." http://www.fda.gov/MedicalDevices/ProductsandMedical Procedures/ObesityDevices/ucm350132.htm. Access date July 15, 2013.

Guidelines for use of bariatric surgery developed by pediatric surgeons and surgery departments include Inge, T., N. Krebs, et al. "Bariatric Surgery for Severely Overweight Adolescents." *Pediatrics* 114 (2004): 217–223; Michalsky, M., R. Kramer, et al. "Developing Criteria for Pediatric/Adolescent Bariatric Surgery Programs." *Pediatrics* 128 (2011): S65–S70.

Reviews of the use of bariatric surgery in children include Sugerman, H. J., E. L. Sugerman, et al. "Bariatric Surgery for Severely Obese Adolescents." *Journal of Gastrointestinal Surgery* 7 (2003): 102–107; Inge, T., M. Zeller, et al. "A Critical Appraisal of Evidence Supporting a Bariatric Surgical Approach to Weight Management for Adolescents." *Journal of Pediatrics* 147 (2005): 10–19; Tsai, W., T. Inge, and R. Burd. "Bariatric Surgery in Adolescents." *Archives of Pediatrics and Adolescent Medicine* 161 (2007): 217–221.

63. "Dieting is a significant risk factor" quotation from Pitman and Kaufman, *All Shapes and Sizes*, 9.

On the contribution of exercise to balancing the obese child's energy equation, see Johnson, M. L., B. Burke, and J. Mayer. "Relative Importance of Inactivity and Overeating in the Energy Balance of Obese High School Girls." *American Journal of Clinical Nutrition* 4 (1956): 37–44; Anderson, R., C. Crespo, and S. Bartlett. "Relationship of Physical Activity and Television Watching with Body Weight and Level of Fatness among Children." *Journal of the American Medical Association* 279 (1998): 938–942; Robinson, T. "Reducing Children's Television Watching to Prevent Obesity." *Journal of the American Medical Association* 282 (1999): 1561–1567; Reilly, J. J., D. M. Jackson, et al. "Total Energy Expenditure and Physical Activity in Young Scottish Children." *The Lancet* 363, no. 17 (2004): 211–212.

9. Summer Slimming

Epigraph: "Overweight—Slight or Quite." *New York Times*, 16 March 1975, SM126.

1. See, for example, *MTV News Presents: Fat Camp*. First broadcast 15 February 2006 by MTV. Directed by James Huang, Kristen Schylinski, and Cheryl Sirulnich; *MTV News Presents: Return to Fat Camp*. First broadcast 1 December 2007 by MTV. Directed by Cheryl Sirulnich and Leslie Appleyard.

2. Peckos, P., and J. Spargo. "For Overweight Teenage Girls." *American Journal of Nursing* 64 (1964): 85–87; David, L. *Slimming for Teen-Agers*. New York: Pocket Books, 1966; Peckos, P. "The Treatment of Adolescent Obesity." *Issues in Comprehensive Pediatric Nursing* 1 (1976): 17–30; Peckos, P. "Interview with Penny Peckos." Conducted by author, September 6 2009, Brewster, MA.

3. Goldman, R. F., B. Bullen, and C. Seltzer. "Changes in Specific Gravity and Body Fat in Overweight Female Adolescents as a Result of Weight Reduction." *Annals of the New York Academy of Sciences* 110 (1961): 913–917; Peckos and Spargo, "For Overweight Teenage Girls"; Peckos, "Treatment of Adolescent Obesity"; David, *Slimming for Teen-Agers*.

4. Klemesrud, J. "These Campers Have a Lot to Lose—And That's Their Goal." *New York Times*, 24 July 1967, 46.

5. Exceptions to directors' lack of medical training were the first camp for overweight boys, Camp Macabee, started in Virginia in 1966 by a pediatric endocrinologist, Graciano P. Gancayco, which ran until the mid-1970s; and Camp Napanoch in Wisconsin, which from 1966 to about 1974 was owned by pediatrician Morton B. Glenn, director of the American College of Nutrition and author of dieting books for adults. Glenn, M. *How to Get Thinner Once and for All.* Greenwich, CT: Fawcett, 1965; Glenn, M. *But I Don't Eat That Much.* New York: Penguin, 1974; Advertisement: "Camp Macabee: Original Camp for Overweight Boys." *New York Times*, 23 April 1972, SM94.

   Directors who pointed to their own slim bodies as evidence that their approach worked include those of Camps Napanoch, Shane, and Kingsmont. "Sending Your Child to 'Fat Camp.'" *Los Angeles Times*, 18 May 1978, L34; "Camp Shane." Camp Shane LLC, http://www.campshane.com/. c2009. Access date 12 October 2009; Advertisement: "Overweight Girls and Boys" (Camp Shane). *New York Times*, 25 February 1973, 301; Advertisement: "Girls for a Summer of Fun" (Camp Napanoch). *New York Times*, 10 March 1974, 326; "Camp Kingsmont History," www.campkingsmont.com/about/history .html. 2008. Access date 21 April 2008; Advertisement: "Overweight Boys Make a Summer of Losing Weight" (Camp Kingsmont). *New York Times*, 10 March 1974, 326.

6. Fat camps were regular items in newspapers. Newspaper articles and camp advertisements provide a contemporary source of information about the camps, such as numbers of attendees and costs. For example, Advertisement: "Overweight?" (Camp Lakecrest). *New York Times*, 2 June 1963, 258; "Miseries of an Overweight Child." *Look Magazine*, 17 November 1967, 36–41; Advertisement: "Weight Watchers Ferosdel Camp." *New York Times*, 23 April 1972, SM94; Klemesrud, J. "Don't Call It a Fat Camp." *New York Times*, 4 August 1975, 34; Advertisement: "The First Weight Control Plan That Uses Your Child's Own Rapid Growth as the Key to 'Growing' Slim!" . *New York Times*, 17 October 1982, BR35; Advertisement: "Is Weight Holding Your Daughter Back?" (Camp Murietta). *New York Times*, 17 March 1985, SM105.

7. On camps' buildings, see, for example, Strauss, M. "Summer Youth Camps Blossom in the Catskills." *New York Times*, 5 May 1968, XX4.

   On Weight Watchers' camps, see, for example, Advertisement: "Weight Watchers' Camps Overweight Girls 10 Years and Up." *New York Times*,

10 March 1974, 326; Advertisement: "Now Weight Watchers' Camps All Girls—Blast." *New York Times,* 3 April 1983, SM61; Berland, T. "Ask the Right Questions About 'Fat Camps.'" *Los Angeles Times,* 13 May 1976, C30.

8. Ellin, A. *Teenage Waistland.* New York: Public Affairs, 2005, 27; American Camp Association, www.acacamps.org. Access dates 29 April 2008, 2 February 2013.

9. On the history of organized camping, see Paris, L. *Children's Nature: The Rise of the American Summer Camp.* New York: New York University Press, 2008; Eels, E. *Eleanor Eels' History of Organized Camping.* Martinsville, IN: American Camping Association, 1986; Van Slyck, A. *A Manufactured Wilderness.* Minneapolis: University of Minnesota Press, 2006.

10. Historians have documented that European and American society felt itself to be in a "crisis of manliness" in the late nineteenth century and early years of the twentieth century. Time spent in the natural world could, however, counter this distressing supposed emasculation. See, for example, Oppenheim, J. *"Shattered Nerves": Doctors, Patients, and Depression in Victorian England.* Oxford: Oxford University Press, 1991; Mosse, G. *The Image of Man: The Creation of Modern Masculinity.* Oxford: Oxford University Press, 1996; Will, B. "The Nervous Origins of the American Western." *American Literature* 70 (1998): 293–316; Gijkswijt-Hofstra, M. "Introduction: Cultures of Neurasthenia from Beard to the First World War." In *Cultures of Neurasthenia,* M Gijkswijt-Hofstra and R. Porter, eds., 1–30. Amsterdam: Rodopi, 2001.

　　"I am now a healthy boy . . ." quoted in Paris, *Children's Nature,* 263.

11. The history of this idea dates from an Enlightenment model of childhood suggested by Jacques Rousseau in his 1762 treatise *Emilie, or On Education,* which argues that, contrary to earlier Christian ideas of children as being full of sin, children were innocent and in a natural state of goodness. Art historians noted that this model strongly influenced how children were depicted in Enlightenment, Romantic, and Victorian sentimental art. Children were often shown in natural settings or with flowers or animals to allude to their pure wholesomeness. See, for example, Higonnet, A. *Pictures of Innocence.* London: Thames and Hudson, 1998; Cook, D., ed. *Symbolic Childhood.* New York: Peter Lang, 2002; Holland, P. *Picturing Childhood.* London: I.B. Tauris, 2004.

12. Camp Murietta used this slogan in its advertisements in the early and mid-1970s. For example, Advertisement: "Overweight? Become a New Girl at Camp Murietta." *New York Times,* 25 February 1973, 301.

13. The dietary prescriptions of fat camps are described in Peckos and Spargo, "For Overweight Teenage Girls"; David, *Slimming for Teen-Agers;* Klemesrud, "These Campers Have a Lot to Lose"; Mason, G. *Help Your Child Lose Weight and Keep It Off.* New York: Grossett and Dunlap, 1975; "Sending Your Child to 'Fat Camp,'" L34; Lywander, L. "A Different Weight Control Program for Youngsters." *The New York Times,* 28 December 1980, NJ14; Mansfield, S. "The Fat Farm." *The Washington Post,* 13 July 1980, A1.

Hiding wrappers in bed frames reported in Peckos, interview with author.

The hidden cache of candy wrappers reported by St. Sure, E., Brewster Town Archivist. Personal communication with author, April 29, 2008.

14. Seascape's offerings described in Advertisement: "Overweight—Slight or Quite." *New York Times,* 5 January 1975, SM17. The advertisement was run repeatedly in 1975 and 1976.

    Gussie Mason's secret weapon patent is Mason, G. Isometric Exercise Boots. US Patent 3,406,968, filed November 24, 1964, and issued October 22, 1968. "Secret weapon" in her "war on fat" from Mason, *Help Your Child Lose Weight,* 107.

    Camp Macabee, in Virginia, took the boys to Washington D.C. and Gettysburg. Camp Seascape took the girls to various sites around Cape Cod, including the theatre at Dennis; on rainy days they went on bus outings. Peckos, interview with author; Advertisement: "Camp Macabee" *New York Times,* 23 April 1972, SM94.

15. Klemesrud, "These Campers Have a Lot to Lose," 46. Mason refers to the "fat environment" in Mason, *Help Your Child Lose Weight,* 4.

16. "Miseries of an Overweight Child," 39.

17. Mansfield, "Fat Farm."

18. "Deeper roots" quotation from Mansfield, S. "A Weighty Problem for Teen-Age Girls." *Los Angeles Times,* 10 August 1980, F2. Camp Shane's program discussed in Ellin, *Teenage Waistland.*

19. Peckos, interview with author.

    Other girls' camps that used this approach included the Allegro Spa, Lakecrest Camp, and Clover Lodge. Advertisement: "The Allegro Spa." *New York Times,* 15 April 1973, 358; Advertisement: "Overweight? Lakecrest Camp/Spa." *New York Times,* 15 April 1973, 358; Advertisement: "Overweight Girls" (Clover Lodge). *New York Times,* 23 April 1972, SM94.

20. "Overweight—Slight or Quite," SM126; Blumenthal, D. "Where Campers Lose Weight and Gain Confidence." *The New York Times,* 11 April 1987, 52; Advertisement: "Overweight Girls" (Clover Lodge), SM94; Klemesrud, "These Campers Have a Lot to Lose."

21. On weighing in, see, for example, Mason, *Help Your Child Lose Weight;* Klemesrud, "These Campers Have a Lot to Lose"; Blumenthal, "Where Campers Lose Weight."

22. Ellin, *Teenage Waistland;* Huang, Schylinski, and Sirulnich., "Fat Camp"; Sirulnich and Appleyard, "Return to Fat Camp; Klein, S. *Moose: A Memoir of Fat Camp.* New York: William Morrow, 2008.

23. Pinkwater, D. *Fat Camp Commandoes.* New York: Scholastic, 2001, 7. See also Manes, S. *Slim Down Camp.* New York: Houghton Mifflin, 1981; Blumenthal, D. *Fat Camp.* New York: NAL Jam, 2006.

    Cartman goes to fat camp in "Fat Camp." *South Park.* Season 4, Episode 15, first broadcast 6 December 2000 by Comedy Central. Directed by T. Parker and written by T. Parker and M. Stone; Bart goes to fat camp in "The Heartbroke Kid." *The Simpsons.* Episode 350, first broadcast May 1, 2005 by Fox. Directed by S. D. Moore and written by I. Maxtone-Graham; *Heavyweights.* Film. Directed by S. Brill. Burbank, CA: Walt Disney Pictures, 1995, 100 min.

24. Mansfield, "Weighty Problem," F2.

25. On the persistence of weight losses and the methods camps employ to extend their influence, see, for example, Peckos and Spargo, "For Overweight Teenage Girls"; Werkman, S., and E. Greenberg. "Personality and Interest Patterns in Obese Adolescent Girls." *Psychosomatic Medicine* 24 (1967): 72–80; Southam, M. A., B. G. Kirkley, A. Murchison, and R. I. Berkowitz. "A Summer Day Camp Approach to Adolescent Weight Loss." *Adolescence* 19 (1984): 855–868; Ellin, *Teenage Waistland.*

26. For example, Advertisement: "Overweight?" (Camp Lakecrest), 258; Advertisement: "Overweight? Become a New Girl at Camp Murietta," 301; Advertisement: "Overweight Girls and Boys" (Camp Shane), 301.

27. Cost of Camps Stanley and Tahoe from Klemesrud, "These Campers Have a Lot to Lose"; "Sending Your Child to 'Fat Camp,'" L34. Adjusted for inflation using Bureau of Labor Statistics CPI Inflation Calculator, http://www.bls .gov/data/inflation_calculator.htm.

   Prices of camps today from American Camp Association," www.acacamps .org. Access dates 29 April 2008, 2 February 2013. Average price $8,990.

   Not-for-profit camps, for example, Pratt, K. J., A. L. Lamson, et al. "Camp Golden Treasures: A Multidisciplinary Weight-Loss and a Healthy Lifestyle Camp for Adolescent Girls." *Family Systems Health* 27 (2009): 116–124.

28. "At camp La Jolla" quotation from "Camp La Jolla: Weight Loss Camps." Camp La Jolla, http://www.camplajolla.com/. c2009. Access date 12 October 2009.

   Examples of attempts to include families in the camp are "Parents Join Kids at Fitness Camp." *Wall Street Journal,* 16 June 2004, D3; Weingarten, T. "Summer Camp for Losers." *Newsweek* 151, no. 20 (2008): 56.

29. Camp Seascape's data was reported in Goldman, Bullen, and Seltzer, "Changes in Specific Gravity and Body Fat."

   Other camps' successes and "it's 50–50" quotation from Ellin, *Teenage Waistland,* 27; Duarte, G. M. "MTV Cameras Follow Overweight Kids at Camp Pocono Trails." *Pocono Record,* 27 February 2006, http://www.newimagecamp .com/poconorecord/poconorecord2.htm.

   Recent studies of the effects of fat camps as obesity treatments are Di Pietro, M., P. Campanaro, et al. "Role of Camping in the Treatment of Childhood Obesity." *Acta Bio Medica Ateneo Parmense* 75 (2004): 118–121; Walker, L. L., P. J. Gately, et al. "Children's Weight-Loss Camps." *International Journal of Obesity and Related Metabolic Disorders* 27 (2003): 748–754; Gately, P. J.,

C. B. Cooke, et al. "Children's Residential Weight-Loss Programs Can Work." *Pediatrics* 116 (2005): 73–77; Cooper, C., Sarvey S., et al. "For Comparison: Experience with a Children's Obesity Camp." *Surgery for Obesity and Related Diseases* 2 (2006): 622–626.

30. Wellspring Academies, http://www.wellspringacademies.com/. 2008. Access date 29 April 2008.

10. Bigger Bodies in a Broken World

Epigraph: Kluger, J. "How America's Children Packed On the Pounds." *Time*, 23 June 2008, 66–69, 66.

1. Dietz, W., S. Gortmaker, et al. "Trends in the Prevalence of Childhood and Adolescent Obesity in the United States." *Pediatric Research* 19 (1985): 198A. A detailed analysis was later published as Gortmaker, Steven, William Dietz, et al. "Increasing Pediatric Obesity in the United States." *American Journal of Diseases of Children* 141 (1987): 535–540.

2. For example, Gortmaker, S., W. Dietz, et al. "Increasing Pediatric Obesity in the United States"; Troiano, R., K. Flegal, R. Kuczmarski, S. Campbell, and C. Johnson. "Overweight Prevalence and Trends for Children and Adolescents: The National Health and Nutrition Examination Surveys, 1963–1991." *Archives of Pediatrics and Adolescent Medicine* 149 (1995): 1085–1091; Ogden, C., R. Troiano, et al. "Prevalence of Overweight among Preschool Children in the United States, 1971 through 1994." *Pediatrics* 99 (1997): e1; Freedman, D., S. Srinivasan, et al. "Secular Increases in Relative Weight and Adiposity among Children over Two Decades:" *Pediatrics* 99 (1997): 420–426; Ogden, C., K. Flegal, et al. "Prevalence and Trends in Overweight among US Children, Adolescents, 1999–2000." *Journal of the American Medical Association* 288 (2002): 1728–1732; Ogden, C., M. Carroll, et al. "Prevalence of Overweight and Obesity in the United States, 1999–2004." *Journal of the American Medical Association* 295 (2006): 1549–1555; Ogden, C., M. Carroll, et al. "Prevalence of High Body Mass Index in US Children and Adolescents, 2007–2008." *Journal of the American Medical Association* 303 (2010): 241–249.

On the patterning of the childhood obesity epidemic by ethnic group and socioeconomic standing, see Strauss, R., and H. Pollack. "Epidemic Increase in Childhood Overweight, 1986–1998." *Journal of the American Medical Association* 286 (2001): 2845–2848; Gordon-Larsen, P., L. S. Adair, and B. Popkin. "The Relationship of Ethnicity, Socioeconomic Factors, and Overweight in US Adolescents." *Obesity Research* 11 (2003): 121–129; Bethell, C., Read D., et al. "Consistently Inconsistent: A Snapshot of across- and within-State Disparities in the Prevalence of Childhood Overweight and Obesity." *Pediatrics* 123, supplement 5 (2009): S277–S286; Wang, Y. "Disparities in Pediatric Obesity in the United States." *Advances in Nutrition* 2 (2011): 23–31.

3. For example, Burdette, H., and R. Whitaker. "A National Study of Neighborhood Safety, Outdoor Play, Television Viewing, and Obesity in Preschool Children." *Pediatrics* 116 (2005): 657–662; Cohen, D., B. Finch, et al. "Collective Efficacy and Obesity: The Potential Influence of Social Factors on Health." *Social Science and Medicine* 62 (2006): 769–778; Lumeng, J., D. Appugliese, et al. "Neighborhood Safety and Overweight Status in Children." *Archives of Pediatrics and Adolescent Medicine* 160 (2006): 25–31; Cecil-Karb, R., and A. Grogan-Kaylor. "Childhood Body Mass Index in Community Context." *Health and Social Work* 34 (2009): 169–177; Pollan, M. *The Omnivore's Dilemma.* New York: Penguin, 2006.

   On how de rigueur such a list is, see, for example, Dietz, W. "Editorial: The Obesity Epidemic in Young Children." *British Medical Journal* 322 (2001): 313–314; Larkin, M. "Defusing the 'Time Bomb' of Childhood Obesity." *The Lancet* 359, no. 16 (2002): 987; Kimm, S. Y. S., and E. Obarzanek. "Childhood Obesity: A New Pandemic of the New Millennium." *Pediatrics* 110 (2002): 1003–1007; Caprio, S., and M. Genel. "Confronting the Epidemic of Childhood Obesity." *Pediatrics* (2005): 494–495. Popular coverage includes Klein, R. "Big Country." *New Republic,* 19 and 26 September 1994, 28–37; Tartamella, L., E. Herscher, and C. Woolston. *Generation Extra Large.* New York: Basic Books, 2004; Okie, S. *Fed Up!* Washington, DC: Joseph Henry Press, 2005; Kluger, "How America's Children Packed On the Pounds"; Walsh, B. "It's Not Just Genetics." *Time,* 23 June 2008, 70–80; Sayre, C. "School Cuisine." *Time,* 23 June 2008, 82–87; Moore, P. "The White House Diet." *Children's Health,* 15 September 2009, 62–69.

4. For a similar idea of the failure of modernity, see Rosenberg, C. E. "Pathologies of Progress: The Idea of Civilization as Risk." *Bulletin of the History of Medicine* 72 (1998): 714–730.

   On healthy living as an ideal, see, for example, Goldstein, M. *The Health Movement.* New York: Twayne, 1992; Brandt, A., and P. Rozin, eds. *Morality and Health.* New York: Routledge, 1997; Schwartz, H. *Never Satisfied: A Cultural History of Diets, Fantasies, and Fat.* New York: Free Press, 1986.

5. Neel, J. "Diabetes Mellitus: A 'Thrifty' Genotype Rendered Detrimental by Progress?" *American Journal of Human Genetics* 14 (1962): 353–362, 354–355. Also Neel, J. "The Thrifty Genotype Revisited." In *The Genetics of Diabetes Mellitus,* J. Köbberling and R. Tattersall, eds., 283–293. New York: Academic Press, 1982.

6. See, for example, the 23 June 2008 edition of *Time* magazine and particularly Kluger, "How America's Children Packed On the Pounds."

7. Ibid., 66–68. For criticism of the thrifty gene idea, see Swinburn, B. A "The Thrifty Gene Hypothesis: How Does It Look after 30 Years?" *Diabetic Medicine* 13 (1996): 695–699; Southam, L. N., Soranzo, S. B. et al. "Is the Thrifty Gene Hypothesis Supported by Evidence Based on Confirmed Type 2 Diabetes- and Obesity-Susceptibility Variants?" *Diabetologia* 52 (2009): 1846–1851.

8. On television and its social impact, see Spigel, L. "Seducing the Innocent: Children and Television in Postwar America." In *The Children's Culture Reader,* H. Jenkins, ed., 110–135. New York: New York University Press, 1998; Signorelli, N. *A Sourcebook on Children and Television.* New York: Greenwood, 1991; Krasnow, E., L. Longley, and H. Terry. *The Politics of Broadcast Regulation.* New York: St. Martin's Press, 1982; Minow, N., and C. LaMay. *Abandoned in the Wasteland: Children, Television, and the First Amendment.* New York: Hill and Wang, 1995.

"Scantily clad leg" quotation from Miller, J. "TV and the Children." *The Nation* 171 (1950): 87. On later worries about the effects of televised violence on children, see Surgeon General's Scientific Advisory Committee on Television and Social Behavior. "Television and Growing Up: The Impact of Televised Violence. Report to the Surgeon General, United States Public Health Service." *Reports of the Surgeon General.* Washington, DC: National Institute of Mental Health, 1972; National Institute of Human Health. "Television and Behavior: Ten Years of Scientific Progress and Implications for the Eighties." Rockville, MD: National Institute of Mental Health, 1982. See also Signorelli, *Sourcebook on Children and Television,* 81–98.

On worries about television's effect on social interaction, see, for example, "Television: The Infant Grows Up." *Time,* 24 May 1948, http://www.time .com/time/magazine/article/0,9171,794400,00.html; Hurlock, E. B. "Television Bugaboo." *Today's Health* 28 (1950): 68.

9. National Association of Radio and Television Broadcasters. "The Television Code." Washington, DC: National Association of Radio and Television Broadcasters, 1952, 1.

10. "Women's services . . ." quotation from NARTB, "The Television Code," 7.
   "Exercise the utmost care" quotation from ibid., 5.

11. On consumer activism, see Kozinets, R., and J. Handleman. "Adversaries of Consumption: Consumer Movements, Activism, and Ideology." *Journal of Consumer Research* 31 (2004): 691–704; Glickman, L. *Buying Power: A History of Consumer Activism in America.* Chicago: University of Chicago Press, 2009. Particularly in relation to TV, see Moody, K. "The Broadcast Reform Movement." *Change* 8 (1976): 54–55; Krasnow, Longley, and Terry, *Politics of Broadcast Regulation.*

On ACT, CSPI, and CCMM, see Feinbloom, R. "Action for Children's Television: How Pediatricians Can Help the ACT." *Pediatrics* 47 (1971): 630–631; Richter, W. "Action for Children's Television: U.S. Citizens' Action Group." Museum of Broadcast Communications. 2009. http://www.museum .tv/archives/etv/A/htmlA/actionforch/actionforch.htm Access date 24 September 2009; Charren, P. "Closing ACT: A Report to the Lilly Endowment." Cambridge, MA: Action for Children's Television, 1992 ; Center for Science in the Public Interest. "A Brief History." CSPI, www.cspinet.org/history /cspihist.htm. c1997. Access date 7 October 2009; Center for Science in the

Public Interest. "Building a Healthier America since 1971." Washington, DC: CSPI, 2006; Choate, R. "The Sugar-Coated Children's Hour." *The Nation* 214 (1972): 146–148.

12. McNeal, J. "Children as Consumers." *Journal of the Academy of Marketing Science* 7 (1979): 346–359; McNeal, J. *Children as Consumers.* Lexington, TX: Lexington Books, 1987; McNeal, J. *Kids as Customers.* Lexington, TX: Lexington Books, 1992; McNeal, J. *The Kids' Market.* New York: Paramount Market, 1999, 17.

On the rise of the child consumer, see Seiter, E. *Sold Separately: Children and Parents in Consumer Culture.* New Brunswick, NJ: Rutgers University Press, 1993; Schor, J. *Born to Buy.* New York: Scribner, 2004; Kapur, J. *Coining for Capital: Movies, Marketing, and the Transformation of Childhood.* New Brunswick: Rutgers University Press, 2005; Zelizer, V. *Pricing the Priceless Child.* New York: Basic Books, 1985; Jacobson, L. *Raising Consumers.* New York: Columbia University Press, 2004.

13. Quotation is from Dr. Frances Horwich, director of children's programming for WFLF-TV, addressing a seminar entitled "Advertising for the Child Consumer." "Horwich Hits Use of Kids in TV Ads Aimed at Adults: 'It Bewilders 'Em.'" *Advertising Age,* 1 May 1967, 3. ACT referred to the quotation in a later petition: Action for Children's Television. "ACT Petition: Before the FTC, Washington DC. In the Matter of Petition to Prohibit Advertisements for Edibles on Children's Television Programs. (Supplemental Filing)," March 22, 1972 and January 1973. Carton 1, ACT Box 2, ACT Collection, Special Collections, Monroe C. Gutman Library, Harvard Graduate School of Education, Cambridge, MA.

14. The study of children's television advertising was Barcus, F. E. "Saturday Children's Television: A Report of TV Programming and Advertising on Boston Commercial Television." Newtonville, MA: Action for Children's Television, 1971.

Choate's advertising code outlined in Choate, R. "Minute from Robert Choate: CCMM Proposal on Code for Advertising Edibles to Children.", 1971. Carton 2, Box 8, ACT Collection, Special Collections, Monroe C. Gutman Library, Harvard Graduate School of Education, Cambridge, MA.

15. ACT lobbied the FCC in 1970 and again in 1974, and the FTC in 1972, all in relation to children's television programming and advertising. Federal Communications Commission. "Children's Television Programs: Report and Policy Statement." *Federal Register* 39, no. 215 (1974) 39396–39409, ; Dixon, W. D. "Presiding Officer's Report on Proposed Trade Regulation Rule Food Advertising," February 21, 1978, 118. Carton 2, ACT Box 8, ACT Collection, Special Collections, Monroe C. Gutman Library, Harvard Graduate School of Education, Cambridge, MA. The announcements of the rule-making were made in the *Federal Register* from 1974 to 1983.

Action for Children's Television. "In the Matter of Petition to Prohibit Advertisements for Edibles on Children's Television Programs." March 22, 1972 and January 1973. Carton 1, ACT Box 2, ACT Collection, Special Collections, Monroe C. Gutman Library, Harvard Graduate School of Education, Cambridge, MA; Federal Trade Commission. "Letter Regarding Petition to Prohibit Advertisements for Edibles on Children's Television Programs." April 3, 1975. Carton 1, ACT Box 2, ACT Collection, Special Collections, Monroe C. Gutman Library, Harvard Graduate School of Education, Cambridge, MA. Italics added.

"Purpose of the proposed rule . . ." quotation from Action for Children's Television. "Petition before the Federal Trade Commission in the Matter of Petition to Promulgate a Rule Prohibiting the Advertising of Candy to Children on Television," April 2, 1977, 51. Carton 1, ACT Box 2, ACT Collection, Special Collections, Monroe C. Gutman Library, Harvard Graduate School of Education, Cambridge, MA.

16. Action for Children's Television, "Petition before the Federal Trade Commission," 41.
17. "Pandemic levels of tooth decay" from "Federal Trade Commission [16 Cfr Part 461] Children's Advertising." *Federal Register* 43, no. 82 (1978): 17967–17972, 17968. ACT and CSPI were joined by the Consumer Federation of America in petitioning the FTC. O'Reilly, K. "Letter to the Federal Trade Commission on the Subject of Food Advertising to Children Rulemaking from the Consumer Federation of America," April, 1977. Carton 1, ACT Box 2, ACT Collection, Special Collections, Monroe C. Gutman Library, Harvard Graduate School of Education, Cambridge, MA.

"Children are extremely susceptible" quotation from Council for Children, Media and Merchandising. "Before the FTC Petition of the Center for Science in the Public Interest for a Rule to Regulate Advertising of Sugared Food Products on Children's Television," 3, April 1977. Carton 1, ACT Box 2, ACT Collection, Special Collections, Monroe C. Gutman Library, Harvard Graduate School of Education, Cambridge, MA.

"Deceptive within Section 5" quotation from Action for Children's Television. "Petition before the Federal Trade Commission," 44. In a follow-up letter, CSPI also suggested that the FTC consider making a ruling on advertising food with high fat content to children on the basis that medical evidence showed a connection between a high-fat diet and heart disease in adulthood. The FTC did not, however, incorporate this suggestion into their statement on the proposed ruling. Jacobson, M. F. "Letter to the Federal Trade Commission on the Subject of Food Advertising to Children Rulemaking from CSPI." January 26, 1978. Carton 36, ACT Collection, Special Collections, Monroe C. Gutman Library, Harvard Graduate School of Education, Cambridge, MA.

"Federal Trade Commission [16 Cfr Part 461] Children's Advertising." *Federal Register* 43, no. 82 (1978): 17967–17972. The announcements of the rule-making process were published in the *Federal Register* from 1978 to 1981.

18. For example, Waters, H., and J. Copeland. "Sugar in the Morning." *Newsweek,* 30 January 1978, 75; Coates, C. "ABC Reform Is Not Enough, Critics of Children's TV Claim." *Advertising Age,* 5 February 1979, 8; "War-Gaming on the Ad-Ban." *Broadcasting,* 13 March 1978, 23.

19. "Jumping the Gun on Washington Children's Ad Proceedings." *Broadcasting,* 5 March 1979, 29–30; "Special Report: Children's Television." *Broadcasting,* 29 October 1979, 39–56; Press clipping: "Raise $30 million to Stop or Delay," *Washington Star,* Undated 1978. ACT Periodical Clippings and Press Releases Box 15, ACT Collection, Special Collections, Monroe C. Gutman Library, Harvard Graduate School of Education, Cambridge, MA; "War-Gaming on the Ad-Ban."

20. Burson-Marsteller also later represented Union Carbide Corporation during the Bhopal disaster (1984); Phillip Morris in its campaigns against second-hand smoke restrictions (early 1990s); and the Indonesian government in regard to military conduct in East Timor (1996). More recently, the company represented Blackwater USA following an incident in which Blackwater employees were alleged to have killed Iraqi citizens (2007).

    Hall, S. Press Clipping: "Angry Public Relations War Erupts over Kids' TV Ads." Undated 1979. ACT Periodical Clippings and Press Releases Box 1, ACT Collection, Special Collections, Monroe C. Gutman Library, Harvard Graduate School of Education, Cambridge, MA.

    "Big thrust" in Congress quotation from "War-Gaming on the Ad-Ban," 23.

    Case against Pertshuck in "ANA Begins Its Court Battle to Alter Children's TV Ad Rule." *Advertising Age,* 9 October 1978, 8; "FTC Entangled in Court-room." *Broadcasting,* 30 October 1978, 40; "Chocolate Manufacturers Association of the US in US District Court, DC Civil Action no. 78–1372 'Complaint for Injunctive Relief.'" 9 May 1978. Carton 1, ACT Box 4, ACT Collection, Special Collections, Monroe C. Gutman Library, Harvard Graduate School of Education, Cambridge, MA; "Federal Trade Commission [16 Cfr Part 461] Children's Advertising (Revisions of Notice of Proposed Trade Regulation Rulemaking)." *Federal Register* 44, no. 12 (1979): 3495–3496.

    "Sparkplug . . ." quotation from press clipping: "FTC Law Suit." *Advertising Age,* undated 1978. Carton 34, ACT Collection, Special Collections, Monroe C. Gutman Library, Harvard Graduate School of Education, Cambridge, MA.

21. Kramer, L. "TV Ads Are Said to Benefit Child by Developing Skepticism." *Washington Post,* 18 January 1979, A5.

22. "Censorship Fears, More Claims That Self-Regulation Is Sufficient Voiced at FTC Children's Hearing." *Broadcasting,* 26 March 1979, 84, 92.

23. The study was Ward, S. "Children's Reactions to Commercials." *Journal of Advertising Research* 12 (1972): 37–45. Ward later left Harvard Business School and took up a position as a professor of marketing at Wharton. His career ended ignominiously when he was arrested for pedophilia in 2006 and jailed for fifteen years.

    The studies showing the effectiveness of advertising were Galst, J. P., and M. A. White. "The Unhealthy Persuaders: The Reinforcing Value of Television and Children's Purchase-Influencing Attempts at the Supermarket." *Child Development* 47 (1976): 1089–1096; Goldberg, M., G. Gorn, and W. Gibson. "TV Messages for Snack and Breakfast Foods: Do They Influence Children's Preferences?" *Journal of Consumer Research* 5 (1978): 73–81; Goldberg, M., and G. Gorn. "Some Unintended Consequences of TV Advertising to Children." *Journal of Consumer Research* 5 (1978): 22–29.

    On methodological bias and its effect in studies assessing the effects of advertising on children, see Goldberg, M., and G. Garn. "Researching the Effects of Television Advertising on Children: A Methodological Critique." In *Learning from Television*, M. Howe, ed., 125–152. New York: Academic Press, 1983.

24. "Summaries of Testimony by Witnesses for ACT Children's Advertising Rulemaking (FTC) Washington DC Mar 5–30 1979." Carton 33, ACT Collection, Special Collections, Monroe C. Gutman Library, Harvard Graduate School of Education, Cambridge, MA.

25. "Up to Their Teeth in Washington over Children's Ads." *Broadcasting,* 12 March 1979, 35–38, 38.

26. "National nanny" quotation from LeRoux, M. "Witnesses Claim Kids Ad Ban Would Shut Down Some Indies." *Advertising Age,* 29 January 1979, 3.

    Keeshan's views reported in "Up to Their Teeth in Washington over Children's Ads," 38. Captain Kangaroo was not averse to advertising to children. He advertised Schwinn bicycles as part of his show. Schwinn sponsored the program.

27. "Free flow of commercial information" from Virginia State Board of Pharmacy v. Virginia Citizens Consumer Council, 425 U.S. 748 1976).

    "First amendment morass" quotation from "ACLU Submission to FTC in Matter of Children's Advertising Hearing." March 1979. Carton 37, ACT Collection Special Collections, Monroe C. Gutman Library, Harvard Graduate School of Education, Cambridge, MA.

    On Massachusetts law seeking to ban tobacco sales in the vicinity of schools, see Lorrilard Tobacco Co. v. Reilly (533 U.S. 525 (2001)); Murphy, L., Director, and M. Johnson, Legislative Counsel, to the Honorable Edward M. Kennedy and the Honorable Judd Gregg, Re. S. 2626, the Youth Smoking Prevention and Public Health Act, 18 September 2002. "Statement for the Record to the Senate Health, Education, Labor and Pensions Committee on FDA Regulation of Tobacco." American Civil Liberties Union, http://www.aclu.org/free

-speech/statement-record-senate-health-education-labor-and-pensions -committee-fda-regulation-tob. Access date 18 September 2002.

"Against the health and well-being" quotation from Pertshuck, M. *Revolt against Regulation: The Rise and Pause of the Consumer Movement.* Berkeley: University of California Press, 1982, 71.

28. On arguments concerning inflation see "Ripple Effect Cited from FTC Ad Ban." *Broadcasting,* 23 July 1979, 44; "Carter Intends to Fight for FTC Control." *Advertising Age,* 29 January 1979, 83; "Nervous Days at the FTC." *Broadcasting,* 24 September 1979, 38–42, 38.

FTC portrayed as "running away with making new laws" in, for example, "Getting Down to It on FTC." *Broadcasting,* 19 November 1979, 70, 72; "Senate Puts the Kibosh on FTC Children's Ad Proceeding." *Broadcasting,* 11 February 1980, 34–37.

29. "Federal Trade Commission [16 Cfr Part 461] Children's Advertising (Termination of Rulemaking Proceeding)." *Federal Register* 46, no. 191 (1981): 48710–48714.

30. Center for Science in the Public Interest. "Building a Healthier America since 1971."

31. Schlosser, E. *Fast Food Nation.* Boston: Houghton Mifflin, 2001; *Supersize Me.* Film. Directed by M. Spurlock. 2004, New York, NY, Samuel Goldwyn Films, 100 min.; Pollan, *Omnivore's Dilemma.*

32. Studies implicating the nature and content of television watching include Dietz, W., and S. Gortmaker. "Do We Fatten Our Children at the Television Set?" *Pediatrics* 75 (1985): 807–812; Pate, R., and J. Ross. "Factors Associated with Health-Related Fitness." *Journal of Physical Education, Recreation and Dance* 58, (1987): 93–95; Gortmaker, S., A. Must, et al. "Television Viewing as a Cause of Increasing Obesity among Children in the United States, 1986–1990." *Archives of Pediatric and Adolescent Medicine* 150 (1996): 356–363; Anderson, R., C. Crespo, and S. Bartlett. "Relationship of Physical Activity and Television Watching with Body Weight and Level of Fatness among Children." *Journal of the American Medical Association* 279 (1998): 938–942.

That television fails to show the realistic outcome of the dietary practices it portrays is discussed in Dietz and Gortmaker, "Do We Fatten Our Children at the Television Set?"

33. U.S. Department of Health and Human Services. "The Surgeon General's Call to Action to Prevent and Decrease Overweight and Obesity." Rockville, MD: Public Health Service, Office of the Surgeon General, 2001, v, xi.

Politicians who had spoken on the issue of regulating junk-food advertising to children included Senator Tom Harkin (D-Iowa), Senator Sam Brownback (R-Kansas), Senator Gordon Smith (R-Oregon), and Senator Hillary Clinton (D-New York).

On research agreement that regulating television advertising could be a useful public health intervention, see Robinson, T., L. Hammer, et al. "Does

Television Viewing Increase Obesity and Reduce Physical Activity?" *Pediatrics*
91 (1993): 273–280; Gortmaker, Must, et al. "Television Viewing"; Robinson,
T. "Reducing Children's Television Watching to Prevent Obesity." *Journal of
the American Medical Association* 282 (1999): 1561–1567; Anderson, Crespo,
and Bartlett, "Relationship of Physical Activity and Television Watching";
Dietz, W., and S. Gortmaker. "Preventing Obesity in Children and Adolescents." *Annual Review of Public Health* 22 (2001): 337–353.

On the support of organized medicine for advertising regulations, see, for
example, National Institute of Human Health, "Television and Behavior";
American Academy of Pediatrics. "The Commercialization of Children's
Television." *Pediatrics* 89 (1992): 343–344.

34. On the place of the workshop within the FTC's overall activities, see
Federal Trade Commission. "The FTC in 2006." In *Chairman's Annual
Report*, 1–54. Washington, DC: Federal Trade Commission, 2006, especially
40–41.

35. Chairman Deborah Platt Majoras addressing Federal Trade Commission.
Federal Trade Commission. "Perspectives on Marketing, Self-Regulation and
Childhood Obesity (Workshop Transcript)." 1–99. http://www.ftc.gov/bcp
/workshops/foodmarketingtokids/transcript.pdf Washington, D.C.: Federal
Trade Commission, 2005. Access date 14 February 2010, 16.

On reminders of the Kid-Vid saga, see, for example, Dick O'Brien (Chairman, American Association of Advertising Agencies), in Federal Trade Commission, "Perspectives on Marketing", 79; Grocery Manufacturers Association.
"Comments of Grocery Manufacturers' Association concerning the FTC
and DHHS Public Workshop on Marketing, Self-Regulation and Childhood Obesity." Federal Trade Commission. http://www.ftc.gov/os/comments
/FoodMarketingtoKids/516960-00057.pdf, 2005. Access date 14 February
2010; MacLeod, W., and J. Oldham. "Kid-Vid Revisited: Important Lessons
for the Childhood Obesity Debate." *Antitrust* (2004): 31–35; Nickelodeon.
"Statement Submitted by Nickelodeon for the 'Food Marketing to Kids
Workshop,' Washington D.C. 8 June 2005." Federal Trade Commission.
http://www.ftc.gov/os/comments/FoodMarketingtoKids/516960-00046.pdf,
2005. Access date 14 February 2010.

36. Federal Trade Commission, "Perspectives on Marketing", 16.

37. "Understand the inherent bias . . ." quotation from Jeff McIntyre, addressing
Federal Trade Commission, "Perspectives on Marketing", 92.

"The best example of self-regulation . . ." quotation from Dick O'Brien
(chairman, AAAA), addressing Federal Trade Commission, "Perspectives on
Marketing", 81.

38. Along with internal guidelines that advertising agencies or their customers
might have, CARU's "Self-Regulatory Program for Children's Advertising"
was the only formal mechanism for self-regulating children's advertising in
2005. The NAB's television code was no longer in existence. In 1982, the

Justice Department had started proceedings against the NAB on the grounds that its television code was a violation of antitrust laws (the Sherman Antitrust Act). Following the decision, the NAB disbanded the code, thus, ironically, ending one of the mainstays of self-regulating children's television.

Children's Advertising Review Unit. "Self-Regulatory Program for Children's Advertising." New York: CARU, Council of Better Business Bureaus 1975; Council of Better Business Bureaus. "About the Children's Advertising Review Unit (CARU)." Children's Advertising Review Unit, www.caru.org /about/index.aspx. 2008. Access date 10 October 2009.

"Self-regulation is the most sensible answer" quotation from "Big Spenders Ask NARB to Set Guidelines for Children's Ads." *Advertising Age*, 21 January 1974, 1, 73.

39. CARU, "Self-Regulatory Program," 4–5.
40. National Advertising Review Council (NARC). "White Paper: Guidance for Food Advertising Self-Regulation." New York: NARC, 2004, 10.
41. Ibid., 38.
42. Senator Harkin addressing Federal Trade Commission, "Perspectives on Marketing", 32.
43. CARU's threefold purpose described in NARC, "White Paper," 18.
44. "Responsible industry-generated action . . ." quotation from Federal Trade Commission. "Press Release: FTC, HHS Release Report on Food Marketing and Childhood Obesity." Release date 2 May 2006, www.ftc.gov/opa/2006/05 /childhoodobesity.shtm.

On the wide support for public education, see for example, Majoras, D. P., P. J. Harbour, et al. "Perspectives on Marketing, Self-Regulation and Childhood Obesity: A Report on a Joint Workshop of the Federal Trade Commission and the Department of Health and Human Services." Washington, DC: Federal Trade Commission, Department of Health and Human Services, 2006; Federal Trade Commission, "Press Release: FTC, HHS Release Report"; Federal Trade Commission. "The FTC in 2007: A Champion for Consumers and Competition." In *Chairman's Annual Report*. 1–55. Washington, DC: Federal Trade Commission, 2007.

45. The FTC's study of advertising to children is Holt, D., P. M. Ippolito, et al. "Children's Exposure to TV Advertising in 1977 and 2004." Washington, DC: Federal Trade Commission (Bureau of Economics Staff Report), 2007. The report compared data from 1977 with data from 2004. For children aged two to eleven, the number of ads children saw had risen since the 1970s, because ads were shorter, but the amount of time and the proportion for food had dropped. For older children, aged six to eleven, both the number of ads and the amount of advertising time seen had increased. The FTC report was disputed by the not-for-profit organization the Kaiser Family Foundation, which had done its own study and found that children of the 2000s were seeing about double the number of ads as they had seen in the 1970s. "The Role

of Media in Childhood Obesity." Menlo Park: Henry J. Kaiser Family Foundation, 2004.

The IOM's report is McGinnis, J. M., J. Goodman, and V. Kraak. "Food Marketing to Children and Youth: Threat or Opportunity." Washington, DC: Committee on Food Marketing and the Diets of Children and Youth, National Academy of Sciences, Institute of Medicine, 2006. "Statistically, there is strong evidence quotation" from ibid., 8–9.

46. "The backlash is building" quotation from Senator Tom Harkin, addressing Federal Trade Commission, "Perspectives on Marketing", 31.

"There is not a government body . . ." quotation from Eggerton, J. "Study: Kids Food Ads Must Change." *Broadcasting and Cable*, 12 December 2005, 7.

11. Fat Kids Go to Court

Epigraph: Banzhaf, J. "Obesity Litigation." *Journal of Law, Economics and Policy* 7 (2010): 249–258, 258.

1. Reported in Banzhaf, J. F., T. H. Frank, et al. "Protecting the Public Health: Litigation and Obesity (Panel)." *Journal of Law, Economics and Policy* 7 (2010): 259–280, 268.

2. For example, MacLeod, W., and J. Oldham. "Kid-Vid Revisited: Important Lessons for the Childhood Obesity Debate." *Antitrust* Summer (2004): 31–35; Frank, T. "Taxonomy of Obesity Legislation." *University of Arkansas at Little Rock Law Review* 28 (2006): 427–441; Price, J. in Banzhaf, J. F., T. H. Frank, et al. "Protecting the Public Health: Litigation and Obesity (Panel)." *Journal of Law, Economics and Policy* 7 (2010): 259–280.

3. Daynard, R. "Legal Approaches to the Obesity Epidemic." *Consumer Policy Review* 13 (2003): 154–158; Mello, M., D. Studdert, and T. Brennan. "Obesity: The New Frontier of Public Health Law." *New England Journal of Medicine* 354 (2006): 2601–2610; Neal, J. "Childhood Obesity Prevention: Is Recent Legislation Enough?" *Journal of Juvenile Law* 27 (2006): 108–122; Pomeranz, J., S. Teret, et al. "Innovative Legal Approaches to Address Obesity." *Milbank Quarterly* 87 (2009): 185–213.

4. Blanck, H., and S. Kim. "Creating Supportive Nutrition Environments for Population Health Impact and Health Equity." *American Journal of Preventive Medicine* 43 (2012): S85–S90; Gortmaker, S., B. Swinburn, et al. "Changing the Future of Obesity." *Lancet* 378, no. 9793 (2011): 838–847; Gostin, L. "Law as a Tool to Facilitate Healthier Lifestyles and Prevent Obesity." *Journal of the American Medical Association* 297 (2007): 87–90; Pomeranz, J. L., and K. D. Brownell. "Advancing Public Health Obesity Policy through State Attorneys General." *American Journal of Public Health* 101 (2011): 425–431.

5. Price in Banzhaf, Frank et al. "Protecting the Public Health," 263.

6. "New frontier" of public health law from Mello, Studdert, and Brennan, "Obesity."

"Sue the bastards" quotation from Banzhaf, "Obesity Litigation," 258. Banzhaf was quoting Supreme Court Justice Benjamin Cardozo (1870–1938) who said "In the end, there was a principle in the legal armory, which when taken down from the wall where it was rusting, was capable of furnishing a weapon for the fight and hewing a path to justice."

Banzhaf in Banzhaf, Frank et al. "Protecting the Public Health," 277.

"Obesity Threat Assessment" package outlined in Womble, Carlyle, Sandridge, and Rice, Pamphlet: *Obesity Lawsuits Threaten Your Company's Future. Are You Ready?* Winston-Salem, NC, 2004.

7. On the use of litigation as threat, see, for example, Parker, L., M. Spear, et al. "Legal Strategies in Childhood Obesity Prevention: Workshop Summary." Washington, DC: National Academy of Sciences, 2011.

8. "Mission to reclaim childhood" from Campaign for a Commercial-Free Childhood. "About CCFC." Campaign for a Commercial-Free Childhood, www.commercialexploitation.org/aboutus.html. 2004. Access date 8 Oct 2009.

"Engaged in acts and practice . . ." from Gardener, S. "Letter to Sumner M. Redstone, Chairman and CEO Viacom Inc and James M. Jenness, Chairman and CEO Kellogg Company." *Notification of Intent to Sue,* Litigation Office Director of Litigation, CSPI. Washington, DC: Center for Science in the Public Interest, 2006.

9. Statistic of 27 percent of Kellogg's marketing directed at six- to eleven-year-olds from Martin, Andrew. "Kellogg to Curb Marketing of Foods to Children." *New York Times,* 14 June 2007, http://www.nytimes.com/2007/06/14/business /media/14kellogg-web.html?ex=1339473600&en=df5a741e078f43b8&ei=51 18&partner=rssaol&emc=rss#.

Gardener, "Letter," 8.

10. Higgins, J. "Junk-Food Suit Gives Nick Bellyache." *Broadcasting and Cable,* 23 January 2006, 12.

11. "Suing the pants" quote from Simon, M. "Suing the Pants off SpongeBob." *AtlerNet,* 1 February 2006, http://www.alternet.org/story/31585/. See also "SpongeBob, Kellogg Get the Big Squeeze." *Brandweek,* 23 January 2006, http://www.commercialexploitation.org/news/spongebobsqueeze.htm.

12. Kellogg Company. "Kellogg Global Nutrient Criteria." Kellogg Company, www.kelloggcompany.com/corporateresponsibility.aspx?id=1524. 2009. Access date 8 October 2009.

13. Center for Science in the Public Interest. "Kellogg Makes Historic Settlement Agreement, Adopting Nutrition Standard for Marketing Foods to Children." CSPI, www.goodnutrition.org/new/200706141.html. 2007. Access date 9 October 2009.

The settlement was covered in a number of media outlets such as Sniffen, M. "Kellogg to Raise Nutrition of Kids' Food." *Associated Press,* 14 June 2007, http://www.usatoday.com/money/economy/2007–06–14–756954327_x.htm; Martin, "Kellogg to Curb Marketing."

14. Kellogg Company. "Kellogg Global Nutrient Criteria."

15. The Academy of Pediatrics also called for a ban on product placement techniques in children's programs and films. American Academy of Pediatrics. "Children, Adolescents, and Advertising." *Pediatrics* 118 (2006): 2563–2569.

16. For example, Nickelodeon and Discovery Kids announced policies in 2007 to become effective in 2009 when previous licensing agreements were due to expire. Albinack, P. "Washington Watch." *Broadcasting and Cable,* 20 August 2007, 12.

    Disney undertook to eliminate trans fats from all its park menus by 2007 and from its licensed products by 2008, and set limits on the number of calories, fats, and sugars in its meals. Mucha, Z. (Walt Disney Company and Affiliated Associates). "Walt Disney Company Introduces New Food Guidelines to Promote Healthier Kids' Diets." news release, 16 October 2006, www .corporate.disney.go.com/news/corporate/2006/2006_1016_food_guidlines .html.

17. Council of Better Business Bureaus. Policy statement: "About the Initiative (Children's Food and Beverage Advertising Initiative)." Better Business Bureau, www.bbb.org.us. 26 October 2009, 1. Access date 30 October 2009.

18. About $870 million of advertising spending in 2006 by major food advertisers was directed at under-twelves, versus $1 billion to adolescents. Kovacic, W., P. Jones Harboud, et al. "Marketing Food to Children and Adolescents." Washington, DC: Federal Trade Commission, 2008.

    Council of Better Business Bureaus, "About the Initiative," 2.

19. Council of Better Business Bureaus. "Food and Beverage Companies Continue to Raise Bar When Advertising to Kids." Better Business Bureaus, www.bbb .org.us. 26 October 2009. Access date 30 October 2009.

20. On the 2007 announcement, see, for example, O'Brien, D. "Special Report: Food Advertising and Children." Washington, DC: American Association of Advertising Agencies, 2007; Eggerton, J. "Industry Self-Regs Could Trump Task Force." *Broadcasting and Cable,* 21 April 2008, 6; Adler, R. "As FTC Convenes 2007 Workshop on Childhood Obesity, ANA Highlights Unprecedented Steps by Private Industry . . ." Washington, DC.: Association of National Advertisers, 2007.

    The 2009 expansion of the initiative is addressed in Council of Better Business Bureaus. "Children's Food and Beverage Advertising Initiative Program and Core Principles Statement (Effective January 1, 2010)." Arlington, VA: CBBB, November 2009. http://cms-admin.bbb.org/storage/0/Shared%20 Documents/Core%20Principles%20Final%20Letterhead%2012-2-09.pdf; Council of Better Business Bureaus. "CFBAI Newsletter." Arlington, VA: CBBB, February ; Council of Better Business Bureaus. "The Children's Food and Beverage Advertising Initiative in Action: A Report of Compliance and Implementation During 2009." Arlington, VA: CBBB, December 2010. http://www.bbb.org/us/storage/0/Shared%20Documents/BBBwithlinks.pdf

"And as for parents . . ." quotation from Editorial. "New Food Ads." *Broadcasting and Cable,* 23 July 2007, 26.

"Congratulations to food marketers . . ." quotation from Editorial. "Food Marketers Make Smart Tactical Move with Ad Ban." *Advertising Age,* 23 July 2007, 12.

21. For example, Daynard, "Legal Approaches"; Kelly, B., and J. Smith. "Legal Approaches to the Obesity Epidemic: An Introduction." *Journal of Public Health Policy* 25 (2004): 346–352; Garson, A., and C. Engelhard. "Attacking Obesity: Lessons from Smoking." *Journal of the American College of Cardiology* 49 (2007): 1673–1675; Gostin, "Law as a Tool"; Parker, Spear, et al., "Legal Strategies"; Pomeranz, Teret, et al., "Innovative Legal Approaches."

22. On Daynard and Banzhaf's roles in tobacco litigation, see Brandt, A. *The Cigarette Century.* New York: Basic Books, 2007.

23. For example, Willette, A. "Where Have All the Parents Gone? Do Efforts to Regulate Food Advertising to Curb Childhood Obesity Pass Constitutional Muster?" *Journal of Legal Medicine* 28 (2007): 561–77; Brooke, C. "Is Obesity *Really* the Next Tobacco? Lessons Learned from Tobacco for Obesity Litigation." *Annals of Health Law* 15 (2006): 61–106; Price in Banzhaf, Frank et al. "Protecting the Public Health."

24. For example Mercer, S., L. Green, et al. "Possible Lessons from the Tobacco Experience for Obesity Control." *American Journal of Clinical Nutrition* 77, supplement (2003): 1073–1082; Munger, L. "Is Ronald McDonald the Next Joe Camel? Regulating Fast Food Advertisements Targeting Children in Light of the American Overweight and Obesity Epidemic." *Connecticut Public Interest Law Journal* 3 (2003–2004): 456–480; Mello, Studdert, and Brennan, "Obesity"; Neal, "Childhood Obesity Prevention"; Pomeranz, Teret, et al., "Innovative Legal Approaches"; Banzhaf in Banzhaf, Frank et al. "Protecting the Public Health."

25. Gardener in Banzhaf, Frank et al. "Protecting the Public Health," 269.

On the vulnerability with respect to children, see, for example, Daynard, "Legal Approaches"; Munger, "Is Ronald McDonald the Next Joe Camel?"; Weiss, R., and J. Smith. "Legislative Approaches to the Obesity Epidemic." *Journal of Public Health Policy* 25 (2004): 379–390; Linn, S. "Food Marketing to Children in the Context of a Marketing Maelstrom." *Journal of Public Health Policy* 25 (2004): 367–378.

26. See, for example, Daynard, "Legal Approaches"; Daynard, R., P. T. Howard, and C. Wilking. "Private Enforcement: Litigation as a Tool to Prevent Obesity." *Journal of Public Health Policy* 25 (2004): 408–417.

27. On "superusers," see, for example, Schlosser, E. *Fast Food Nation.* Boston: Houghton Mifflin, 2001.

Research into obesity metabolism funded by Kellogg's and the Sugar Foundation includes Marshall, N. B., and J. Mayer. "Energy Balance in Goldthioglucose Obesity." *American Journal of Physiology* 178 (1954): 271–274; Bates, M., C. Zomzely, and J. Mayer. "Fat Metabolism in Experimental Obesity." *American Journal of Physiology* 181 (1955): 187–190.

On the potential distastefulness of marketing strategies directed at children, see, for example, Weiss, E. B. "What Youth Market?" *Advertising Age,* 28 June 1965, 74–75.

"Any person who seeks to present . . ." quotation from "Federal Trade Commission [16 Cfr Part 461] Children's Advertising." *Federal Register* 43, no. 82 (1978): 17967–17972, 17971.

28. "Chocolate Manufacturers Association of the US in US District Court, DC Civil Action no. 78–1372 'Complaint for Injunctive Relief.'" 9 May 1978. Carton 1, ACT Box 4, ACT Collection, Special Collections, Monroe C. Gutman Library, Harvard Graduate School of Education, Cambridge, MA.

29. Banzhaf in Banzhaf, Frank et al. "Protecting the Public Health," 278.

30. Ingredients in french fries outlined in Pelman v. McDonald's Corp., 237 F. Supp. 2d 512 (S.D.N.Y. 2003) ("Pelman I"). This challenge rests on what is called "consumer expectation theory."

31. The pleadings went through a number of stages (pleadings, appeals, amendments, and repleadings). Pelman v. McDonald's Corp., 237 F. Supp. 2d 512 (S.D.N.Y. 2003) ("Pelman I"); Pelman v. McDonald's, no. 02 Civ. 7821(RWS), 2003 U.S. Dist. LEXIS 15202 (S.D.N.Y. 2003) ("Pelman II"); Pelman v. McDonald's Corp., 396 F. 3d 508 (2d Cir. 2005) ("Pelman III"); Pelman v. McDonald's Corp., 396 F. Supp. 2d 439 (S.D.N.Y. 2005) ("Pelman IV"); Pelman v. McDonald's Corp., 452 F. Supp. 2d 320 (S.D.N.Y. 2006) ("Pelman V").

32. "Defendants' Consolidated Opposition to Plaintiff's Motion to Remand and Reply in Support of Defendant's Motion to Dismiss Pelman v. McDonald's Corporation." United States District Court, S.D. New York: Westlaw (2002 WL 32495997), 2002, 3. See also "Defendant's Memorandum of Law in Opposition to Plaintiff's Motion for Partial Summary Judgment Pelman V. McDonald's Corporation." United States District Court, S.D. New York: Westlaw (WL 23474945), 2003.

33. Goldman, D. "Common Sense May Not Be McDonald's Ally for Long." *Adweek,* 2 December 2002, http://www.adweek.com/aw/esearch/article_display.jsp?vnu_content_id=1771751.

34. "Amended Verified Complaint Pelman V. McDonald's Corporation." United States District Court, S.D. New York: Westlaw (WL 23474873), 2003, 10.

35. Pelman, et al. v. McDonald's Corp. 02 Civ. 07821 (DCP)1.

36. Reiter, A., Strategy and Policy Associate Director, National Restaurant Association. Personal communication with author, re: Commonsense Consumption Acts, 13 October 2009. On Cheeseburger Acts, see, for example,

Burnett, D. "Fast-Food Lawsuits and the Cheeseburger Bill." *Virginia Journal of Social Policy and Law* 14 (2006–2007): 357–417; Brooke, "Is Obesity *Really* the Next Tobacco?"

37. Price in Banzhaf, Frank et al. "Protecting the Public Health," 260–261.
38. Pelman v. McDonald's Corp., 237 F. Supp. 2d 512 (S.D.N.Y. 2003) ("Pelman I").
39. Frank, "Taxonomy of Obesity Legislation"; Banzhaf, John. "Ten Fat Law Suits (Including 2 Threatened Ones) Have Been Successful." Professor John Banzhaf III website http://banzhaf.net/suefat.html. 2010. Access date 26 January 2012; Banzhaf, "Obesity Litigation."
40. See Nestle, M. *Food Politics*. Berkeley: University of California Press, 2002, 202–206.
41. Banzhaf, J. "Letters from Two Attorneys Warn Seattle School Board about Legal Liability for 'Coke for Kickbacks' Contract." Professor John Banzhaf III website http://banzhaf.net/docs/seattleltrs.html. 2003. Access date 26 January 2012; Banzhaf, J. "Copy of Email Sent to Major School Board Associations, School Boards, and Their Attorneys." Professor John Banzhaf III website http://banzhaf.net/docs/sodawarn.html. 2005. Access date 26 January 2012.
42. "Unfortunate . . . ineffective . . ." quotation from Dezio, K. "American Beverage Association Statement on California Legislation Imposing Restriction on Beverages Sold in High Schools." American Beverage Association www .ameribev.org/nutrition—science/school-beverage-guidelines/newsreleases. 2005. Access date 26 January 2012.

    Elementary schools may sell eight-ounce servings of no/low fat milk and 100 percent juice; middle schools may sell ten-ounce servings; high schools may sell eight-ounce no/low-cal sodas and sports drinks, twelve-ounce servings of no/low-fat milks and 100 percent juices, and more than 50 percent of the product mix must be made up of water and no/low-cal options. Alliance for a Healthier Generation, American Heart Foundation, et al. "Memorandum of Understanding—School Beverage Guidelines." 2006. http://www.ameribev .org/files/336_MOU%20Final%20(signed).pdf
43. On how extensively the guidelines have been implemented, compare American Beverage Association. "Alliance School Beverage Guidelines Final Progress Report." 8 March 2010 http://www.ameribev.org/files/240_School%20 Beverage%20Guidelines%20Final%20Progress%20Report.pdf; Turner, L., and F. Chaloupka. "Wide Availability of High-Calorie Beverages in US Elementary Schools." *Archives of Pediatrics and Adolescent Medicine* 165 (2011): 223–228.

    Studies on the medical effects of soda and the correlation of soda consumption with levels of obesity include Harnack, L., J. Stang, and M. Story. "Soft Drink Consumption among US Children and Adolescents: Nutritional Consequences." *Journal of the American Dietetic Association* 99 (1999): 436–441; Ludwig, D., K. Peterson, and S. Gortmaker. "Relation between Consumption of Sugar-Sweetened Drinks and Childhood Obesity." *The Lancet* 357, no. 17 (2001): 505–508; Berkey, C. S., Helaine R., et al. "Sugar-Added Beverages and Adolescent Weight Gain." *Obesity Research* 12 (2004): 778–788.

Public health and activist interest in soda taxes and school restrictions includes Jacobson, M. "Soft Drinks: Time to Tax." *Nutrition Action Healthletter,* March 2009, 2; Brownell, K., and T. Frieden. "Ounces of Prevention." *New England Journal of Medicine* 360 (2009): 1805–1808; Pomeranz, J. "Advanced Policy Options to Regulate Sugar-Sweetened Beverages to Support Public Health." *Journal of Public Health Policy* 33 (2012): 75–88.

On state taxation measures, see Bridging the Gap Program. "State Sales Tax on Regular, Sugar-Sweetened Soda (as of January 1, 2011)." University of Illinois at Chicago, www.bridgeingthegapresearch.org. 2011. Access date 25 January 2012.

44. Dezio, K. "Beverage Industry Committed to Responsible Marketing." American Beverage Association www.ameribev.org/nutrition—science/school -beverage-guidelines/newsreleases. 2005. Access date 26 January 2012.

45. Antler, A. "The Role of Litigation in Combating Obesity among Poor Urban Minority Youth." *Cardozo Journal of Law and Gender* 15 (2008–2009): 275–301; Gardener in Banzhaf, Frank et al. "Protecting the Public Health," 266.

Conclusion

1. Recent prevalence estimates from Ogden, C., M. Carroll, et al. "Prevalence of High Body Mass Index in US Children and Adolescents, 2007–2008." *Journal of the American Medical Association* 303 (2010): 241–249.

2. For example, Wang, G., and W. Dietz. "Economic Burden of Obesity in Youths Aged 6 to 17 Years: 1979–1999." *Pediatrics* 109 (2002): e81–e86.

   On *global* costs, see, for example, Walpole, S., D. Prieto-Merino, et al. "The Weight of Nations: An Estimation of Adult Human Biomass." *Biomed Central Public Health* 12 (2012): 439–445.

3. On the failure to distinguish between treatment and prevention through diet and exercise, see, for example, Let's Move!, which is "dedicated to solving the problem of obesity." "Let's Move!" White House, http://www.letsmove.gov/. 2013. Access date 10 July 2013.

4. Nickelodeon's approach outlined in Nickelodeon. "Statement Submitted by Nickelodeon for The 'Food Marketing to Kids Workshop,' Washington D.C. 8 June 2005." Federal Trade Commission 2005, 2. http://ftc.gov/os/comments/ FoodMarketingtoKids/516960-00046.pdf.

5. "Within a generation" quotation from Obama, B. "Presidential Memorandum: Establishing a Task Force on Childhood Obesity." The White House, Office of the Press Secretary, www.whitehouse.gov/the-press-office/presidential -memorandum-establishing-a-task-force-childhood-obesity. 9 February 2010. Access date 1 June 2011.

White House Task Force on Childhood Obesity. "Solving the Problem of Childhood Obesity within a Generation." Washington, D.C., May 2010. www.letsmove.gov/white-house-task-force-childhood-obesity-report -president

6. The Council for Better Business Bureaus (CBBB), which hosts, monitors, and promotes the Children's Food and Beverage Advertising Initiative, is keen to retain self-regulation. In response to the task force's paper, the CBBB proposed in 2011 to develop uniform nutrition criteria for all pledging companies' food advertising to children under twelve. The criteria will be implemented by the end of 2013. Council of Better Business Bureaus. "The Children's Food and Beverage Advertising Initiative—White Paper on CFBAI's Uniform Nutrition Criteria." Arlington, VA: CBBB, 2011.

The White House Task Force reported at the one-year mark in February 2011. At that time, actions had been "focused on putting infrastructure in place," such as by passing the Healthy, Hunger-Free Kids Act 2010 to improve school nutrition standards. Since then, certain food companies have announced new policies on children's meals and on food labeling, and there have been initiatives with sport and physical education organizations to improve children's exercise opportunities. The First Lady has been prominent in the press as a spokeswoman for Let's Move! and especially for her efforts in schools to encourage healthy eating and activity. White House Task Force on Childhood Obesity. "One-Year Progress Report." Washington, D.C., February 2011. http://www.letsmove.gov/sites/letsmove.gov/files/Obesity_update_report .pdf; "Let's Move!" White House, http://www.letsmove.gov/. 2013. Access date 10 July 2013.

7. "National grassroots movement" from United States Department of Health and Human Services. "The Surgeon General's Vision for a Healthy and Fit Nation." Rockville, MD: Public Health Service, Office of the Surgeon General, 2010, 2.

There was significant press coverage of Congress's handling of the Agriculture Department's proposal on improving the nutritional standards of the National School Lunch program. See, for example, Nixon, R. "School Lunch Proposals Set Off a Dispute." *New York Times,* 1 November 2011, http://www.nytimes.com/2011/11/02/us/school-lunch-proposals-set-off-a -dispute.html?pagewanted=1; Nixon, R. "Congress Blocks New Rules on School Lunches." *New York Times,* 15 November 2011, http://www.nytimes .com/2011/11/16/us/politics/congress-blocks-new-rules-on-school-lunches .html?_r=0.

Acknowledgments

It is a great pleasure to come to the stage in writing this book of thanking all the people who helped along the way. My special thanks to my editorial team for their skill, knowledge, patience, and kindness—both my editor at Harvard University Press, Elizabeth Knoll, and her assistant, Joy Deng, and my editor at home, my husband, Russell Miles.

I particularly thank Professor Charles Rosenberg and Professor Allan Brandt, who were sources of guidance and intellectual motivation and who watered the seeds of this project.

Other thanks to Gordon Harvey at Harvard for his interest and encouragement; Deborah Kelley-Milburn, the oracle on the end of Widener Library's "Ask a librarian" e-mail; Jan Bourneuf of Widener Research Services; Edward Copenhagen, curator of Gutman Library's Special Collections; the librarians at Harvard Business School's de Gaspé Beaubien and Stamps reading rooms; Joshua Kantor at the Harvard Law Library; the librarians at Harvard Medical School's Countway Library and especially Jack Eckert of the rare books collection for his help with sources and with scanning images; Pam Cornell and Alethea Drexler of the Texas Medical Center Library; Ken Rose and his staff at the Rockefeller Archive Center; John P. Swann of the Federal Drug Agency's History Office; Penny Peckos, who met with me in Brewster, Massachusetts, to talk about her work at Camp Seascape; Berit Schumaker, who helped organize our meeting; Ellen St. Sure, the Brewster Town Archivist; Teresa Lamperti from the Brewster Historical Society; John Occhipinti, who most kindly replied to my letter and talked with me about his childhood, and the other John Occhipintis, including "my" John's cousin, who helped me find him; Karl Procaccini for the time he spent tracking down legal sources for my final chapter and for his understanding of state and federal tort law; Brenda Umberger from the National Center for Standards and Certification Information for her help with children's clothing standards; Amanda Reiter, Associate Director of the National Restaurant Association, for her data on Commonsense Consumption Acts; the good people behind the Frank Knox

295

Fellowship and at the Warren Center for American Studies for their financial support; Deborah Levine for sharing her thesis chapter on scales and weighing with me; Tamara Hug, Aga Lanucha, Louisa Russell, and David Thompson in the front office for their title brainstorming; Linda Waldman from NewBay Media for her charitable and insightful help with pictures; David Gleeson from American Radio Heritage for his help with magazine photos; and the generosity of Abbott Pharmaceuticals in allowing the free use of their advertisement.

And to end with the person who was really the beginning, I give many, many, many thanks to my mother, Irene, who has always inspired me with her own scholarly pursuits. Mom helped edit the chapters and said nice things about how proud and impressed she was of her daughter's work—a truly excellent mother in all respects. To you, most especially, thank you.

Index

Academy of the Sierras. *See* Wellspring Academy

Action for Children's Television (ACT), 177–182, 184

adiposity rebound, 66

adiposity. *See* fat (body component)

advertising, 146–147, 151, 169, 174, 176, 199, 200; agencies 176, 178, 179, 180, 186–190, 201; children's understanding of, 181–182, 200; code, 176–177, 178, 196–198; deceptive, 179, 182, 184, 187, 193, 194, 200, 203–205; depiction of children in, 43–44; industry associations, 174, 176–183, 186–190; of unhealthy food, 174–190, 193–207; on television, 175–190, 193–198; regulation of, 175–190, 195–198; unfair, 183–184, 190, 193, 216; use of cartoon characters in, 193–195

African American children. *See* ethnicity

American Academy of Pediatrics (AAP), 79, 106–107, 185–186, 195

American Beverage Association (ABA), *See* soda, manufacturers of

American Camping Association, 160–161

American Medical Association (AMA), 34, 38, 49, 79, 88, 94, 102–103, 106–107, 146, 160

amphetamines, 2, 87, 88, 100–109, 212. *See also* diet pills

anhedonia, 103. *See also* emotions

anorexia. *See* eating disorder

anthropometry, 73, 74. *See also* height; skinfold thickness; weight

appearance, 41, 44, 47, 60, 148–149, 163–164, 166, 168. *See also* attractiveness

appetite, 23, 42, 91, 101–104, 109, 112, 139

Asian children. *See* ethnicity

Association for the Study of Internal Secretions. *See* Endocrine Society

Atkins diet, 42, 144

Atkins, Robert, 144. *See also* Atkins diet

attractiveness, 2, 4, 16, 21–22, 35–36, 42–44, 141, 148–149, 152, 165. *See also* appearance

Atwater, Wilbur, 133. *See also* calories

Bacon, Linda, 10

Baldwin-Wood tables, 47, 49

Bancroft Elementary School, 15–16

Banting, William, 42; *Letter on Corpulence, Addressed to the Public,* 42

Banzhaff, John, III., 191–192, 198, 206

bariatric surgery, 157

basal metabolic rate (BMR), 7, 53, 97–98, 112, 117

Beach, Francis, 1–2

behavioral modification therapy, 124–126, 165. *See also* behaviorism